I0428849

Contents

Introduction

Underage drinking and associated problems have profound negative consequences for underage drinkers, their families, their communities, and society as a whole. Underage drinking contributes to a wide range of costly health and social problems, including motor vehicle crashes (the greatest single mortality risk for underage drinkers); suicide; interpersonal violence (e.g., homicides, assaults, rapes); unintentional injuries such as burns, falls, and drowning; brain impairment; alcohol dependence; risky sexual activity; academic problems; and alcohol and drug poisoning. On average, alcohol is a factor in the deaths of approximately 4,700 youths in the United States per year, shortening their lives by an average of 60 years (Centers for Disease Control and Prevention [CDC] Alcohol-Related Disease Impact [ARDI] application, 2011).

National data show meaningful reductions in underage drinking, particularly among younger age groups. From 2004 to 2011, young people ages 12 to 20 showed statistically significant declines in both past-month alcohol use and binge alcohol use. These encouraging results were most significant in the 12- to 17-year-old age group, where past-month alcohol use declined by 24.4 percent and past-month binge drinking declined by 33.3 percent.

But there is still cause for concern. For example, in 2011, 36.6 percent of 20-year-olds reported binge drinking (drinking at levels substantially increasing the risk of injury or death) in the past 30 days; about 12 (11.8) percent of 20-year-olds had, in those 30 days, binged five or more times. Furthermore, although drinking levels are lower at younger ages, patterns of consumption across the age spectrum pose significant threats to health and well-being. Particularly troubling is the erosion of the traditional gap between underage males and females in binge drinking. This gap is disappearing as females' drinking practices converge with those of males.

Still, there is reason for optimism and hope for continued progress. As discussed in Chapters 3 and 4 of this report, states are increasingly adopting comprehensive policies and practices to alter the individual and environmental factors that contribute to underage drinking and its consequences; these can be expected to reduce alcohol-related death and disability and associated health care costs. These efforts can potentially reduce underage drinking and its consequences and change norms that support underage drinking in American communities.

Characteristics of Underage Drinking in America

Alcohol Is the Most Widely Used Substance of Abuse among American Youth

Alcohol continues to be the most widely used substance of abuse among America's youth, and a higher proportion use alcohol than use tobacco or other drugs. For example, according to the 2011 Monitoring the Future (MTF) study, 27.2 percent of 10th graders reported using alcohol in the past 30 days, 17.6 percent reported marijuana use, and 11.8 percent reported cigarette use in the same period (Johnston et al., 2012a).[1]

---

[1] For comparability with data from the 2011 National Survey on Drug Youth and Health (NSDUH) and 2011 Youth Risk Behavior Surveillance System (YRBSS), the latest MTF data included in this report are also from 2011. The 2012 MTF data, which became available in December 2012, will be included in the next report.

Binge Drinking[2]

Binge drinking is the most common underage consumption pattern. High blood alcohol concentrations (BACs) and impairment levels associated with binge drinking place binge drinkers and those around them at substantially elevated risk for negative consequences. Accordingly, reducing binge drinking has become a primary public health priority.

Binge rates increase rapidly with age (Exhibit E.1). In 2011, approximately 6.1 million youths 12 to 20 years old (15.8 percent) reported binge drinking in the past month (SAMHSA, 2012a). Although youth generally consume alcohol less frequently than adults and consume less alcohol overall than adults, when they do drink they are much more likely to binge drink (Exhibit E.2). Accordingly, most youth alcohol consumption occurs in binge-drinking episodes. For example, 92 percent of the alcohol consumed by 12- to 14-year-olds is through binge drinking (Pacific Institute for Research and Evaluation [PIRE], 2002). A significant proportion of underage drinkers consume substantially more than the five-drink binge criterion. For example, averaged 2010 and 2011 data show that 10.7 percent of underage drinkers had nine or more drinks during their last drinking occasion (SAMHSA, Center for Behavioral Health Statistics and Quality [CBHSQ][3], National Survey on Drug Use and Health [NSDUH], 2012a). It is important to note that very young adolescents, because of their smaller size, reach binge-drinking BACs with fewer drinks (three to four drinks for persons ages 12 to 15) than do older adolescents (e.g., age 18 or older) (Donovan, 2009).

Female Youth Drinking Rates Are Converging With Male Youth Rates

The convergence of female youth rates of consumption with those of male youth and the implications of this trend are causes for concern. Although older adolescent rates of consumption and binge drinking are higher for males than females, the gap is closing. In 2011, 25.5 percent of male 12th graders reported binge drinking (defined as consumption of five or more drinks in a row) at least once in the prior 2-week period compared with 17.6 percent of female 12th graders (Exhibit E.3) (Johnston et al., 2012a). This difference of just 7.9 percentage points contrasts with the 23 percent difference found in 1975. Younger adolescent females (e.g., 8th graders) now exhibit rates of drinking, binge drinking, and getting drunk similar to rates for adolescent males (Johnston et al., 2012a).

The literature on gender-specific effects of alcohol use suggests that the health status of young women may be adversely affected by current trends in their alcohol consumption. Alcohol use is associated, for example, with an increased risk of unintended pregnancy, sexually transmitted disease, and violence victimization among women, adverse health outcomes that may increase

---

[2] Binge drinking is the consumption of a large amount of alcohol over a relatively short period of time. No common terminology has been established to describe different drinking patterns. Based on National Survey on Drug Use and Health (NSDUH) data, SAMHSA defines binge drinking as five or more drinks on one occasion on at least 1 day in the past 30 days, and heavy drinking as five or more drinks on at least 5 different days in the past 30 days. However, NSDUH can provide binge-drinking estimates based on the NIAAA gender-specific definition. Some studies, including Wechsler's (2002) survey of college students, define binge drinking as five or more drinks in a row for men and four or more for women. Other sources use "frequent heavy drinking" to refer to five or more drinks on at least five occasions in the last 30 days. Appendix A discusses these differences in more detail. See Courtney and Polich (2009) for further discussion of the definition issues.

[3] In August 2010, the SAMHSA Office of Applied Studies (OAS) was renamed the Center for Behavioral Health Statistics and Quality (CBHSQ).

Exhibit E.1: Current and Binge Alcohol Use among Persons Ages 12 to 20: 2011 (SAMHSA, 2012 detailed tables)

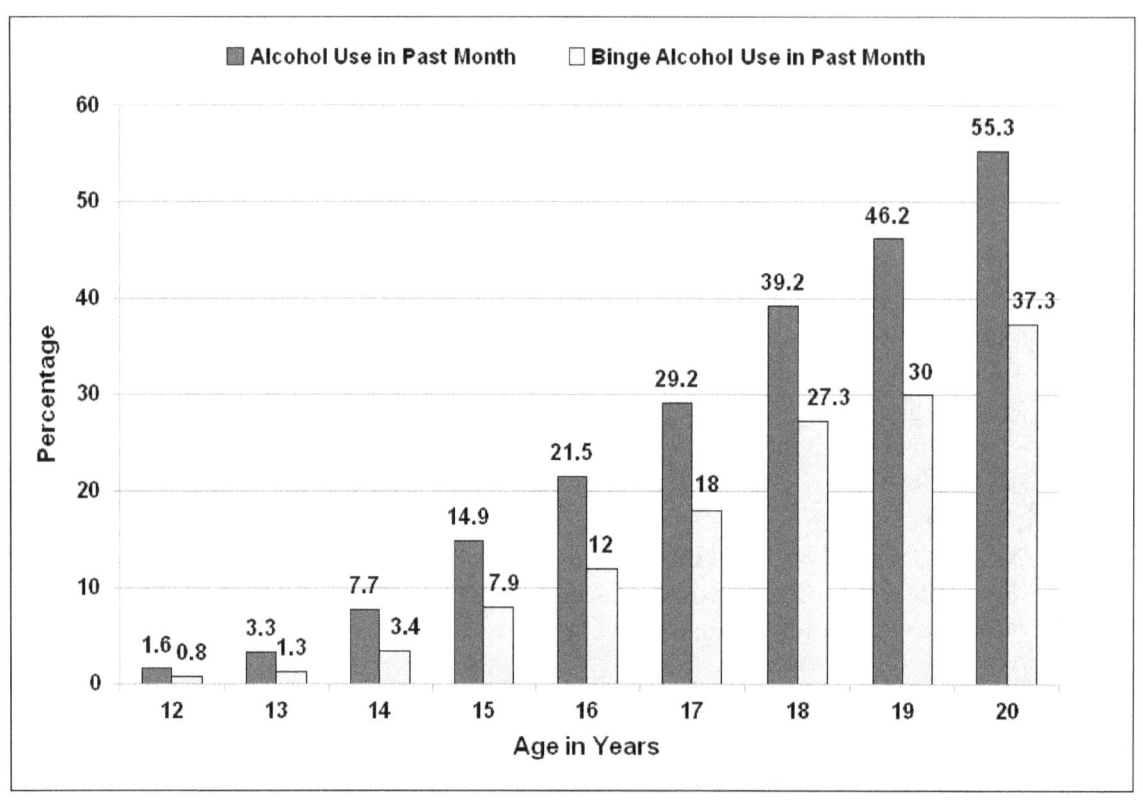

Exhibit E.2: Drinking Days per Month and Number of Drinks per Occasion for Youth (12–20), Young Adults (21–25), and Adults (≥26): 2011 (SAMHSA, CBHSQ, NSDUH, Special Data Analysis, 2012)

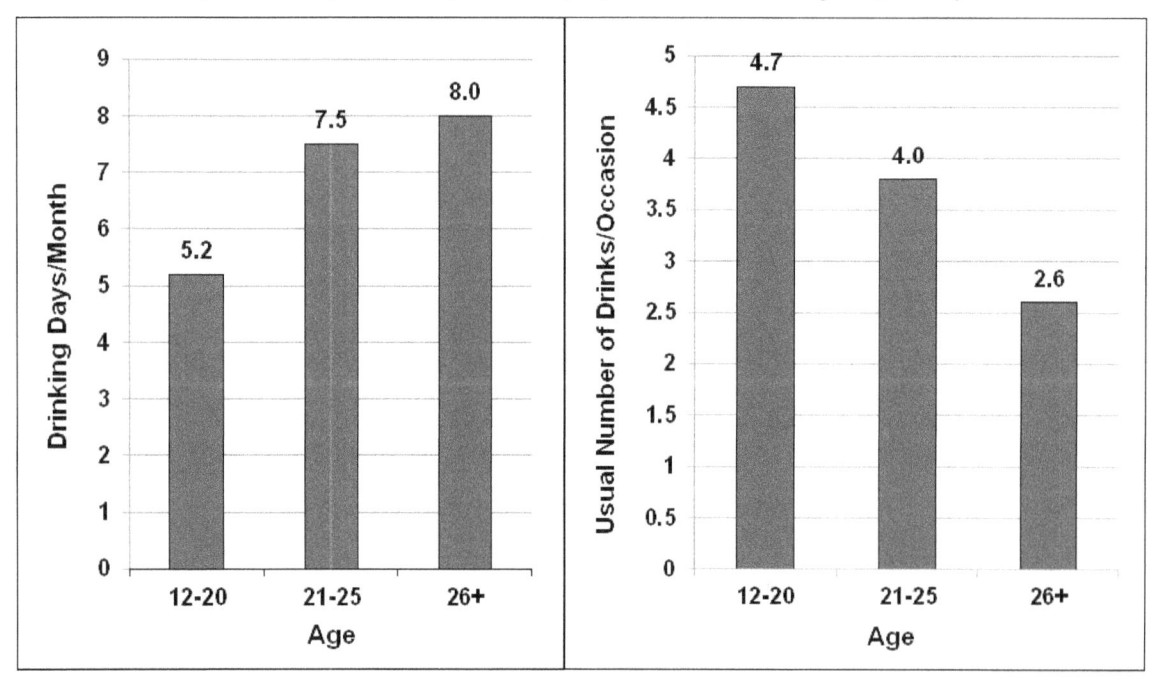

Exhibit E.3: Rates of Binge Drinking in the Past 2 Weeks among Male and Female 8th, 10th, and 12th Graders, 1991–2011 (Johnston et al., 2012a)

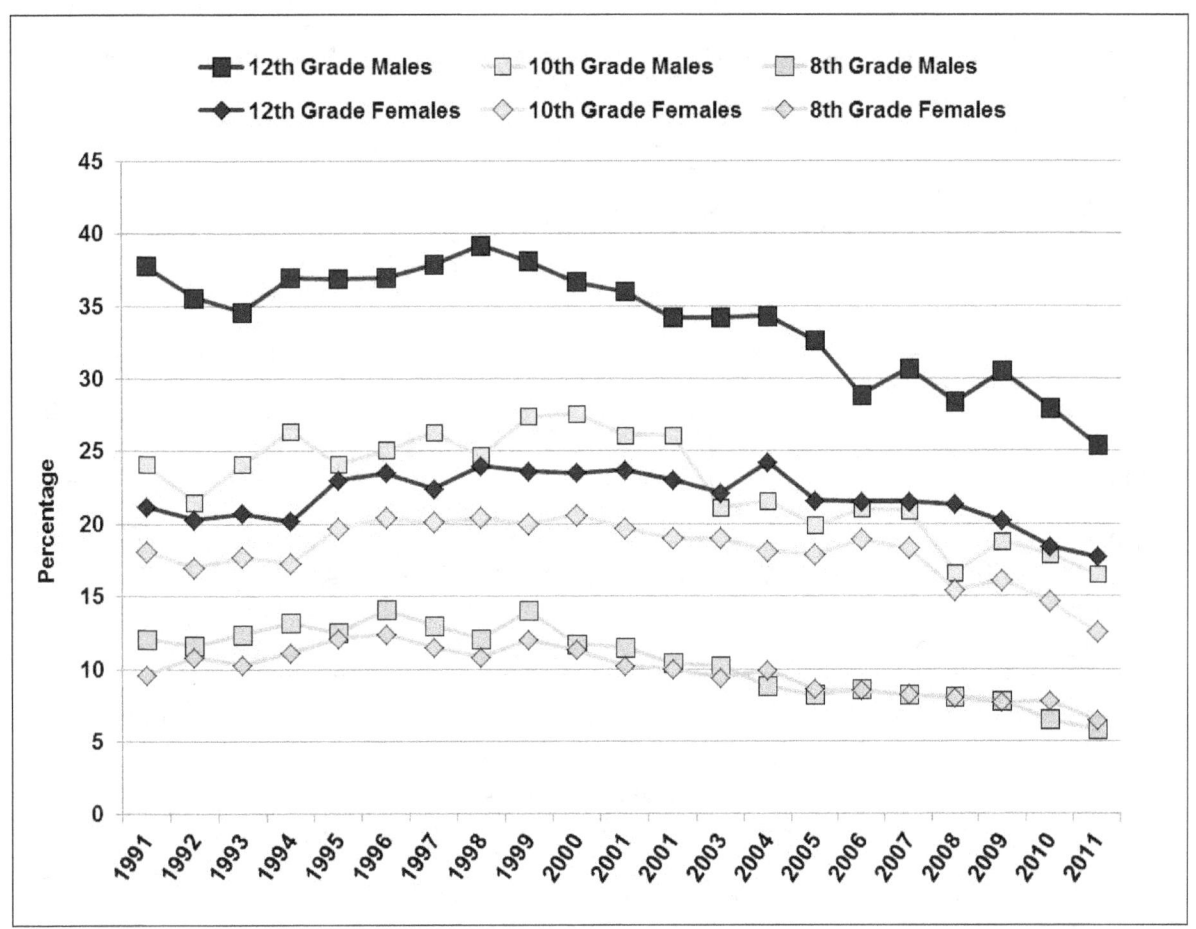

with higher rates of alcohol use (Abbey, 2011; Maisto et al., 2002; Norris et al., 2009; Sugarman et al., 2009; Testa and Livingston, 2009).

Adolescents' Beverage Preferences Are Shifting From Beer to Distilled Spirits

Different alcohol beverage types may be associated with different patterns of underage consumption. Ease of concealment, palatability, alcohol content, marketing strategies, media portrayals, parent modeling, and economic and physical availability may all contribute to the quantity of and settings for consumption. Similarly, beverage types may affect the policies and enforcement strategies that are most effective in reducing underage drinking (CDC, 2007). Tracking beverage preferences among young people is, therefore, an important aspect of prevention policy.

Distilled spirits are becoming more popular among adolescents, and are challenging beer as the beverage most likely to be consumed by underage drinkers, especially those who report binge drinking. Flavored alcoholic beverages are also popular with adolescents. Females, in particular, have shifted their beverage preference from beer to these other alternatives (Exhibit E.4). However, wine remains a relatively unpopular beverage among younger drinkers.

Exhibit E.4: Drinking Trends in the Percentage of Male and Female 12th Graders Using Alcoholic Beverages by Beverage Type, 1988–2011 (Johnston et al., 2012a)

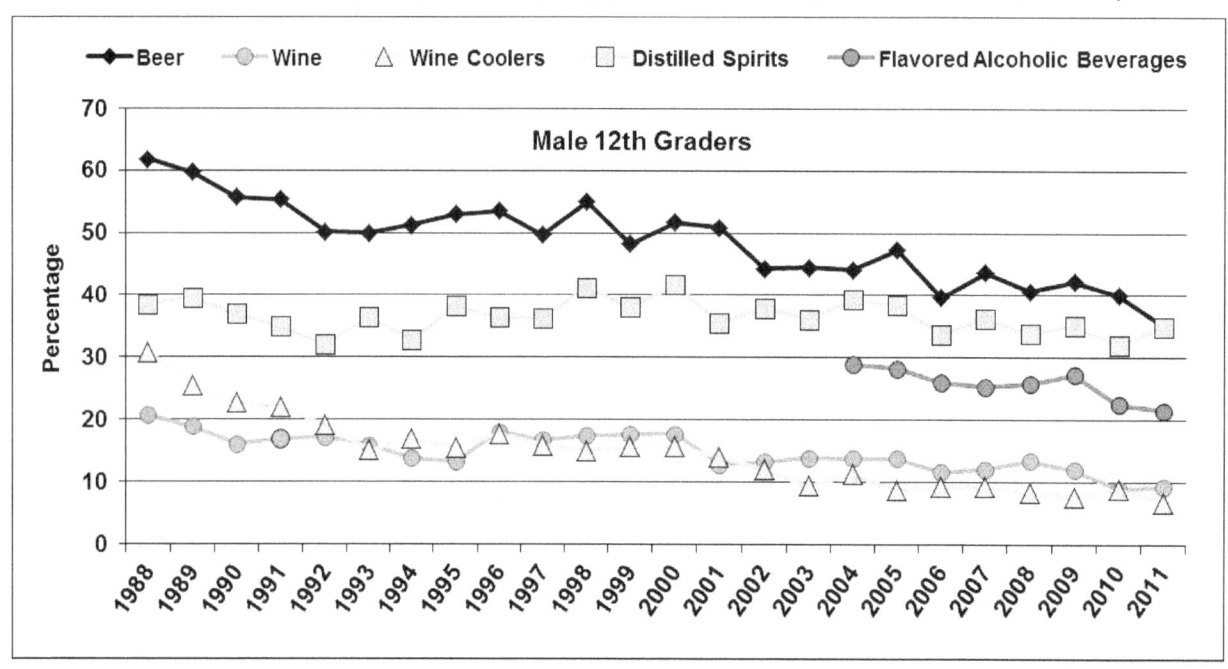

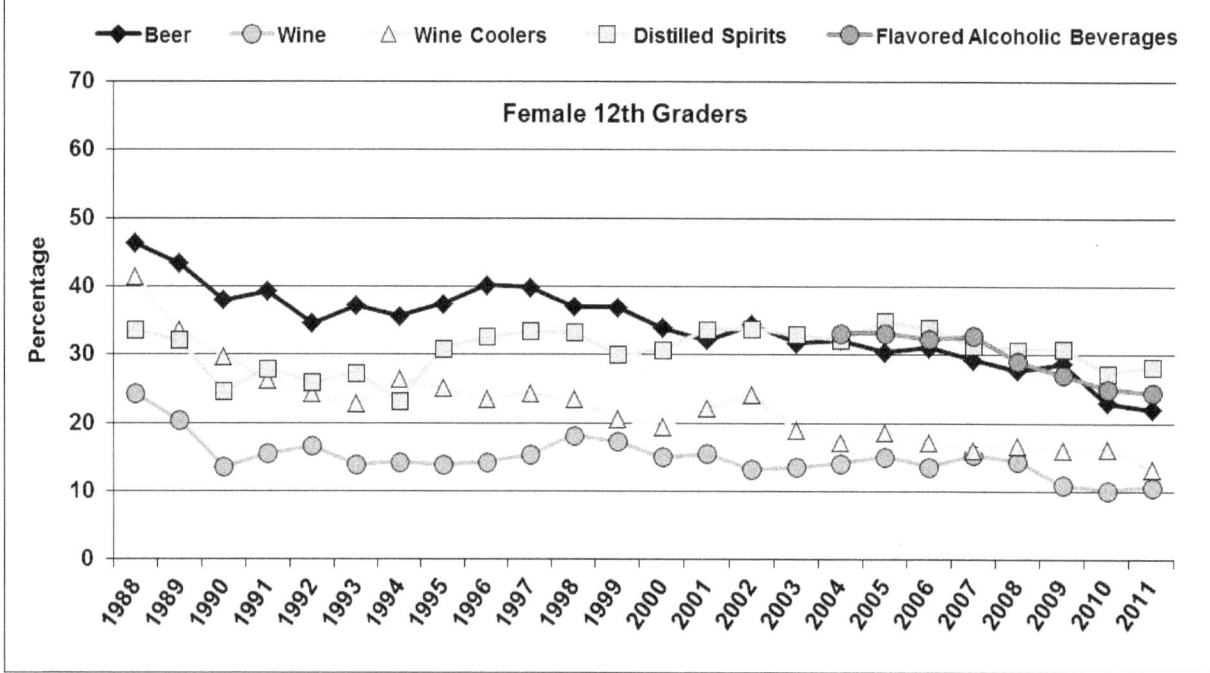

Data from eight states indicated that, among students in 9th through 12th grades who reported binge drinking, liquor was the most prevalent beverage type (Siegel, Naimi, Cremeens, & Nelson, 2011).

Youth Start Drinking at an Early Age

As discussed below, early initiation to alcohol use increases the risk of a variety of developmental problems during adolescence and problems later in life. Early initiation is often an important indicator of future substance use (NSDUH, 2012). Accordingly, delaying the onset of alcohol initiation may significantly improve later health. Although the peak years of initiation to alcohol are 7th to 11th grades, 10 percent of 9- to 10-year-olds have already started drinking (Donovan et al., 2004), and about one fifth of underage drinkers begin before they are 13 years old (CDC, 2012). Slightly fewer than 1 million (972,000) persons who initiated alcohol use in the past year reported they were ages 12 to 14 when they initiated. This translates to approximately 2,660 youths ages 12 to 14 who initiated alcohol use per day in 2011 (SAMHSA, CBHSQ, NSDUH, Special Data Analysis, 2012).

Drinking Rates Vary Significantly by Racial and Ethnic Group

White youths who are 12 to 20 years old are more likely to report current alcohol use and binge drinking than any other racial or ethnic group. Asian and Black youths had the lowest rates (Exhibit E.5) (SAMHSA, CBHSQ, NSDUH, Special Data Analysis, 2012); however, data indicate that prevalence of drinking before age 13 is higher among Black and Hispanic youths than among White youths (CDC, 2012).

These ethnic and racial differences must be viewed with caution. As Caetano, Clark, and Tam (1998) note, there are important differences in alcohol use and related problems among ethnic and racial subgroups of Whites, Blacks, Hispanics, Asians, and Native Americans/Alaska Natives. Moreover, the authors stress that the patterns of consumption for any group or subgroup represent a complex interaction of psychological, historical, cultural, and social factors that are not adequately captured by a limited set of labels. With these cautions in mind, however, the data in Exhibit E.5 highlight the importance of considering race and ethnicity in planning underage drinking countermeasures in specific communities.

Underage Drinking Is More Likely To Occur in Private Residences Where Three or More People Are Present

The social and physical settings for underage drinking affect patterns of alcohol consumption. For a young person, the usual number of drinks consumed is substantially higher when two or more other people are present than when drinking with one person or alone (Exhibit E.6). Drinking in the presence of others is by far the most common setting for young drinkers. More than 80 percent of youth who had consumed alcohol in the past month reported doing so when at least two others were present (SAMHSA, 2012a). Thus, most young people are drinking in social contexts that appear to promote heavy consumption, and where people other than the drinker may be harmed by the drinker's behavior.

As shown in Exhibit E.7, private residences are the most common setting for youth alcohol consumption, although age differences are reported. Most underage drinkers reported drinking in either someone else's home or their own. The next most popular drinking locations are at a restaurant, bar, or club; at a park, on a beach, or in a parking lot; or in a car or other vehicle (SAMHSA, CBHSQ, NSDUH, Special Data Analysis, 2012). Youths 18 to 20 years old are

Exhibit E.5: Alcohol Use and Binge Drinking in the Past Month among 12- to 20-Year-Olds by Race/Ethnicity and Gender: Annual Averages Based on 2002–2011 Data (SAMHSA, CBHSQ, NSDUH, Special Data Analysis, 2012)

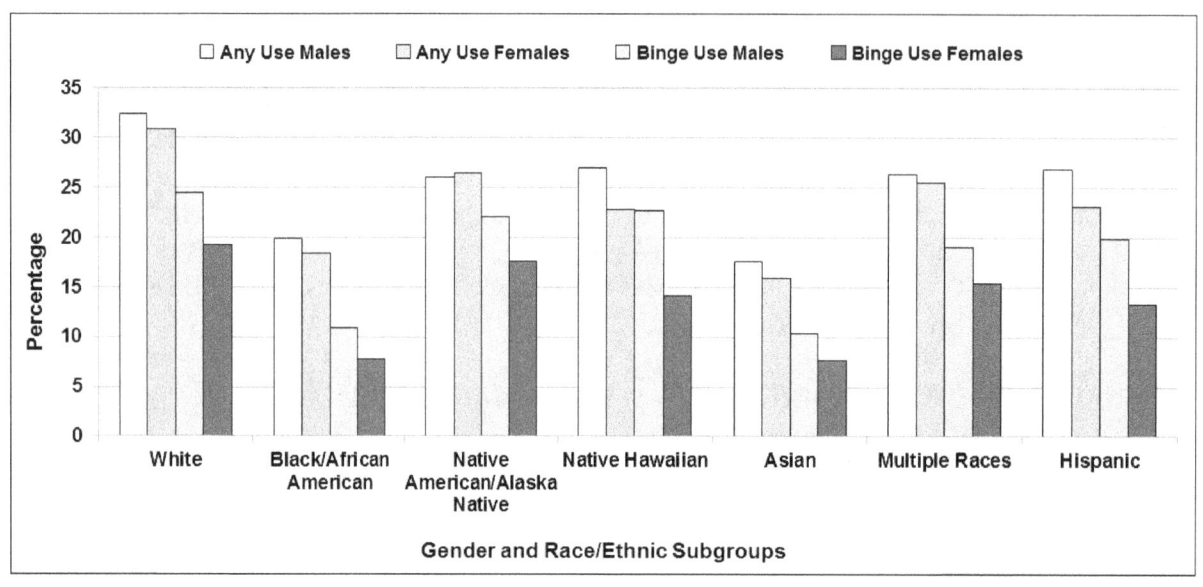

Exhibit E.6: Average Number of Drinks Consumed on Last Occasion of Alcohol Use in the Past Month among Past-Month Alcohol Users Ages 12–20, by Social Context and Age Group: Annual Averages Based on 2010–2011 Data (SAMHSA, CBHSQ, NSDUH, Special Data Analysis, 2012)

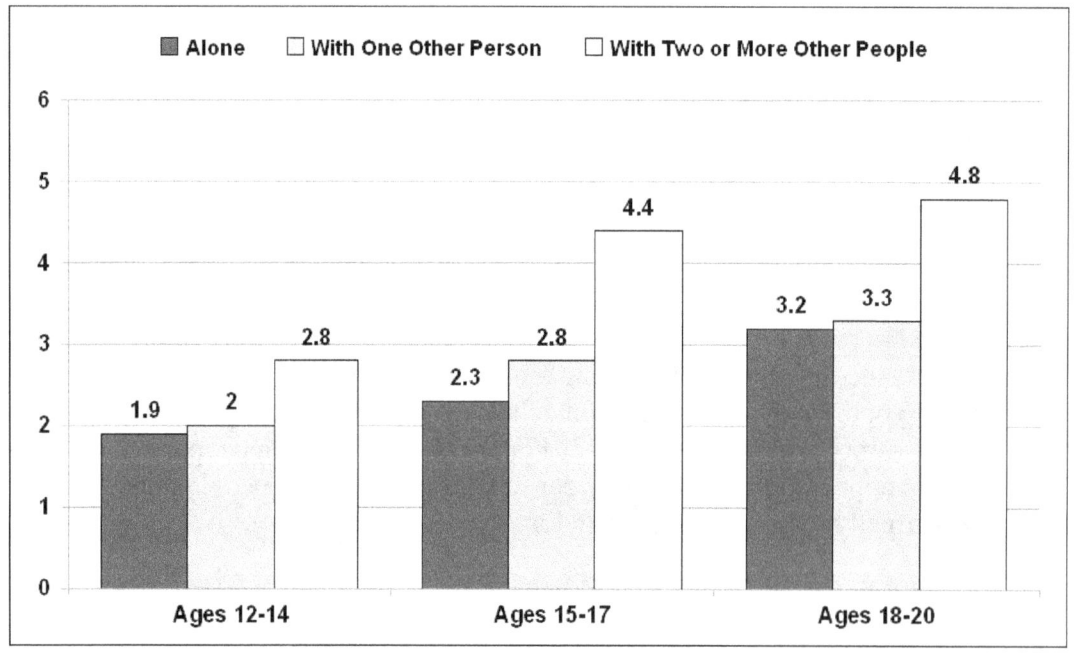

Exhibit E.7: Drinking Locations of Last Alcohol Use among Past-Month Alcohol Users Ages 12–20 by Age Group: Annual Averages Based on 2010–2011 Data (SAMHSA, CBHSQ, NSDUH, Special Data Analysis, 2012)

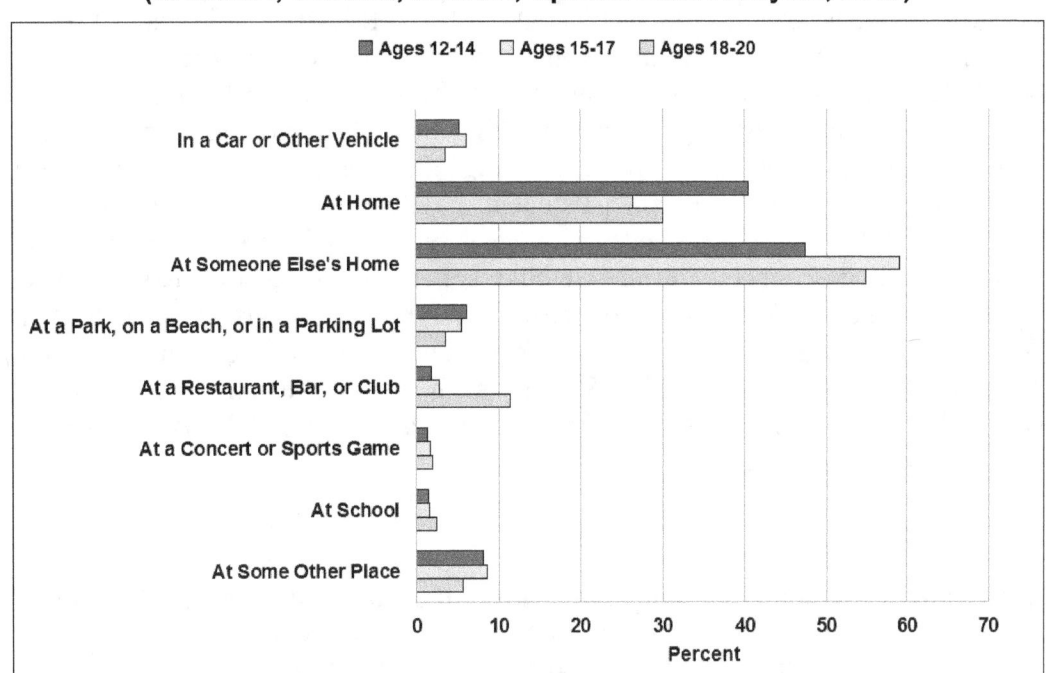

more likely than their younger peers to report drinking in restaurants, bars, or clubs, although the absolute rates of such drinking are low compared with drinking in private residences. These data suggest that underage drinking occurs primarily in social settings (three or more drinkers) at a private residence. This conclusion is consistent with research findings that underage drinking parties, where large groups of underage people gather at private residences, are high-risk settings for binge drinking and associated alcohol problems (Mayer, Forster, Murray, & Wagenaar, 1998). Similar findings exist for college students' binge drinking (Clapp, Shillington, & Segars, 2000).

Young People Perceive Alcohol To Be Readily Available

Since 1993, youth have reported declines in alcohol availability. However, the number of young people who report that alcohol is fairly easy or very easy to obtain remains high. For example, in 2011, 89.9 percent of 12th graders reported that it was easy or very easy to obtain (Johnston et al., 2012a). Very young drinkers are most likely to obtain alcohol at home from parents or siblings, or drink alcoholic beverages stored in the home. In addition, new data suggest that retailer interstate shipping of alcohol has opened up a potentially important avenue of alcohol access for underage persons (see below). Please note that some of the methods young people use to obtain alcohol do not violate underage drinking laws in some states (see Chapter 4).

Drinking Continues To Be Prevalent in Campus Culture at Many Universities

A total of 80.5 percent of college students drink; 36.1 percent report drinking five or more drinks on an occasion in the past 2 weeks (Johnston et al., 2012b). Research indicates that some college students' drinking far exceeds the minimum binge criterion of five drinks per occasion (Wechsler et al., 1999). Although colleges and universities vary widely in student binge-drinking rates, overall rates of college student drinking and binge drinking exceed those of non-college-age peers (Johnston et al., 2012b). Unlike high school students and non-college-age peers, rates of binge drinking among college students have shown little decline since 1993 (Johnston et al., 2012b). These differences are not easily attributable to differences between college- and non-college-bound students. Although college-bound 12th graders are consistently less likely than their non-college-bound counterparts to report occasions of heavy drinking, college students report higher rates of binge drinking than college-age youth not attending college (Johnston et al., 2011b) (Exhibit E.8). This suggests that the college environment influences drinking practices (Hingson, Heeren, Levenson, Jamanka, & Voas, 2002; Kuo, Wechsler, Greenberg, & Lee, 2003).

Exhibit E.8: Prevalence of Binge Drinking in the Past 2 Weeks by 12th Graders with and without College Plans, College Students, and Others 1 to 4 Years Past High School: 1991–2011 (Johnston et al., 2012a,b)

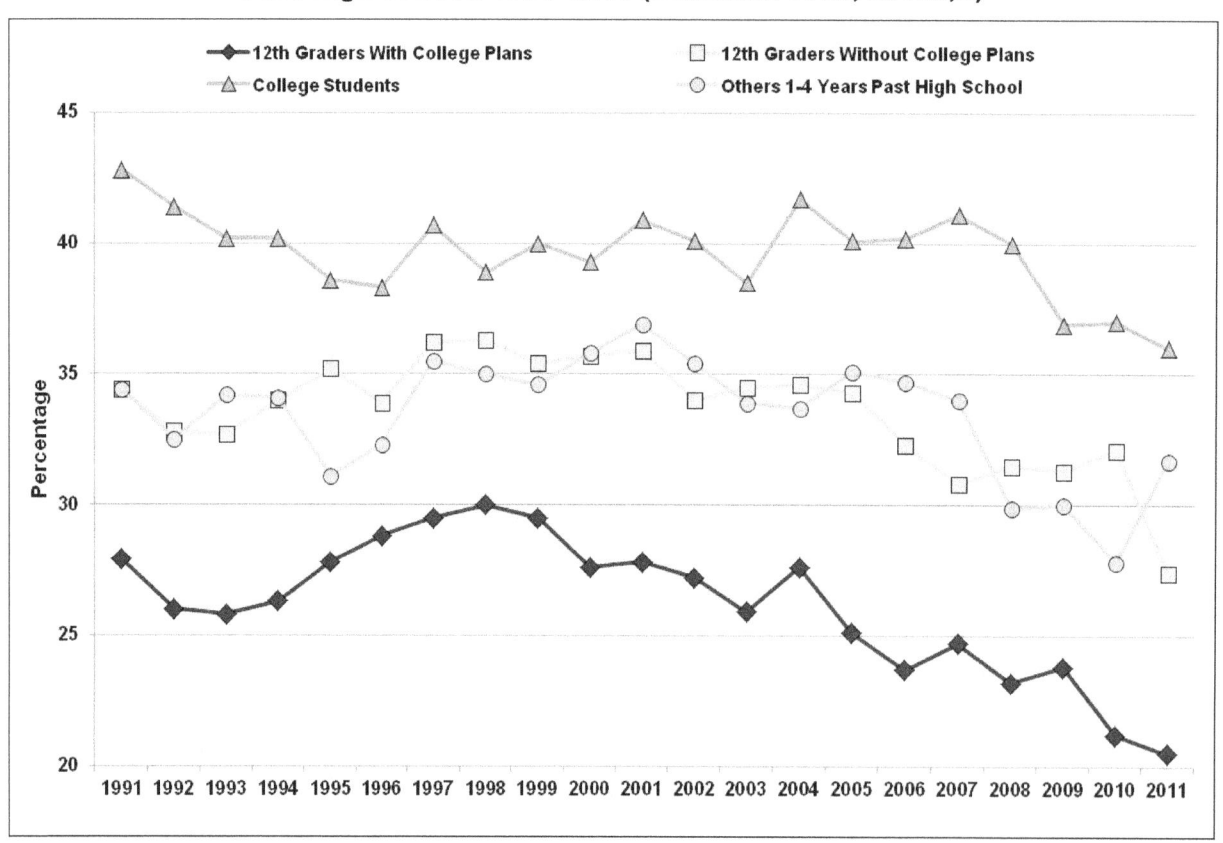

Youth Drinking Is Correlated with Adult Drinking Practices

Generational transmission has been widely hypothesized as one factor shaping the alcohol consumption patterns of young people. For example, children of parents who binge are twice as likely to binge themselves and to meet alcohol-dependence criteria. Whether through genetics,

social learning, or cultural values and community norms, researchers have repeatedly found a correlation between youth drinking and the drinking practices of parents (Pemberton, Colliver, Robbins, & Gfroerer, 2008). Nelson, Naimi, Brewer, and Nelson (2009) demonstrated this relationship at the population (state) level. State estimates of youth and adult current and binge drinking from 1993 through 2005 were significantly correlated when pooled across years. The results suggest that some policies primarily affecting adult drinkers (e.g., pricing and taxation, hours of sale, on-premises drink promotions) may also affect underage drinking.

Consequences and Risks of Underage Drinking

Alcohol-Related Motor Vehicle Traffic Crashes

The greatest single mortality risk for underage drinkers is motor vehicle crashes (Exhibit E.9). All drivers who have been drinking are at greater risk of injury because such drivers are less likely to use restraints (http://www-nrd.nhtsa.dot.gov/Pubs/811622.pdf). Mile for mile, teenagers are involved in three times as many fatal crashes as all other drivers (National Center for Statistics and Analysis [NCSA], 2009). Younger drivers are frequently inexperienced in hazard recognition and often take unnecessary risks due to a combination of poor decisionmaking and an illusion of invulnerability (Williams, 2006). One study found that at 0.08 BAC, adult drivers in all age and gender groups—compared with sober drivers—were 11 times more likely to die in a single-vehicle crash. Among those 16 to 20 years old at 0.08 percent BAC, male drivers were 52 times more likely than sober male drivers the same age to die in a single-vehicle fatal crash (Zador, 1991). In 2010, of the 1963 young drivers ages 15 to 20 killed in motor vehicle crashes, 490 (25 percent) had a BAC of .08 g/dL or higher (National Highway Traffic Safety Administration [NHTSA] Fatality Analysis Reporting System [FARS], 2010).

Exhibit E.9: Leading Causes of Death for Youth Ages 12–20: 2009 (CDC WISQARS, 2012)[4]

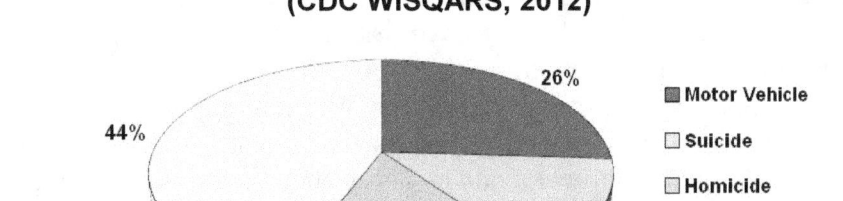

_____

[4] CDC's web-based Injury Statistics Query and Reporting System (WISQARS) is an interactive database system that provides customized reports of injury-related data.

According to 2011 survey data, about 3.6 percent of 16-year-olds, 6.7 percent of 17-year-olds, 10.0 percent of 18-year-olds, 14.2 percent of 19-year-olds, and 16.5 percent of 20-year-olds reported driving under the influence of alcohol in the past year (SAMHSA, 2012b, detailed tables). The Community Preventive Services Task Force recommends maintaining current minimum legal drinking-age laws based on strong evidence of their effectiveness in reducing alcohol-related crashes and associated injuries among 18- to 20-year-old drivers (http://www.thecommunityguide.org/mvoi/AID/mlda-laws.html).

Unintentional and Intentional Injuries and Other Trauma

As Exhibit E.9 shows, homicide and suicide follow motor vehicle crashes as the second and third leading causes of death among teenagers. In 2009, 2,652 young people who were 12 to 20 years old died from homicide; 2,383 died from suicide (CDC, 2011). In addition, 2,410 people who were 12 to 20 years old died from unintentional injuries other than motor vehicle crashes, such as poisoning, drowning, falls, and burns (CDC, 2011).

At present, it is unclear how many of these deaths are alcohol related. One study (Smith, Branas, & Miller, 1999) estimated that for all ages combined, nearly one third (31.5 percent) of homicides are alcohol related. Data from 17 states shows that among suicide decedents tested who were ages 10 to 19 (all of whom were under the legal drinking age in the United States), 12 percent had BACs >0.08 g/dL (Crosby et al., 2009). Another study focusing on youth suicide estimated that 9.1 percent of hospital-admitted suicide acts by those under age 21 involved alcohol and that 72 percent of these cases were attributable to alcohol (Miller et al., 2006).

Police and child protective services records suggest that those under age 21 commit 31 percent of rapes, 46 percent of robberies, and 27 percent of other assaults (Miller et al., 2006). As the authors note, relying on victim reports rather than agency records would yield higher estimates. For the population as a whole, an estimated 50 percent of violent crime is related to alcohol use by the perpetrator (Harwood, Fountain, & Livermore, 1998). The degree to which violent crimes committed by those younger than 21 are alcohol related is as yet unknown.

Underage Drinking Increases the Likelihood of Risky Sexual Activity

According to the Surgeon General (U.S. Department of Health and Human Services [HHS], 2007), underage drinking plays a significant role in risky sexual behavior, including unwanted, unintended, and unprotected sexual activity, and sex with multiple partners. Such behavior increases the risk of unplanned pregnancy and sexually transmittable diseases (STDs), including infection with HIV, the virus that causes AIDS (Cooper & Orcutt, 1997). When pregnancies occur, underage drinking may result in fetal alcohol spectrum disorders, including fetal alcohol syndrome, a leading cause of mental retardation (Warren & Bast, 1988; Stratton, Howe, & Battaglia, 1996). Abbey (2011) notes that approximately half of all reported and unreported college sexual assaults involve alcohol consumption by the perpetrator, victim, or both. Estimates of perpetrators' intoxication during the incident ranged from 30 to 75 percent.

Early Initiation of Alcohol Use Increases the Risk of Alcohol Dependence and Other Negative Consequences Later in Life

It is increasingly clear that early initiation to alcohol use is associated with a variety of developmental problems during adolescence in later life. Grant and Dawson (1997) found that more than 40 percent of people who initiated drinking before age 13 were classified with alcohol dependence at some time in their lives. By contrast, rates of alcohol dependence among those who started drinking at age 17 or 18 were 24.5 percent and 16.6 percent, respectively (Exhibit E.10). Only 10 to 11 percent who started at age 21 or older met the criteria. Early initiation is also associated with intentional and unintentional injury to self and others after drinking (Hingson & Zha, 2009; Hingson, Heeren, Jamanka, & Howland, 2000); violent behavior, including predatory violence and dating violence (Blitstein, Murray, Lytle, Birnbaum, & Perry, 2005; Ellickson, Tucker, & Klein, 2003; Swahn, Bossarte & Sullivent, 2008); criminal behavior (Eaton, Davis, Barrios, Brener, & Noonan, 2007); prescription drug misuse (Hermos et al., 2008); unplanned and unprotected sex (Hingson, Heeren, Winter, & Wechsler, 2003); motor vehicle crashes (Hingson et al., 2002); and physical fights (Hingson, Heeren, & Zakocs, 2001).

Adverse Effects on Normal Brain Development Are a Potential Long-Term Risk of Underage Alcohol Consumption

Research suggests that early, heavy alcohol use may affect the physical development and functioning of the brain. Some cross-sectional neurological studies suggest decreased ability among heavy alcohol users in planning, executive function, memory, spatial operation, and attention. These deficits, in turn, may put alcohol-dependent adolescents at risk for falling farther behind in school, putting them at an even greater disadvantage relative to nonusers (Brown, Tapert, Granholm, & Dellis, 2000). Some of these cross-sectional findings have been supported by longitudinal analyses (Squeglia, Jacobus, & Tapert, 2009).

Exhibit E.10: Ages of Initiation and Levels of DSM Diagnoses for Alcohol Abuse and Dependence (Grant & Dawson, 1997)

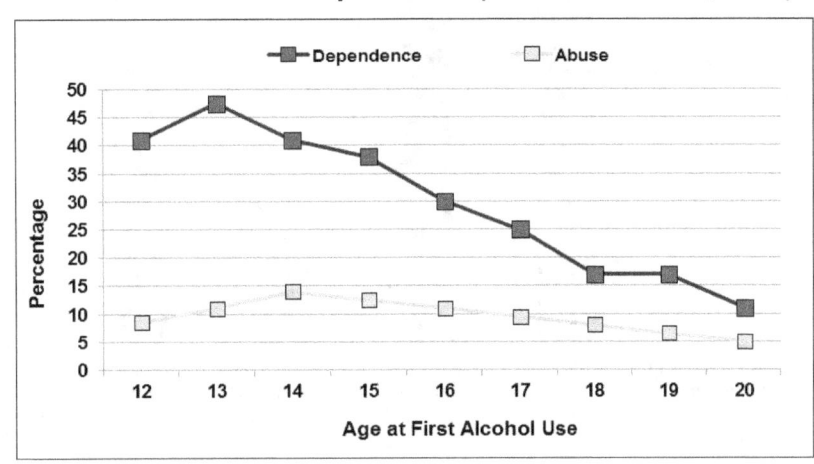

Underage Drinking Is Associated with Reduced Performance

Underage drinking, including binge drinking, is associated with reduced academic performance. Students who reported binge drinking were three times more likely than non–binge drinkers to report earning mostly Ds and Fs on their report cards (Miller, Naimi, Brewer, & Jones, 2007).

College Drinking Has Numerous Adverse Consequences

As noted in Exhibit E.8, overall rates of college students' drinking and binge drinking exceed those of their age peers who do not attend college. These alcohol consumption rates on college campuses constitute a significant public health problem, as shown in Exhibit E.11. One NIAAA-funded study (Abbey et al., 1996) reported that over half of college women respondents had experienced some form of sexual assault. Slightly fewer than one third of these assaults were characterized by respondents as attempted or completed rapes. However, the incidence of college sexual assaults is difficult to measure, and different studies report different rates. A review by Abbey (2011) of three relevant studies (Abbey et al, 2004; Seto & Barbaree, 1995; Testa, 2002) concludes that approximately half of all reported and unreported sexual assaults involve alcohol consumption by the perpetrator, victim, or both. Abbey further reports that, typically, if the victim consumes alcohol, the perpetrator does as well. Estimates of perpetrators' intoxication during the incident ranged from 30 to 75 percent. Approximately 25 percent of college students report academic consequences of their drinking, including missing class, falling behind, doing poorly on exams or papers, and receiving lower grades overall.

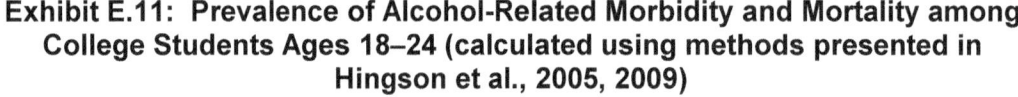

Exhibit E.11: Prevalence of Alcohol-Related Morbidity and Mortality among College Students Ages 18–24 (calculated using methods presented in Hingson et al., 2005, 2009)

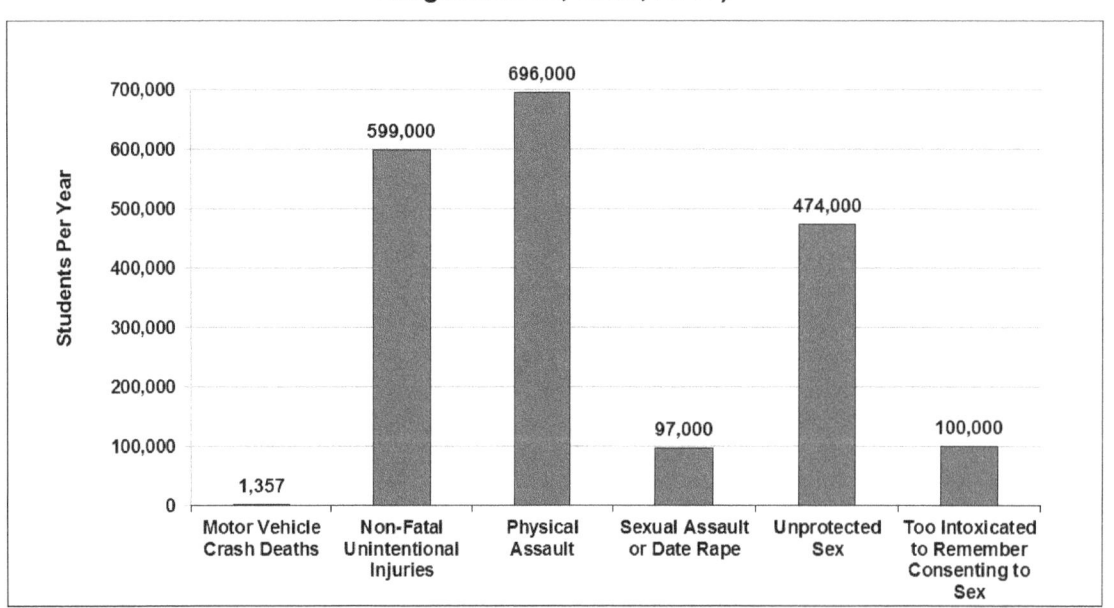

The National Effort To Reduce Underage Drinking

Underage drinking has been recognized as a public health problem for many years. Recently, however, the national effort to prevent alcohol use by America's young people has intensified as the multifaceted consequences associated with underage drinking have become more apparent. A brief summary of key milestones over the last two decades follows:

- 1992—Congress created SAMHSA "to focus attention, programs, and funding on improving the lives of people with or at risk for mental and substance abuse disorders."

- 1998—Congress mandated that the Department of Justice, through the Office of Justice Programs' Office of Juvenile Justice and Delinquency Prevention (OJJDP), establish and implement the Enforcing the Underage Drinking Laws (EUDL) program, a state- and community-based initiative.

- 2004—Congress directed the Secretary of the HHS to establish the Interagency Coordinating Committee on the Prevention of Underage Drinking (ICCPUD) and to issue an annual report summarizing all federal agency activities related to the problem.

- 2006—Congress passed the Sober Truth on Preventing (STOP) Underage Drinking Act, Public Law 109-422, popularly known as the STOP Act. The act states, "a multi-faceted effort is needed to more successfully address the problem of underage drinking in the United States. A coordinated approach to prevention, intervention, treatment, enforcement, and research is key to making progress. This Act recognizes the need for a focused national effort, and addresses particulars of the Federal portion of that effort as well as Federal support for state activities." The STOP Act also calls for two annual reports: (1) a Report to Congress from the HHS Secretary (the "Annual Report to Congress") and (2) a report on state underage drinking prevention and enforcement activities (the "State Report"). Chapters 1 through 3 of this document constitute the Annual Report to Congress; Chapter 4 constitutes the State Report. Together, they fulfill the STOP Act mandate and are designed to build on the efforts that precede it.

- 2007—The Surgeon General's *Call to Action To Prevent and Reduce Underage Drinking* (HHS, 2007) (henceforth termed *Call to Action*), the first on that subject, was issued. Based on the latest and most authoritative research, particularly on underage drinking as a developmental issue, the *Call to Action* outlines a comprehensive national effort to prevent and reduce underage alcohol consumption. The strategies for implementing the goals of the *Call to Action* are presented in the full *Call to Action*, which is available at http://www.surgeongeneral.gov/topics/underagedrinking/calltoaction.pdf.

The STOP Act requires the HHS Secretary to report to Congress on "the extent of progress in preventing and reducing underage drinking nationally." Data presented in Chapter 1 of this report demonstrate that meaningful progress has been made in reducing underage drinking prevalence. The factors that have contributed to this progress are varied and complex. However, one clear factor has been the increased attention to this issue at all levels of society. Federal initiatives have raised underage drinking to a prominent place on the national public health agenda, created a policy climate in which significant legislation has been passed by states and localities, raised awareness of the importance of aggressive enforcement, and stimulated coordinated citizen action. These changes are mutually reinforcing and have provided a framework for a sustained national commitment to reducing underage drinking.

Nevertheless, the rates of underage drinking are still unacceptably high, resulting in preventable and tragic health and safety consequences for the nation's youth, families, communities, and society as a whole. Therefore, ICCPUD remains committed to an ongoing, comprehensive approach to preventing and reducing underage drinking. This document, with its yearly updates to the State Report and survey responses, is part of that sustained effort to reduce underage drinking in America.

Below we highlight national efforts to address underage college drinking (further described in Chapter 1). The rates of alcohol consumption on college campuses constitute a significant public health problem.

Best Practices for Prevention of Underage College Drinking

To change the college drinking culture, the NIAAA-supported Task Force on College Drinking, composed of researchers, administrators, and students (NIAAA, 2002a), recommends that schools intervene with best practices at three levels: the individual student, including at-risk or alcohol-dependent drinkers; the entire student body; and the college and surrounding community. The Task Force also developed a "3-in-1" framework of college drinking prevention best practices. This framework is described in Chapter 1. In 2007, after an updated review of the college intervention literature, NIAAA issued "What Colleges Need to Know Now: An Update on College Drinking Research."

In 2011, the National College Health Improvement Project (NCHIP) launched the Learning Collaborative on High-Risk Drinking, to develop strategies for reducing alcohol problems on college campuses. For a description of the Learning Collaborative, see Chapter 1.

Research on college drinking prevention is ongoing, as is innovation on campuses across the country. Evidence for college-specific best practices is growing, and practices known to be effective with the general youth population are being tested in college settings. The Learning Collaborative on High-Risk Drinking may represent an important step forward in the commitment of colleges and universities to address underage drinking on campus. It also suggests a new effort to develop effective collaborations among college campuses, federal agencies, and researchers.

Report on State Programs and Policies Addressing Underage Drinking

Recognizing the importance of state programs and policies in preventing underage drinking, the STOP Act directs HHS and ICCPUD to provide an annual report on state underage drinking prevention activities. It defines specific categories of prevention programs, policies, enforcement activities related to those policies, and state expenditures to guide the report's development.

The annual State Report (Chapter 4) provides the following information for the 50 states and the District of Columbia (henceforth referred to as "states"):

1. Information on 25 underage drinking prevention policies focused on reducing youth access to alcohol and youth involvement in drinking and driving

2. Data from a survey addressing underage drinking enforcement programs; programs targeted to youth, parents, and caregivers; collaborations, planning, and reports; and state expenditures on the prevention of underage drinking

The 25 policies included in Chapter 4 can be grouped under four general headings:

- Laws Addressing Minors in Possession of Alcohol
- Laws Targeting Underage Drinking and Driving
- Laws Targeting Alcohol Suppliers
- Alcohol Pricing Policies

Laws Addressing Minors in Possession of Alcohol

1. Underage possession
2. Underage consumption
3. Internal possession by minors
4. Underage purchase and attempted purchase
5. False identification

Laws and the penalties associated with them are designed to raise the costs to underage people of obtaining and/or consuming alcohol. Such laws provide a primary deterrent (preventing underage drinking among nondrinkers) and a secondary deterrent (reducing the probability that adjudicated youth will drink again before reaching age 21). In addition, laws addressing internal possession facilitate enforcement and laws regarding false identification for obtaining alcohol make obtaining alcohol more difficult.

Laws Targeting Underage Drinking and Driving

6. Youth blood alcohol concentration limits (underage operators of noncommercial motor vehicles)
7. Loss of driving privileges for alcohol violations by minors ("use/lose" laws)
8. Graduated driver's licenses

Like laws addressing minors in possession of alcohol, these laws seek to deter underage driving after drinking by raising the cost of this behavior. In addition, graduated driver's licenses restrict driving privileges to reduce the incidence of a variety of risky driving behaviors, including driving while intoxicated.

Laws Targeting Alcohol Suppliers

9. Furnishing alcohol to minors
10. Compliance check protocols
11. Penalty guidelines for sales to minors
12. Responsible beverage service
13. Minimum ages for off-premises sellers
14. Minimum ages for on-premises servers and bartenders
15. Outlet siting near schools
16. Dram shop liability
17. Social host liability
18. Hosting underage drinking parties

19. Retailer interstate shipments of alcohol
20. Direct sales/shipments
21. Keg registration
22. Home delivery

These laws serve to reduce alcohol availability to minors, and hence reduce underage drinking. Some of the laws increase the costs to adults and thus deter furnishing alcohol to minors (e.g., compliance checks and social host and dram shop liability). Other laws directly impede furnishing (e.g., responsible beverage service, minimum age for servers and sellers, direct shipment, and home delivery).

Alcohol Pricing Policies

23. Alcohol taxes
24. Drink specials
25. Wholesaler pricing

These policies serve to decrease the "economic availability" of alcoholic beverages through increases in retail price and thus decrease underage drinking and a wide variety of related consequences. The effects of these policies may be direct (e.g., increased taxes, minimum wholesale prices, banning reduced-price drink specials) or indirect (e.g., limiting serving size).

Chapter 4 includes a description of each policy's key components, the status of the policy across states, and trends over time. Summaries are followed by a state-by-state analysis of each policy.

Two of these policies appear in this year's report for the first time: outlet siting near schools and retailer interstate shipments. Of particular note are the findings on retailer interstate shipments, which involve retailers shipping alcohol directly to consumers located across state lines, usually in response to internet orders. This relatively recent phenomenon may provide an important source of alcohol for underage persons and has been the focus of legislative action in 43 states, with 32 states banning these shipments entirely. For more information on this policy and other policies, see the individual state reports and policy summaries in Chapter 4.

State Survey

This section of Chapter 4 provides both the complete responses of the states to the 2012 State Survey (state summaries), and the Cross-State Report. This is the second wave of data collection for the State Survey (which was initiated in 2011). Comparisons for selected enforcement activities are presented between data collected in 2011 and data collected in 2012.

The survey content was derived directly from the STOP Act, covering topics and using terminology from the act. The survey questions were structured to allow states maximum flexibility in deciding which initiatives to describe and how to describe them. Open-ended questions were used whenever possible to allow states to "speak with their own voices." As noted earlier, the survey addressed four main areas:

1. Enforcement programs
2. Programs targeted to youth, parents, and caregivers
3. Collaborations, planning, and reports
4. State expenditures on the prevention of underage drinking

The Cross-State Report presents data about variables amenable to quantitative analysis. Overall, the 2012 data reveal a wide range of activity in the areas studied, although these vary in scope and intensity from state to state. All states have areas of strength and all have areas where improvements could be realized. The inadequacy of some state data systems to respond to the data requested in the survey is a recurrent theme. This is especially the case in local law enforcement and expenditures. Accurate and complete data are essential both for describing current activities to prevent underage drinking and to monitor progress in future state surveys.

Comparisons of 2011 and 2012 enforcement data suggest trends. Sixty percent of the states reporting for both years indicated that minors in possession arrests increased, whereas 53 percent of the states reported a decrease in the number of state compliance checks. Larger percentages of the states reported reductions in the use of retailer penalties than reported increases. These results must be viewed with caution. In many cases, substantial missing data decrease the extent to which meaningful conclusions can be drawn. Caution must also be exercised in interpreting the 2011–2012 changes. Single-year trends are rarely stable and may not hold up over time.

Conclusion

Data in this report demonstrate that meaningful progress has been made in reducing underage drinking prevalence. The factors contributing to this progress are varied and complex. One clear factor has been increased attention to this issue at all levels of society. Federal initiatives, together with efforts by the national media, state and local governments, and interested private organizations, have raised underage drinking to a prominent place on the national public health agenda, created a policy climate in which significant legislation has been passed by states and localities, raised awareness of the importance of aggressive enforcement, and stimulated coordinated citizen action. These changes are mutually reinforcing and have provided a framework for a sustained national commitment to reducing underage drinking.

Nevertheless, the rates of underage drinking are still unacceptably high, resulting in preventable and tragic health and safety consequences for the nation's youth, families, communities, and society as a whole. Therefore, ICCPUD remains committed to an ongoing, comprehensive approach to preventing and reducing underage drinking.

CHAPTER 1
Preventing and Reducing Underage Drinking: An Overview

Introduction

Alcohol remains the most widely used substance of abuse among America's youth. According to the Substance Abuse and Mental Health Services Administration (SAMHSA) through a special analysis based on 2011 data, a higher percentage of youth who are 12 to 20 years old used alcohol in the past month (25.1 percent) than tobacco (19.6 percent) or illicit drugs (14.9 percent) (SAMHSA, 2012). The extent of alcohol consumption by those younger than the legal drinking age of 21 constitutes a serious threat to both public health and public safety. In response, governments at the federal, state, and local levels have sought to develop effective approaches to reduce underage drinking and its associated costs and consequences. The actions of government alone, however, cannot solve this serious problem. Only a broad, committed collaboration among governments, parents of underage youth, other adults, caregivers (people who provide services to youth, such as teachers, coaches, health and mental health care providers, human services workers, and juvenile justice workers), prevention professionals, youth, and private-sector organizations and institutions can reach an effective solution to this national challenge.

Underage drinking is a complex and challenging social problem that has defied an easy solution. Although selling alcohol to youth under age 21 is illegal in all 50 states and the District of Columbia, some states make it legal to provide (but not sell) alcohol to youth under special circumstances, such as at religious ceremonies, in private residences, or in the presence of a parent or guardian. Despite such broad restrictions, underage youth find it relatively easy to acquire alcohol, often from adults. Alcohol use often begins at a young age; the average age of first use for youths who initiated before age 21 is about 15.9 years old, and 10 percent of 9- to 10-year-olds have already started drinking (Donovan et al., 2004). Alcohol use increases with each additional year of age, and by age 20, more than half (55.3 percent) of youths report having had one or more drinks in the past 30 days (SAMHSA, 2012a). Underage drinkers are much more likely than adults to drink heavily and recklessly. Studies consistently indicate that about 80 percent of college students—of whom 48 percent are underage—drink alcohol, and about 40 percent of all college students engage in binge drinking (i.e., when men consume five or more drinks in a row and women consume four or more drinks in a row (National Institute on Alcohol Abuse and Alcoholism [NIAAA], 2002a)). [6]

Scientific research over the past decade has broadened our understanding of the ways and extent to which underage alcohol use threatens the immediate and long-term development, well-being, and future mental development of young people. Alcohol is a leading contributor to fatal injuries, a major cause of death for people younger than 21. The potential consequences of underage drinking include alcohol-related traffic crashes and fatalities, other unintentional injuries such as burns and drowning, increased risk of suicide and homicide, physical and sexual assault, academic and social problems, inappropriate and/or risky sexual activity, and adverse effects on the developing brain (NIAAA, 2005a). The consequences of underage alcohol use

---

[6] Binge drinking is the consumption of a large amount of alcohol over a relatively short period of time. No common terminology has been established to describe different drinking patterns. Based on National Survey on Drug Use and Health (NSDUH) data, SAMHSA defines "binge drinking" as five or more drinks on one occasion on at least 1 day in the past 30 days and "heavy drinking" as five or more drinks on at least 5 different days in the past 30 days. However, NSDUH can provide binge-drinking estimates based on the NIAAA gender-specific definition. Some studies, including Wechsler's (2002) survey of college students, define "binge drinking" as five or more drinks in a row for men and four or more for women. Other sources use "frequent heavy drinking" to refer to five or more drinks on at least five occasions in the last 30 days. Appendix A discusses these differences in more detail. See Courtney and Polich (2009) for further discussion of the definition issues.

extend beyond underage drinkers: society also pays. For example, in 2010, 50 percent of all deaths in traffic crashes involving a 15- to 20-year-old driver with a blood alcohol concentration (BAC) of .08 or higher were people other than the drinking driver (National Center for Statistics and Analysis, National Highway Traffic Safety Administration [NHTSA] Fatality Analysis Reporting System [FARS], 2010). In 2006, almost $27 billion (about 12 percent) of the total $223.5 billion economic costs of excessive alcohol consumption were related to underage drinking (Bouchery, Harwood, Sacks, Simon, & Brewer, 2011).

As noted below, the problems associated with college drinking include sexual assault or date rape, violent crime on college campuses, and academic consequences including missing class, falling behind, doing poorly on exams or papers, and receiving lower grades overall. Campus alcohol use also affects the academic performance of nondrinkers by contributing to a noisy and disruptive environment that is not conducive to studying.

The National Effort To Reduce Underage Drinking

Underage drinking has been recognized as a public health problem for many years. Recently, however, the national effort to prevent alcohol use by America's young people has intensified as the multifaceted consequences associated with underage drinking have become more apparent.

After Prohibition ended in 1933, states assumed authority for alcohol control, including the enactment of laws restricting youth access to alcohol. The majority of states designated 21 as the minimum legal drinking age (MLDA) for the "purchase or public possession" of alcohol. Beyond setting a minimum drinking age, the nation's alcohol problems were largely ignored through the 1960s (NIAAA, 2005b). However, on December 31, 1970, Congress established NIAAA "to provide leadership in the national effort to reduce alcohol problems through research."

Between 1970 and 1976, 29 states lowered their MLDAs to 18, 19, or 20 years old, in part because the voting age had been lowered (Wagenaar, 1981). However, studies conducted in the 1970s found that motor vehicle crashes increased significantly among teens, resulting in more traffic injuries and fatalities (Cucchiaro, Ferreira, & Sicherman, 1974; Douglass, Filkins, & Clark, 1974; Wagenaar, 1983, 1993; Whitehead, 1977; Whitehead et al., 1975; Williams, Rich, Zador, & Robertson, 1974). As a result, 24 of the 29 states raised their MLDAs between 1976 and 1984, although to different minimum ages. Some placed restrictions on the types of alcohol that could be consumed by persons younger than 21. Only 22 states set an MLDA of 21 years old. In response, the federal government enacted the National Minimum Drinking Age Act of 1984, which mandated reduced federal highway funds to states that did not raise their MLDAs to 21. By 1987, all remaining states had raised their MLDAs to 21 in response to the federal legislation.

In 1992, Congress created SAMHSA "to focus attention, programs, and funding on improving the lives of people with or at risk for mental and substance abuse disorders." In 1998, Congress mandated that the Department of Justice, through the Office of Justice Programs' Office of Juvenile Justice and Delinquency Prevention (OJJDP), establish and implement the Enforcing the Underage Drinking Laws (EUDL) program, a state- and community-based initiative.

As national concern about underage drinking grew, in part because of advances in science that increasingly revealed adverse consequences, Congress appropriated funds for a study by The National Academies to examine the relevant literature to "review existing Federal, state, and nongovernmental programs, including media-based programs, designed to change the attitudes and health behaviors of youth." The National Research Council (NRC) and the Institute of Medicine (IOM) issued that report in 2004. Since then, a number of programs aimed at preventing and reducing underage drinking have been initiated at the federal, state, and local levels. Chapter 3 describes major programs at the federal level; Chapter 4 describes initiatives at the state level.

The conference report accompanying H.R. 2673, the "Consolidated Appropriations Act of 2004," directed the Secretary of the U.S. Department of Health and Human Services (HHS) to establish the Interagency Coordinating Committee on the Prevention of Underage Drinking (ICCPUD) and to issue an annual report summarizing all federal agency activities related to the problem. The HHS Secretary directed the SAMHSA Administrator to convene ICCPUD in 2004. ICCPUD includes representatives from HHS's Office of the Surgeon General (OSG), Centers for Disease Control and Prevention (CDC), Administration for Children and Families (ACF), Office of the Assistant Secretary for Planning and Evaluation (ASPE), and National Institutes of Health (NIH), including NIAAA and NIDA; Department of Justice, Office of Juvenile Justice and Delinquency Prevention (OJJDP); Office of Safe and Healthy Students (OSHS); Department of Transportation, National Highway Traffic Safety Administration (NHTSA); White House Office of National Drug Control Policy (ONDCP); Department of the Treasury; Department of Defense; and Federal Trade Commission (FTC).

ICCPUD coordinates federal efforts to reduce underage drinking and served as a resource for the development of *A Comprehensive Plan for Preventing and Reducing Underage Drinking*, which Congress called for in 2004. ICCPUD received input from experts and organizations representing a wide range of parties, including public health advocacy groups, the alcohol industry, ICCPUD member agencies, and the U.S. Congress. The latest research available at the time was analyzed and incorporated into the plan, which HHS reported to Congress in January 2006. It included three goals, a series of federal action steps, and three measurable performance targets for evaluating national progress in preventing and reducing underage drinking.

In December 2006, Congress passed the Sober Truth on Preventing (STOP) Underage Drinking Act, Public Law 109-422, popularly known as the STOP Act. The Act states, "a multi-faceted effort is needed to more successfully address the problem of underage drinking in the United States. A coordinated approach to prevention, intervention, treatment, enforcement, and research is key to making progress. This Act recognizes the need for a focused national effort, and addresses particulars of the federal portion of that effort as well as federal support for state activities." The STOP Act requires the HHS Secretary, in collaboration with other federal officials enumerated in the Act, to "formally establish and enhance the efforts of the interagency coordinating committee (ICCPUD) that began operating in 2004."

The STOP Act also calls for two annual reports:

1. A report to Congress from the HHS Secretary (the "Annual Report to Congress") that includes:

   – A description of all programs and policies of federal agencies designed to prevent and reduce underage drinking.

- The extent of progress in preventing and reducing underage drinking nationally.
- Information related to patterns and consequences of underage drinking.
- Measures of the exposure of underage populations to messages regarding alcohol in advertising and the entertainment media, as reported by FTC.
- Surveillance data, including information about the onset and prevalence of underage drinking, consumption patterns, and the means of underage access, and certain other data included in the report.
- Such other information regarding underage drinking as the Secretary determines to be appropriate.

2. A report on state underage drinking-prevention and enforcement activities (the "State Report") that includes:

- A set of measures to be used in preparing the report on best practices.
- Categories of underage-drinking-prevention policies, enforcement practices, and programs (see Chapter 4 for list of specific categories).
- Additional information on state efforts or programs not specifically included in the Act.

Chapters 1 through 3 of this document constitute the Annual Report to Congress; Chapter 4 constitutes the State Report. Together, they fulfill the STOP Act mandate and are designed to build on the efforts that precede it. For example, the State Report provides the second wave of data for a substantial new resource for state and local coalitions and policymakers. It reports on comprehensive assessments of state underage drinking laws, policies, and programs, including individual state reports. This is critical information for states as a foundation for enhancing their underage drinking prevention efforts.

In fall 2005, ICCPUD sponsored a national meeting of the states to prevent and reduce underage alcohol use. At the meeting, the Surgeon General announced his intent to issue a *Call to Action* on the prevention and reduction of underage drinking. Subsequently, OSG worked closely with SAMHSA and NIAAA to develop the report. In 2007, *The Surgeon General's Call to Action to Prevent and Reduce Underage Drinking* (HHS, 2007) (henceforth termed *Call to Action*), the first on that subject, was issued. Based on the latest and most authoritative research, particularly on underage drinking as a developmental issue, the *Call to Action* outlines a comprehensive national effort to prevent and reduce underage alcohol consumption. It includes six goals and describes the rationale, challenges, and strategies of each goal, including specific actions for parents and other caregivers, communities, schools, colleges and universities, the criminal and juvenile justice systems, law enforcement, the alcohol industry, and the entertainment and media industries.

ICCPUD agencies collaborated to provide information and data for the *Call to Action*. The 2006 Federal Comprehensive Plan set forth three general goals:

1. Strengthening a national commitment to address underage drinking
2. Reducing demand for, availability of, and access to alcohol by persons younger than 2 years
3. Using research, evaluation, and scientific surveillance to improve the effectiveness of policies and programs designed to prevent and reduce underage drinking

The six specific goals and associated strategies in the *Call to Action* for the nation build on these three general goals.

As the nation's leading medical spokesperson, the Surgeon General is in a unique position to call attention to national health problems. By issuing the *Call to Action,* the Surgeon General has sought to raise public awareness and foster changes in American society—goals similar to those described to Congress in the Comprehensive Plan. The *Call to Action* has incorporated—and, therefore, superseded—the Comprehensive Plan.

As with the Comprehensive Plan, ICCPUD agencies are implementing a variety of federal programs to support the *Call to Action*'s goals. For example, SAMHSA and NIAAA worked with OSG to support rollouts of the *Call to Action* in 13 states; SAMHSA collaborated with ICCPUD to support more than 7,000 town hall meetings, using the *Call to Action*'s *Guide to Action for Communities* (HHS, 2007) as a primary resource; and SAMHSA has asked community coalitions funded under the STOP Act to implement strategies contained in the *Call to Action.* These and other programs are described in more detail in Chapter 3.

Principles and Goals of the *Call to Action*

The national effort to prevent and reduce underage drinking outlined in the *Call to Action* is based on the following principles from which its goals were derived:

- *Underage alcohol use is a phenomenon directly related to human development.* Because of the nature of adolescence, alcohol poses a powerful attraction to adolescents and can have unpredictable outcomes that put every child at risk.

- *Factors that protect adolescents from alcohol use, as well as put them at greater risk, change during the course of adolescence.* Individual characteristics, developmental issues, and shifting factors in adolescents' environments all play a role.

- *Protecting adolescents from alcohol use requires a comprehensive, developmentally based approach* that is initiated prior to puberty and continues throughout adolescence with support from families, schools, colleges, communities, the health care system, and government.

- *Prevention and reduction of underage drinking is the collective responsibility of the nation.* "Scaffolding the Nation's youth"[7] is the responsibility of all people in all of the social systems with which adolescents interact: family, schools, communities, health care systems, religious institutions, criminal and juvenile justice systems, all levels of government, and society as a whole. Each social system has a potential effect on the adolescent, and the active involvement of all systems is necessary to fully maximize existing resources to prevent underage drinking and its related problems. When all of the social systems work together toward the common goal of preventing and reducing underage drinking, they create a powerful synergy that is critical to realizing the vision.

- *Underage alcohol use is not inevitable, and parents and society are not helpless to prevent it.* The *Call to Action* proposes a vision for the future wherein each child is free to develop to his or her potential without the impairment of alcohol's negative consequences. The fulfillment of

---

[7] Scaffolding the nation's youth is the Surgeon General's term for a structured process through which parents and society facilitate positive adolescent development and minimize risk by protecting against adolescents' natural risk-taking, sensation-seeking tendencies. It is a fitting metaphor for the support and protection that parents and society provide children and youth to help them function in a more mature way until they are ready to function without that extra support. This external support system—or scaffold—around the adolescent promotes healthy development and protects against alcohol use and other risky behaviors by facilitating good decisionmaking, mitigating risk factors, and buffering potentially destructive outside influences that draw adolescents to use alcohol.

that vision rests on the achievement of six goals that the *Call to Action* sets for the nation, listed below.

Goal 1: Foster changes in American society that facilitate healthy adolescent development and help prevent and reduce underage drinking.

Goal 2: Engage parents and other caregivers, schools, communities, all levels of government, all social systems that interface with youth, and youth themselves in a coordinated national effort to prevent and reduce underage drinking and its consequences.

Goal 3: Promote an understanding of underage alcohol consumption in the context of human development and maturation that takes into account individual adolescent characteristics as well as ethnic, cultural, and gender differences.

Goal 4: Conduct additional research on adolescent alcohol use and its relationship to development.

Goal 5: Work to improve public health surveillance on underage drinking and on population-based risk factors for this behavior.

Goal 6: Work to ensure that laws and policies at all levels are consistent with the national goal of preventing and reducing underage alcohol consumption.

The strategies for implementing these goals for parents and other caregivers, communities, schools, colleges and universities, businesses, the health care system, juvenile justice and law enforcement, and the alcohol and entertainment industries are included in the full *Call to Action*, which is available at http://www.surgeongeneral.gov/topics/underagedrinking/calltoaction.pdf.

Best Practices for Prevention of Underage Drinking among College Students

Introduction: Extent of the Problem

As noted in Chapter 2, overall rates of college student drinking and binge drinking exceed those of their age peers who do not attend college (Johnston et al., 2012b). Of college students, 80.5 percent drink and 36.1 percent report drinking five or more drinks on an occasion in the past 2 weeks. Research indicates that some college students' drinking far exceeds the minimum binge criterion of five drinks per occasion (Wechsler et al., 1999; White, Kraus, & Swartzwelder, 2006). Underage college students consume about 48 percent of the alcohol consumed by students at 4-year colleges (Wechsler, Lee, Nelson, & Kuo, 2002; Wechsler & Nelson, 2008).

As further described in Chapter 2, the rates of alcohol consumption on college campuses constitute a significant public health problem. Abbey (2011) notes that approximately half of all reported and unreported college sexual assaults involve alcohol consumption by the perpetrator, victim, or both. Estimates of perpetrators' intoxication during the incident ranged from 30 to 75 percent. Alcohol use is also involved in a large percentage of violent crime on college campuses (Commission on Substance Abuse at Colleges and Universities, 1994). Approximately 25 percent of college students report academic consequences resulting from their drinking, including missing class, falling behind, doing poorly on exams or papers, and receiving lower grades overall. Campus alcohol use also affects the academic performance of nondrinkers by contributing to a noisy and disruptive environment that is not conducive to study.

In its 2002 report, *A Call to Action: Changing the Culture of Drinking at U.S. Colleges*, NIAAA noted the following, which remains the case 10 years later:

> The tradition of drinking has developed into a kind of culture—beliefs and customs—entrenched in every level of college students' environments. Customs handed down through generations of college drinkers reinforce students' expectation alcohol is a necessary ingredient for social success. These beliefs and the expectations they engender exert a powerful influence over students' behavior toward alcohol.[8]

College Drinking Prevention Best Practices

In 1998, NIAAA convened its Task Force on College Drinking, composed of college presidents, students, and alcohol research experts on college drinking. During a 3-year research and outreach project, the Task Force produced a landmark report, *A Call to Action: Changing the Culture of Drinking at U.S. Colleges,* which highlighted the magnitude of the problem and made specific recommendations for addressing the problem based on existing research evidence.

The Task Force encouraged school administrators to address college drinking issues in a broad and comprehensive fashion. The report recommended that schools use a "3 in 1 Framework" to develop comprehensive programs that integrate multiple complementary strategies. Such programs focus simultaneously on (1) individuals, including at-risk or alcohol-dependent drinkers; (2) the student population as a whole; and (3) the college and surrounding community. Specific recommendations were grouped into four tiers based on the degree of research evidence to support or refute them. At the time, the strongest research evidence showing effectiveness among college students supported strategies that targeted individual students. A number of environmental strategies showed evidence of effectiveness with similar populations, whereas other strategies were listed as either promising or ineffective. Exhibit 1.1 outlines the strategies examined by the NIAAA Task Force, grouped according to the supporting evidence for them and the levels at which they operate.

Since the Task Force report was issued in 2002, research on college drinking has continued to yield important information about the potential effectiveness of these and additional intervention strategies. In 2007, after an updated review of the college intervention literature, NIAAA issued "What Colleges Need to Know Now: An Update on College Drinking Research." Current research confirms that interventions targeting individual students, including those at risk for alcohol problems, are effective. In addition, research now more clearly supports the use of environmental interventions, particularly campus–community partnerships, as part of a comprehensive program to address harmful college drinking.

---

[8] For many students, alcohol use is not a tradition. Students who drink the least attend 2-year institutions, religious schools, commuter schools, and historically Black colleges and universities (Meilman et al., 1994, 1995, 1999; Presley et al., 1996a,b).

Exhibit 1.1: 3-in-1 Framework

3-IN-1 FRAMEWORK

Tier	Strategy	Individuals, including At-Risk and Dependent Drinkers	Student Population as Whole	Community
		Level of Operation		
1: Effective among college students	Combining cognitive-behavioral skills with norms clarification & motivational enhancement intervention	Yes	No	No
	Offering brief motivational enhancement interventions in student health centers and emergency rooms	Yes	No	No
	Challenging alcohol expectancies	Yes	No	No
2: Effective with general populations	Increased enforcement of minimum drinking age laws	No	Yes	Yes
	Implementation, increased publicity, and enforcement of other laws to reduce alcohol-impaired driving	No	Yes	Yes
	Restrictions on alcohol retail density	No	No	Yes
	Increased price and excise taxes on alcoholic beverages	No	No	Yes
	Responsible beverage service policies in social & commercial settings	No	Yes	Yes
	The formation of a campus/community coalition	No	Yes	Yes
3: Promising	Adopting campus-based policies to reduce high-risk use (e.g., reinstating Friday classes, eliminating keg parties, establishing alcohol-free activities & dorms)	No	Yes	No
	Increasing enforcement at campus-based events that promote excessive drinking	No	Yes	No
	Increasing publicity about enforcement of underage drinking laws/eliminating "mixed" messages	No	Yes	Yes
	Consistently enforcing disciplinary actions associated with policy violations	No	Yes	No
	Conducting marketing campaigns to correct student misperceptions about alcohol use on campus	No	Yes	No
	Provision of "safe rides" programs	No	Yes	Yes
	Regulation of happy hours and sales	No	Yes	Yes
	Enhancing awareness of personal liability	Yes	Yes	No
	Informing new students and parents about alcohol policies and penalties	Yes	Yes	No
4: Ineffective	Informational, knowledge-based or values clarification interventions when used alone	N/A	N/A	N/A

The *Call to Action* also provided best practices recommendations for college drinking prevention, including fostering a culture in which alcohol does not play a central role in college life or the college experience. About a quarter of the recommendations of the *Call to Action* specifically overlap the 3-in-1 framework. The *Call to Action* also recommends:

- Providing frequent alcohol-free late-night events, extending hours of student centers and athletics facilities, and increasing public service opportunities.
- Offering alcohol-free dormitories that promote healthy lifestyles.
- Restricting or eliminating alcohol sales at concerts and at athletic and other campus events.
- Reinstating Friday classes to shorten the extended weekend.

The Community Preventive Services Task Force (2010) and the Institute of Medicine (*Reducing Underage Drinking: A Collective Responsibility*, 2004), although not specifically focused on college drinking, both support the 3-in-1 framework strategies of aggressive enforcement of underage drinking laws, increasing alcohol prices, and excise tax. Exhibit 4.1.1, "Underage Drinking Prevention Policies – Best Practices," presented in Chapter 4.1 lists additional policies that may contribute to a reduction in college drinking, especially drinking that occurs in the surrounding community. The policies include dram shop and social host liability, bans on direct sales (internet/mail order); keg registration; minimum age for servers, sellers, and bartenders; internal possession laws; and restrictions on alcohol advertising. Much of this information is still very helpful today.

For many years, NIAAA has invested substantial resources in supporting studies on individual and environmental interventions to address college drinking. As a result, knowledge about best practices continues to grow. A few recent highlights follow:

1. At the individual level, screening and brief intervention in the college student health center can be effective in reducing high-risk drinking and alcohol-related consequences (Schaus et al., 2009; Fleming et al., 2010).

2. At the environmental level, a large-scale trial showed the effectiveness of community–college partnerships in reducing alcohol problems in off-campus settings through heavily publicized and highly visible alcohol policy and enforcement activities (Saltz, Paschall, McGaffigan, & Nygaard, 2010).

3. An online alcohol education course for incoming freshmen showed benefits through the first semester in reducing binge drinking and alcohol-related problems (Paschall, Antin, Ringwalt, & Saltz, 2011).

These results reinforce the findings in the 2002 *Call to Action* and the 2007 Update of College Drinking Research, that intervening with problem drinking and its associated consequences can occur at different levels and times during college, and that implementing a combination of interventions may be especially helpful.

Moving Forward—The NIAAA Matrix Tool

NIAAA-supported research has resulted in evidence-based practices that can be used to address harmful drinking and related consequences on college campuses, several of which are mentioned above. To foster the implementation of these strategies, NIAAA convened a new College Presidents Working Group in 2011. Its goals are to bring renewed, vigorous national attention to college drinking; encourage the translation of college prevention research findings into practice; and provide a platform for sharing and disseminating evidence-based information. In FY 2012, NIAAA continued to work with the group of 11 college presidents first convened in FY 2011. Among the many practical recommendations the presidents made to NIAAA, one stood out: the need for a clear, easy-to-understand tool to help them evaluate and select interventions that are effective, best fit their schools, and feasible to implement. In response, NIAAA is developing a matrix-based decision tool that organizes what is known about college drinking interventions by important parameters such as the strength of the research evidence and ease of implementation. NIAAA enlisted a team of six college drinking research experts to develop the matrix. Next, 10 additional scientific experts reviewed the draft matrix. Their comments were collated and shared with the developers, who have revised the matrix in response. The matrix will form the centerpiece of a guide for college administrators on intervening to prevent harmful drinking on campus. A searchable online decision tool is envisioned as well.

College Learning Collaborative on High-Risk Drinking

The National College Health Improvement Project (NCHIP) was founded in 2010 by Dr. Jim Yong Kim, then President of Dartmouth College. Its mission is to improve the health of college students through the application of population health solutions coupled with a quality improvement framework in bringing evidence into practice and measuring outcomes.

In February 2011, NCHIP convened a panel of experts on drinking to discuss the current evidence on how to best address the problem, along with the measurement strategies that could be used to track outcomes and effectiveness of campus efforts. Two months later, NCHIP formally launched the Learning Collaborative on High-Risk Drinking.

Membership in the initiative totals 32 institutions. Each participating school has a campus improvement team with multidisciplinary representation, including students, administrators, health services and health promotion professionals, student affairs staff members, faculty members, and other key stakeholders. The collaborative is a 24-month-long process devoted to implementing policies and programs to reduce college high-risk drinking and its associated harms using measurement-based improvement. The goal is to discover what works well, how, and why, and to broadly disseminate these findings so that others can adapt and replicate them on their campuses.

The collaborative used the Institute for Healthcare Improvement's Breakthrough Series framework as the foundation for testing and implementing harm prevention strategies across participating institutions. The framework relies on rapid-cycle tests of change in adapting and implementing existing evidence across multiple settings to accomplish a common aim. Developed in the early 1990s, the Breakthrough Series has been shown effective in many clinical and public health settings.

The following infrastructure supports the work of the 32 schools and universities involved in the collaborative.

- *Learning sessions:* Three face-to-face learning sessions were held (June 2011, January 2012, and July 2012). Each focused on a specific domain: individual drinker, campus environment, and the larger system. Prior to the sessions, teams collected and analyzed data relative to these domains, and prepared storyboards on initiatives targeting these areas on their individual campuses. The sessions enabled participants to share their knowledge and work results on reducing high-risk drinking and its associated harms.

- *Action periods:* Between each learning session, teams tested and implemented new initiatives and interventions while concurrently measuring outcomes and relevant processes. The NCHIP Leadership Team, composed of measurement and quality improvement experts and nationally recognized experts on high-risk drinking, facilitated this process through virtual meetings, monthly conference calls, and review and analysis of team online reporting of progress and measures.

- ***Summative Congress and Dissemination:*** A Summative Congress held in June 2013 synthesized and summarized results of the 2-year collaborative, and discussed sustainability of gains over the long term and possible research opportunities emanating from this work. The collaborative expects to publish its findings and add to the body of knowledge about high-risk drinking on college campuses.

Conclusion

Research on college drinking prevention is ongoing, as is innovation on campuses across the country. Evidence supporting college-specific best practices is growing, and practices known to be effective with the general population of youth are being tested in college settings. The College Learning Collaborative on High-Risk Drinking may represent a step forward in the commitment of colleges and universities to address underage drinking on their campuses. It also suggests a new effort to develop effective collaboration among college campuses, federal agencies, and researchers. If so, there is reason for optimism.

Federal and State Actions Regarding Caffeinated Alcoholic Beverages

Caffeinated alcoholic beverages (CABs) are premixed beverages that combine alcohol, caffeine, and other stimulants. Research suggests that including caffeine in such beverages poses public health and safety risks because the caffeine can mask the depressant effects of alcohol without changing alcohol's intoxicating properties (http://www.cdc.gov/alcohol/fact-sheets/cab.htm). This could lead some to believe they are more capable of operating a vehicle and presents other risks such as encouraging binge drinking, particularly among young drinkers.

These health and safety risks prompted members of the National Association of Attorneys General Youth Access to Alcohol Committee to initiate investigations and negotiations with the Anheuser-Busch and MillerCoors Brewing Companies in 2007. In 2008, those companies agreed to remove caffeine and other stimulants from their products. In 2009, the Federal Drug Administration (FDA) initiated an investigation into the marketing and distribution of other caffeinated malt-based alcoholic beverages and, on November 17, 2010, issued warning letters to four companies that the caffeine added to their alcoholic malt beverages is an "unsafe food additive." The letters stated that further action, including seizure of their products, was possible under federal law.[9] In response, the four companies ceased using added caffeine in their products, and, by summer 2011, it appeared that, with few if any exceptions, malt-based beverages with added caffeine were no longer available in the United States.[10]

In parallel with the federal actions against caffeinated alcoholic beverages, 9 states enacted statutory or administrative bans on such beverages, and 21 states considered such bans.

---

[9] See http://www.fda.gov/ForConsumers/ConsumerUpdates/ucm233987.htm#2. The FDA investigation and warning letters involved companies that produce malt-based alcoholic beverages and did not include wine- and spirits-based products. The investigation did not address products that contain naturally brewed caffeine (e.g., coffee-based drinks).

[10] For more references and details on health and safety risks associated with caffeinated alcoholic beverages and successful efforts to remove them from the marketplace, see the 2012 Report to Congress on the Prevention and Reduction of Underage Drinking (http://www.stopalcoholabuse.gov/media/ReportToCongress/2012/report_main/report_to_congress_2012.pdf), Appendix E.

Extent of Progress

The STOP Act requires the HHS Secretary to report to Congress on "the extent of progress in preventing and reducing underage drinking nationally." An examination of trend data reported in federally sponsored surveys suggests that meaningful progress is being made in reducing the extent of underage drinking. It is generally inadvisable to draw conclusions based on changes from one year to the next because of natural fluctuations. Examining trends over a multiyear period is much more informative. The following exhibits provide estimates of past-year alcohol use from 2004 through 2011 based on NSDUH data.[11] All age groups showed a statistically significant decline in both past-month alcohol use and binge alcohol use in 2011 compared with 2004.

As shown in the last column in Exhibits 1.2 and 1.3, for most age groups the declines have been substantial. Not unexpectedly, changes among 18- to 20-year-olds were smaller but still statistically significant. The large number of 18- to 20-year-olds using alcohol also accounts for the smaller percent change among 12- to 20-year-olds compared with 12- to 17-year olds. As shown in Exhibit 1.4, there was a statistically significant increase in average age at first use over the same time period (SAMHSA, CBHSQ, NSDUH, Special Data Analysis, 2012).

Exhibit 1.2: Past-Month Alcohol Use for 12- to 20-Year-Olds, 2004–2011

Age	2004	2005	2006	2007	2008	2009	2010	2011	% Change 2004 to 2011
12-13	4.3%	4.2%	3.9%	3.5%*	3.4%*	3.5%*	3.2%*	2.5%*	-41.9%
14-15	16.4%	15.1%	15.6%	14.7%*	13.3%*	13.1%*	12.4%*	11.3%*	-31.1%
16-17	32.5%	30.1%*	29.8%*	29.2%*	26.3%*	26.5%*	24.6%*	25.3%*	-22.2%
18-20	51.1%	51.1%	51.6%	50.8%	48.6%*	49.5%	48.5%*	46.8%*	-8.4%
12-17	17.6%	16.5%*	16.7%*	16.0%*	14.7%*	14.8%*	13.6%*	13.3%*	-24.4%
12-20	28.7%	28.2%	28.4%	28.0%	26.5%*	27.2%*	26.2%*	25.1%*	-12.5%

*Difference between 2004 estimate and this estimate is statistically significant at the 0.05 level.

Exhibit 1.3: Past-Month Binge Alcohol Use for 12- to 20-Year-Olds, 2004–2011

Age	2004	2005	2006	2007	2008	2009	2010	2011	% Change 2004 - 2011
12-13	2.0%	2.0%	1.5%	1.5%	1.5%	1.6%	1.0%*	1.1%*	-45.0%
14-15	9.1%	8.0%	9.0%	7.8%*	7.0%*	7.0%*	6.7%*	5.7%*	-37.4%
16-17	22.4%	19.7%*	20.1%*	19.5%*	17.2%*	17.1%*	15.3%*	15.0%*	-33.0%
18-20	36.8%	36.1%	36.2%	35.9%	33.9%*	34.9%	33.1%*	31.2%*	-15.2%
12-17	11.1%	9.9%*	10.3%	9.7%*	8.9%*	8.9%*	7.9%*	7.4%*	-33.3%
12-20	19.6%	18.8%	19.0%	18.7%	17.5%*	18.2%*	16.9%*	15.8%*†	-19.4%

*Difference between 2004 estimate and this estimate is statistically significant at the 0.05 level.
†Difference between 2010 and 2011 estimate is statistically significant at the 0.05 level.

---

[11] The 2006–2010 estimates are based on data files revised in March 2012.

**Exhibit 1.4: Average Age at First Use among Past-Year Initiates of Alcohol Use
Who Initiated Before Age 21, 2004–2011**

Year	2004	2005	2006	2007	2008	2009	2010	2011
Average Age at First Use	15.6	15.6	15.8*	15.8*	15.8*	15.9*	16.0*	15.9*

*Difference between 2004 estimate and this estimate is statistically significant at the 0.05 level.

Data from the Monitoring the Future (MTF) survey and Youth Risk Behavior Survey (YRBS) also suggest positive movement.[12] This alignment within and across surveys, even without statistical significance across all three surveys, is a good sign.

These data demonstrate that meaningful progress has been made in reducing underage drinking prevalence. The factors that have contributed to this progress are varied and complex. However, one clear factor has been increased attention to this issue at all levels of society. Federal initiatives have raised underage drinking to a prominent place on the national public health agenda, created a policy climate in which significant legislation has been passed by states and localities, raised awareness of the importance of aggressive enforcement, and stimulated coordinated citizen action. These changes are mutually reinforcing and have provided a framework for a sustained national commitment to reducing underage drinking.

Nevertheless, the rates of underage drinking are still unacceptably high, resulting in preventable and tragic health and safety consequences for the nation's youth, families, communities, and society as a whole. Therefore, ICCPUD remains committed to an ongoing, comprehensive approach to preventing and reducing underage drinking. This report, with its yearly updates to the State Report and survey responses, is part of that sustained effort to reduce underage drinking in America.

---

[12] Please note for comparability with the 2011 NSDUH and 2011 YRBS data, the latest MTF data included in the report are also from 2011. The 2012 MTF data, which became available in December 2012, will be included in the next report.

CHAPTER 2
The Nature and Extent of Underage Drinking in America

Introduction

Underage drinking and its associated problems have profound negative consequences for underage drinkers themselves, their families, their communities, and society as a whole. Underage drinking contributes to a wide range of costly health and social problems including motor vehicle crashes (the greatest single mortality risk for underage drinkers); suicide; interpersonal violence (e.g., homicides, assaults, and rapes); unintentional injuries such as burns, falls, and drowning; brain impairment; alcohol dependence; risky sexual activity; academic problems; and alcohol and drug poisoning. Alcohol is a factor related to approximately 4,700 deaths among underage youths in the United States every year, shortening their lives by an average of 60 years (http://www.cdc.gov/alcohol/fact-sheets/underage-drinking.htm).

Despite laws against underage drinking in all 50 states; the efforts of federal, state, and local governments spanning decades; and the dedicated work of many private groups and organizations, alcohol is the most widely consumed substance of abuse among America's youth, used more often than tobacco or marijuana. Underage alcohol use remains a challenging public health and public safety problem with severe consequences for youth and their families, communities, and society. For those under 21 years old, alcohol accounts for more deaths than all other illicit drugs combined. Nevertheless, a lack of public recognition of the devastating consequences of underage alcohol use and its personal, economic, and social costs hampers implementation of a comprehensive prevention effort.

Still, there is cause for optimism. As discussed in Chapters 3 and 4 of this report, states are increasingly adopting comprehensive policies and practices that can alter the individual and environmental factors that contribute to underage drinking and its consequences and can be expected to reduce alcohol-related deaths and disability and associated health care costs.

Federal Surveys Used in This Report

The federal government funds three major national surveys that collect data on underage drinking and its consequences: the annual National Survey on Drug Use and Health (NSDUH), formerly called the National Household Survey on Drug Abuse (NHSDA); the annual Monitoring the Future (MTF) survey;[13] and the biennial Youth Risk Behavior Survey (YRBS). Each makes a unique contribution to an understanding of the nature of alcohol use.

Four additional surveys used by the government to obtain data on underage drinkers ages 18 and older are the Behavioral Risk Factor Surveillance System (BRFSS); National Epidemiologic Survey on Alcohol and Related Conditions (NESARC); National Health Interview Survey (NHIS); and Survey of Health Related Behaviors Among Active Duty Military Personnel (formerly called the Worldwide Surveys of Substance Abuse and Health Behaviors Among Military Personnel). A more detailed description of each of these surveys and its unique contribution to research can be found in Appendix A.

---

[13] Please note for comparability with the 2011 NSDUH and 2011 YRBS data, the latest MTF data included in the report are also from 2011. The 2012 MTF data, which became available in December 2012, will be included in the next report.

Characteristics of Underage Drinking in America

Underage alcohol use in America is a public health problem because of the number of children and adolescents who drink, when and how much they drink, and the negative consequences that result from that drinking. Some of the principal findings of governmental surveys and other research related to underage alcohol use in America are described in the following paragraphs.

Underage Alcohol Use Is Widespread

Underage alcohol use in America is a widespread and serious problem:

- *Current Use:* The 2011 NSDUH reported that approximately 25.1 percent of Americans ages 12 through 20 (about 9.7 million people) reported having at least one drink in the 30 days prior to the survey interview. Of this age group, 15.8 percent (6.1 million) were binge drinkers (five or more drinks on the same occasion, e.g., at the same time or within a couple of hours) on at least 1 day in the past 30 days. Approximately 4.4 percent of this age group (1.7 million) were heavy drinkers (five or more drinks on the same occasion on each of 5 or more days in the past 30 days). Thus (by definition), all heavy alcohol users are also binge alcohol users (Substance Abuse and Mental Health Services Administration [SAMHSA], 2012a).

- *Lifetime Use:* MTF 2011 showed that 70.0 percent of 12th, 56.0 percent of 10th, and 33.1 percent of 8th graders have had alcohol at some point in their lives[14] (Johnston, O'Malley, Bachman, & Schulenberg, 2012a). See Exhibit 2.1.

- *Binge Use:* The 2011 NSDUH showed that 3.4 percent of 14-year-olds, 12.0 percent of 16-year-olds, 27.3 percent of 18-year-olds, and 36.6 percent of 20-year-olds engaged in binge drinking within the past 30 days (SAMHSA, 2012, detailed tables).

- *Heavy Use:* The 2011 NSDUH data showed that 2.7 percent of 16-year-olds, 7.7 percent of 18-year-olds, and 11.8 percent of 20-year-olds consumed alcohol heavily in the past 30 days (SAMHSA, 2012, detailed tables).

- *Use to Intoxication:* In MTF 2011, 51.0 percent of 12th, 35.9 percent of 10th, and 14.8 percent of 8th graders reported having been drunk[15] at least once (Johnston et al., 2012a).

- *Past-Month Intoxication:* In MTF 2011, 25.0 percent of 12th, 13.7 percent of 10th, and 4.4 percent of 8th graders reported being drunk in the past month (Johnston et al., 2012a).

Alcohol Is the Most Widely Used Substance of Abuse among American Youth

As indicated in Exhibit 2.2, a higher percentage of youth in 8th, 10th, and 12th grades used alcohol in the month prior to being surveyed than used marijuana (the illicit drug most commonly used by adolescents) or tobacco (Johnston et al., 2012a).

---

[14] Lifetime alcohol use in this survey is defined as "having more than a few sips."
[15] MTF asks "On how many occasions (if any) have you been drunk or very high during the past 30 days?"

Exhibit 2.1: Lifetime Alcohol Use, Use to Intoxication, and Use to Intoxication within the Past Month among 8th, 10th, and 12th Graders: 2011 (Johnston et al., 2012a)

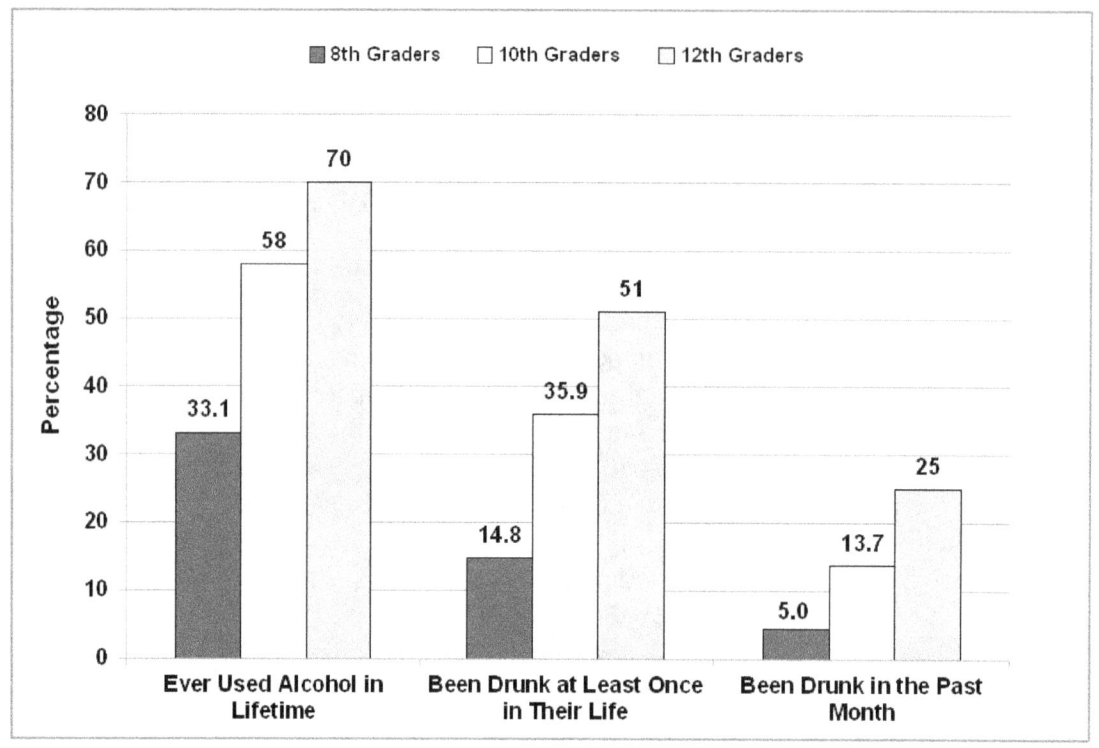

Exhibit 2.2: Past-Month Adolescent Alcohol, Cigarette, and Marijuana Use by Grade: 2011 (Johnston et al., 2012a)

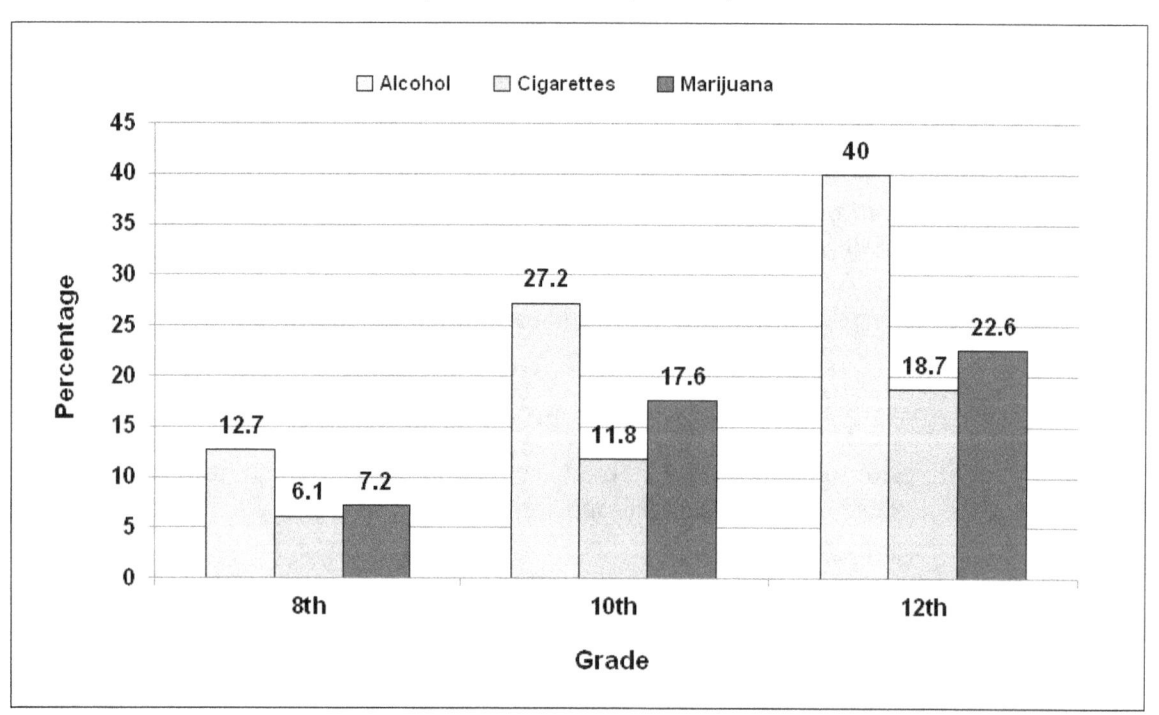

Youths Start Drinking at an Early Age

Drinking often begins at very young ages. Surveys indicate that approximately:

- Ten percent of 9- to 10-year-olds have already started drinking[16] (Donovan et al., 2004).

- More than one fifth of underage drinkers begin drinking before age 13 (CDC, 2012).

- Peak years of initiation are 7th through 11th grades based on data from high school seniors (Johnston, O'Malley, Bachman, & Schulenberg, 2009a).

Slightly fewer than 1 million (972,000) persons who initiated alcohol use in the past year reported being ages 12 to 14 when they initiated. This translates to approximately 2,660 youths ages 12 to 14 who initiated alcohol use per day in 2011 (SAMHSA, CBHSQ, NSDUH, Special Data Analysis, 2012). Youths who report drinking before age 15 are more likely to experience problems including intentional and unintentional injury to self and others after drinking (Hingson & Zha, 2009; Hingson, Heeren, Jamanka, & Howland, 2000); violent behavior, including predatory violence and dating violence (Blitstein, Murray, Lytle, Birnbaum, & Perry, 2005; Ellickson, Tucker, & Klein, 2003; Ramisetty-Mikler, et al., 2006); criminal behavior (Eaton, Davis, Barrios, Brener, & Noonan, 2007); prescription drug misuse (Hermos et al., 2008); unplanned and unprotected sex (Hingson, Heeren, Winter, & Wechsler, 2003); motor vehicle crashes (Hingson, Heeren, Levenson, Jamanka, & Voas, 2002); and physical fights (Hingson, Heeren, & Zakocs, 2001). Early-onset drinking is thus a marker for future problems, including heavier use of alcohol and other drugs during adolescence (Robins & Przybeck, 1985; Hawkins et al., 1997) and alcohol dependence in adulthood (Grant & Dawson, 1998).

Delaying the age of first alcohol use can ameliorate some of the negative consequences of underage alcohol consumption, which means that trends in age of initiation of alcohol use are important to follow. MTF data show that the proportion of 8th, 10th, and 12th graders who had ever used alcohol and the proportion of those who started using alcohol before 7th grade generally declined from 1998 to 2011, suggesting a possible delay in the age at first use (Johnston et al., 2012a).

SAMHSA revised its methodology to provide more timely estimates that more accurately assess trends in average age at first use and other measures of initiation, such as incidence rates. Average age of first use is now calculated based on initiation within the past 12 months. Using this new method, NSDUH data indicate no difference in the average age of first use (15.6 years) among those who initiated alcohol use before age 21 between 2004 and 2005, but a significant increase to 15.8 years in 2006. The average age of first use then remained nearly the same in 2007 (15.8 years), 2008 (15.8 years), and 2009 (15.9 years) before a statistically significant increase in 2010 (16.0 years), which remained nearly the same in 2011 (15.9 years) (SAMHSA, CBHSQ, NSDUH, Special Data Analysis, 2012). Average age of first use for all drinkers, including those who started drinking at age 21 or older, was 16.6 in 2006, 17.0 in 2007, 17.7 in 2008, 17.1 in 2009, 18.0 in 2010, and 17.3 in 2011 (SAMHSA, CBHSQ, NSDUH, Special Data Analysis, 2012). Appendix A further discusses methodological issues in measuring age at first use and other indicators of alcohol initiation.

---

[16] Drinking is defined as having more than a few sips.

For Underage Drinkers, Alcohol Use and Binge Drinking Increase with Age

Drinking becomes increasingly common through the teenage years (O'Malley, Johnston, & Bachman, 1998). Frequent, heavy use by underage drinkers also increases each year from age 12 to age 20 (Flewelling, Paschall, & Ringwalt, 2004). The 2011 NSDUH reports that underage alcohol consumption in the past month increased with age in a steady progression from 1.6 percent for 12-year-olds to 55.3 percent for 20-year-olds and peaked at 70.1 percent for 23-year-olds (SAMHSA, 2012b). As shown in Exhibit 2.3, binge drinking also increased steadily between the ages of 12 and 20, peaking at age 23 (46.7 percent), and then decreased beyond young adulthood (data not shown) (SAMHSA, 2011, detailed tables). Approximately 6.1 million (15.8 percent) 12- to 20-year-olds reported past-month binge alcohol use (SAMHSA, 2012b).

Youth Binge More and Drink More Than Adults When They Drink

Young drinkers tend to drink less often than adults, but they drink more heavily when they do drink. For example, 92 percent of the alcohol consumed by 12- to 14-year-olds is via binge drinking (Pacific Institute for Research and Evaluation [PIRE], 2002). Underage drinkers consume, on average, about five drinks per occasion, about five times a month (SAMHSA, CBHSQ, NSDUH, Special Data Analysis, 2012), whereas adult drinkers 26 and older average three drinks per occasion, eight times a month (SAMHSA, CBHSQ, NSDUH, Special Data Analysis, 2012) (Exhibit 2.4). It is important to note that very young adolescents, because of their smaller size, reach blood alcohol concentrations (BACs) achieved by older binge-drinking

Exhibit 2.3: Current and Binge Alcohol Use among Persons Ages 12–20 by Age: 2011 (SAMHSA, 2012 detailed tables)

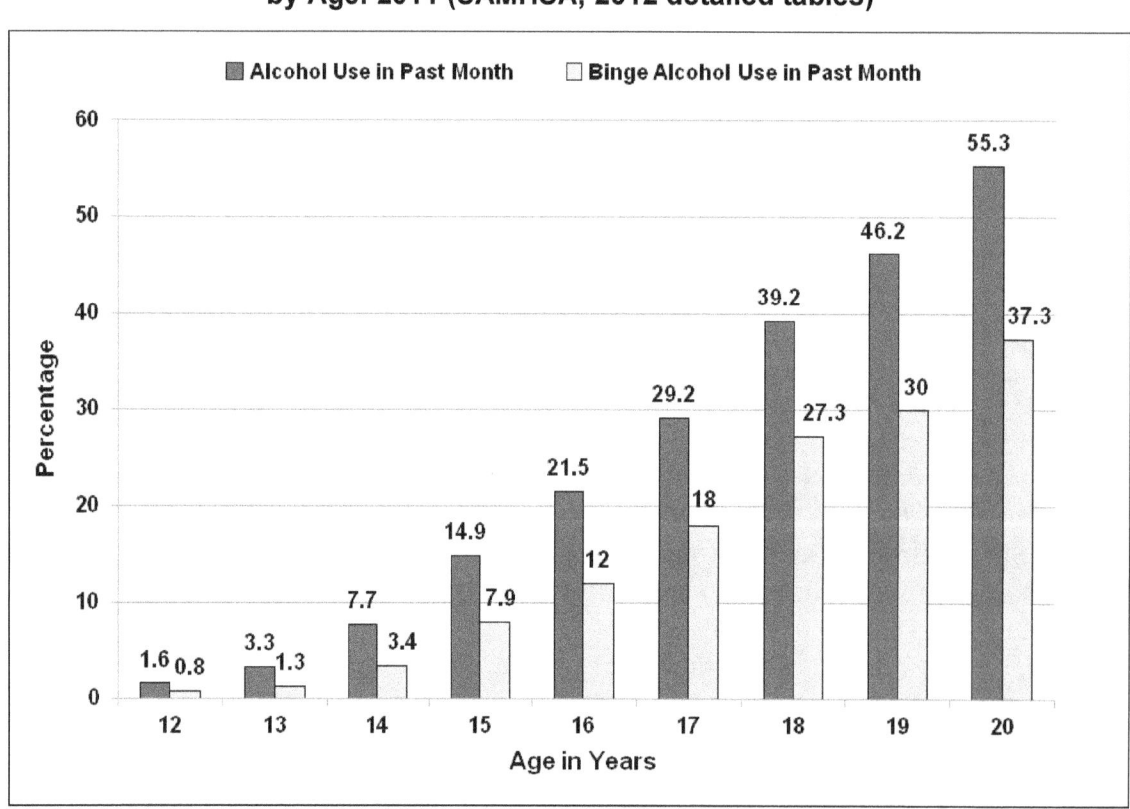

Exhibit 2.4: Number of Drinking Days per Month and Usual Number of Drinks per Occasion for Youth (12–20), Young Adults (21–25), and Adults (≥26): 2011 (SAMHSA, CBHSQ, NSDUH, Special Data Analysis, 2012)

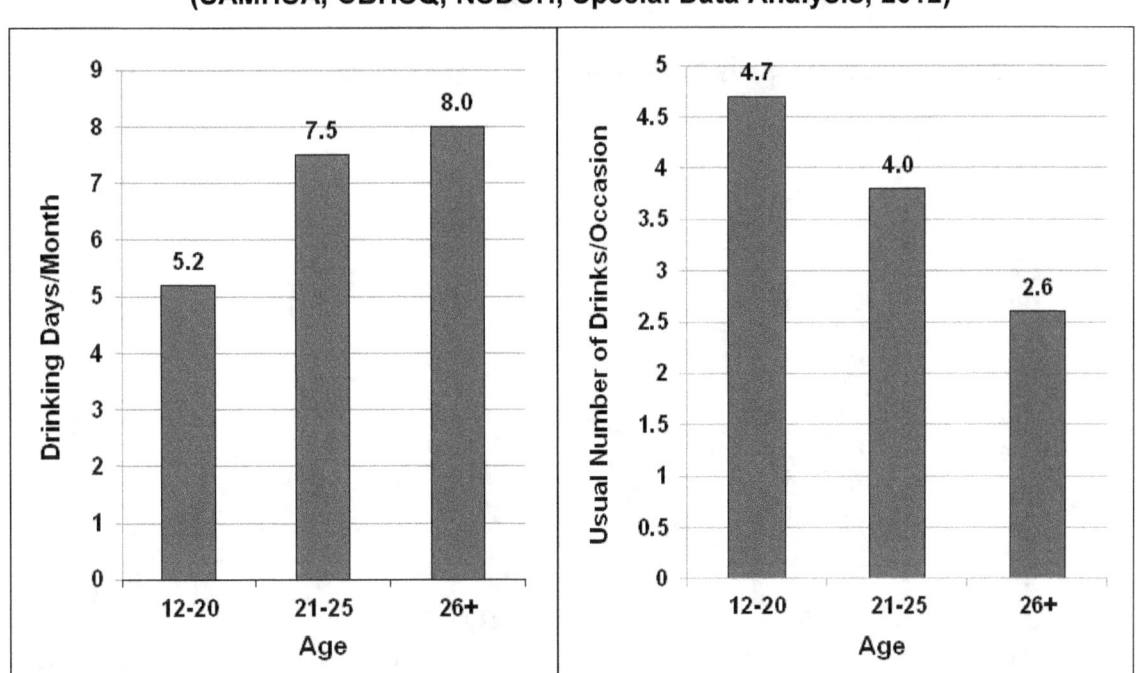

adolescents (e.g., age 18 or older) with fewer drinks (3 to 4 drinks for persons ages 12 to 15) (Donovan, 2009).

When asked about the number of drinks consumed on their last occasion of alcohol use in the past month, 22.2 percent of underage drinkers reported one drink; 18.2 percent, two drinks; 24.3 percent, three or four drinks; 24.6 percent, five to eight drinks; and 10.7 percent, nine or more drinks for 2010 and 2011 combined (SAMHSA, CBHSQ, NSDUH, Special Data Analysis, 2012). The number of drinks consumed differs by gender (Exhibit 2.5); underage females are more likely to report consuming one to four drinks, and underage males, five to nine drinks or more. The number of drinks reported on the last occasion tends to increase with increasing age.

Particularly worrisome is the high prevalence among underage drinkers of binge drinking, which MTF defines as five or more drinks in a row in the past 2 weeks and calls "heavy episodic drinking." In 2011, 6.4 percent of 8th, 14.7 percent of 10th, and 21.6 percent of 12th graders reported heavy episodic drinking (Johnston et al., 2012a). In 2011, about 1.7 million youth ages 12 through 20 (4.4 percent) drank five or more drinks on a single occasion[17] 5 or more days a month (SAMHSA, 2012a).

---

[17] If a typical 160-pound male drinks five standard drinks over a 2-hour period, he would reach a blood alcohol content of 0.08, making him legally intoxicated in all 50 states.

Exhibit 2.5: Number of Drinks Consumed on Last Occasion of Alcohol Use in the Past Month among Past-Month Alcohol Users Ages 12–20, by Gender and Age Group: 2010–2011 (SAMHSA, CBHSQ, NSDUH, Special Data Analysis, 2012)

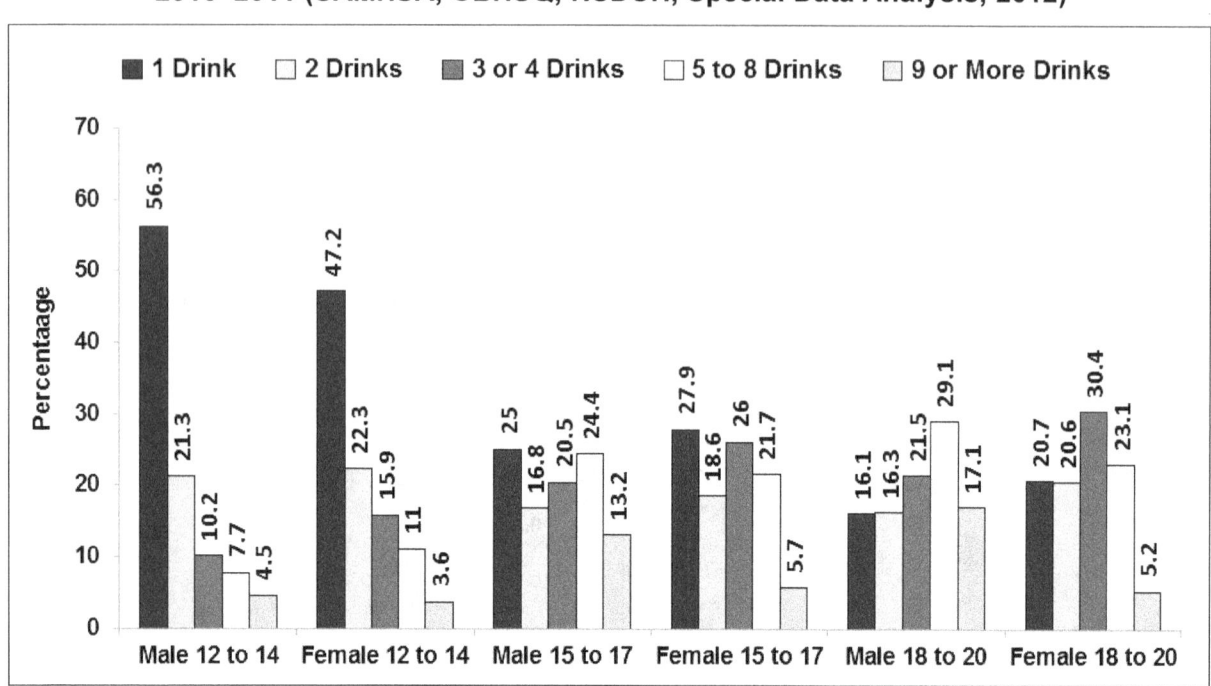

Faden and Fay (2004) used statistical trend analyses to examine underage drinking data from 1975 to 2002. Among 12th graders, drinking five or more drinks in a row in the past 2 weeks declined 7.6 percent, from 36.8 percent in 1975 to 29.2 percent in 2004. Analysis of data from the intervening years showed that the prevalence of drinking five or more drinks in a row in the past 2 weeks rose from 1975 to 1980, fell from 1980 to 1987, steeply declined from 1987 to 1993, rose from 1993 to 1997, and declined from 1997 to 2002 (Faden & Fay, 2004). Subsequent statistical trend analyses showed that among 12th graders the prevalence of drinking five or more drinks in a row in the past 2 weeks continued to fall between 2002 and 2009 (Chen, Yi, & Faden, 2011).

Information on the prevalence of drinking five or more drinks in a row in the past 2 weeks among 8th and 10th graders first became available in 1991. In 1991, 10.9 percent of 8th graders and 21 percent of 10th graders reported engaging in this behavior compared with 9.4 percent and 19.9 percent, respectively, in 2004. Rates in the intervening years oscillated heavily for 8th graders and rose steadily for 10th graders, for whom rates peaked in 2000 and have since gradually declined (Johnston, O'Malley, Bachman, & Schulenberg, 2005). Since 2002, there have been statistically significant declines in binge drinking for all three grades (Johnston et al., 2012a).

Binge Drinking by Teens Is Not Limited to the United States

In many European countries, a significant proportion of young people ages 15 to 16 report binge drinking (Exhibit 2.6). In all countries listed in Exhibit 2.6, the minimum legal drinking age is lower than in the United States. These data call into question the suggestion that having a lower minimum legal drinking age results in less problem drinking by adolescents.

Exhibit 2.6: Percentage of European Students Ages 15–16 Who Reported Being Drunk in the Past 30 Days* Compared with American 10th Graders (Hibell et al., 2012; Data from the 2011 European School Survey Project on Alcohol and Drugs)

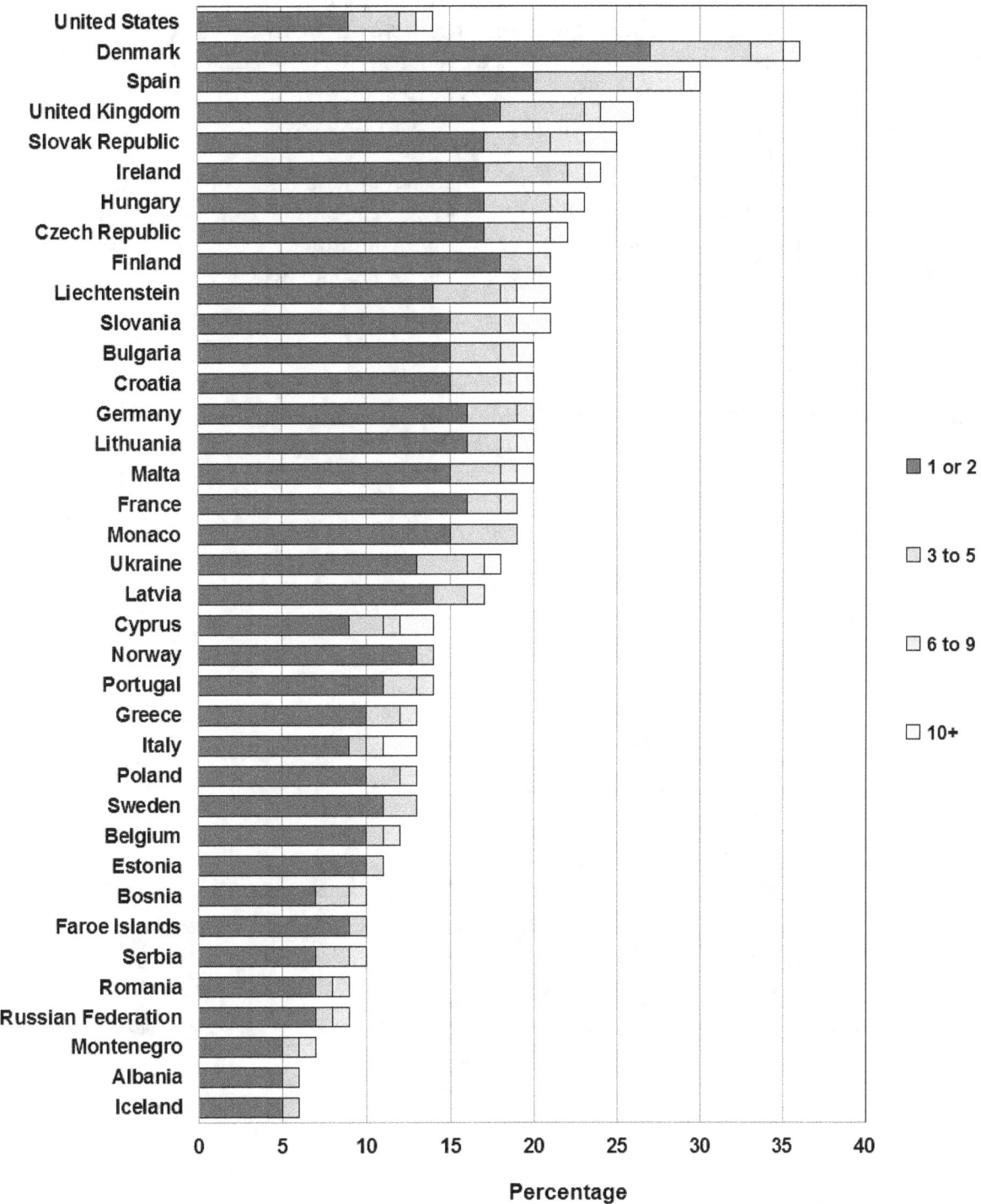

* The 2011 European School Survey Project on Alcohol and Drugs question is: "On how many occasions (if any) have you been intoxicated from drinking alcoholic beverages (staggered when walking, not able to speak properly, throwing up or not remembering what happened)?"

There Is a High Prevalence of Alcohol Use Disorders among Youth

The prevalence of alcohol abuse or dependence among underage drinkers is quite high. Because the *Diagnostic and Statistical Manual of Mental Disorders, Fourth Edition, text revision* (DSM-IV-TR) (APA, 2000) criteria for abuse and dependence were originally developed for use with adults, using them to assess abuse and dependence in adolescents may lead to inconsistencies.[18] As shown in Exhibit 2.7, according to the combined 2010 and 2011 NSDUH data, prevalence of alcohol dependence or abuse is highest among those ages 18 to 29.

About one in seven (13.6 percent) 18- to 20-year-olds met criteria for alcohol dependence or abuse, a prevalence rate second only to that for 21- to 24-year-olds (16.4 percent) and slightly higher than that for 25- to 29-year-olds (12.2 percent). In addition, 1.3 percent of 12- to 14-year-olds and 6.9 percent of 15- to 17-year-olds met criteria for alcohol dependence or abuse.

Exhibit 2.7: Prevalence of Past-Year DSM-IV Alcohol Dependence or Abuse by Age: 2010–2011 NSDUH (SAMHSA, CBHSQ, Special Analyses, 2012)

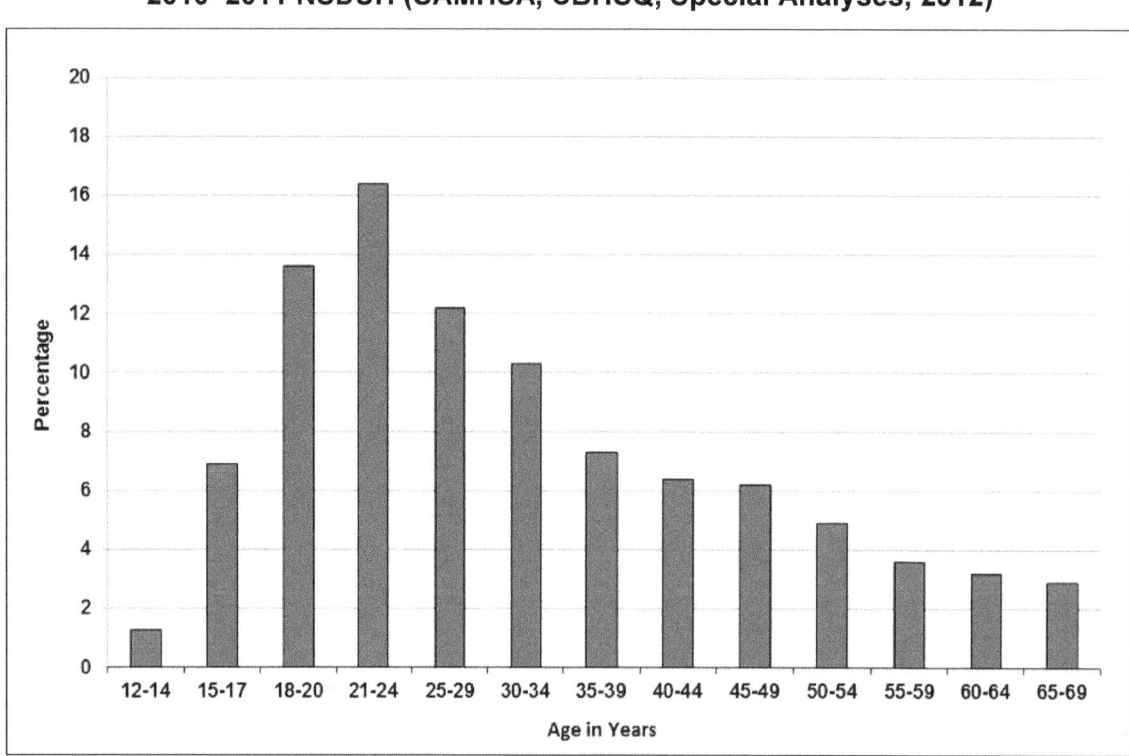

---

[18] Several researchers are actively investigating this important issue (Harford, Yi, Faden, & Chen, 2009; Mewton, Teesson, Slade, & Grove, 2010). The American Psychiatric Association (APA) is also addressing the appropriateness of the current DSM-IV-TR criteria for measuring alcohol abuse and dependence in the young as it prepares to launch DSM-V in 2013. See American Psychiatric Association DSM-V Development at http://www.dsm5.org/Pages/Default.aspx.

Underage Drinking Differs by Gender

Although underage males and females tend to start drinking at about the same age and have approximately the same prevalence of any past-month alcohol use, males are more likely to drink with greater frequency and to engage in binge and heavy drinking. According to the 2011 NSDUH data, 56.8 percent of males ages 12 and older were current drinkers compared with 47.1 percent of females in that age group. However, among underage drinkers, there were significant gender differences only in the 18- to 20-year-old age group. Among individuals ages 12 to 13, rates of current drinking were very similar: 2.2 percent for males and 2.7 percent for females. Among 14- and 15-year-olds, 12.1 percent of females and 10.5 percent of males reported current use. Among those ages 16 to 17, 26.4 percent of males and 24.1 percent of females reported being current drinkers. By ages 18 to 20, 48.6 percent of males reported past-month alcohol use compared with 44.9 percent of females (SAMHSA, CBHSQ, NSDUH, Special Data Analysis, 2012).

Binge-drinking prevalence is the most significant gender difference, at least among older adolescents. In 2011, 25.5 percent of male 12th graders reported binge drinking (having five or more drinks in a row) at least once in the prior 2-week period, whereas 17.6 percent of female 12th graders did (Johnston et al., 2012a). However, the gender gap is closing. In 1975, there was a 23 percentage point spread between the rates; in 2011, it was 7.9 points (Johnston et al., 2012a).

Female binge-drinking rates are comparable to those for males among younger age groups, whereas male rates increase more rapidly with age. The 2011 NSDUH showed past-month binge drinking in 0.8 percent of male and 1.3 percent of female 12- to 13-year-olds, 5.5 percent of male and 5.8 percent of female 14- to 15-year olds, 16.8 percent of male and 13.0 percent of female 16- to 17-year-olds, and 35.5 percent of male and 27.0 percent of female 18- to 20-year-olds (SAMHSA, 2011). MTF, which began collecting data from 8th and 10th graders in 1991, reports similar results. For 8th graders, female binge-drinking rates began converging with male rates in 1991, with equal rates for both genders since 2004 (Exhibit 2.8) (Johnston et al., 2009c, 2012a).

Underage Drinking by Race and Ethnicity

According to 2002–2011 NSDUH data,[19] Whites ages 12 to 20 were more likely to report current alcohol use than any other race or ethnic group. An estimated 32.1 percent of White males and 30.6 percent of White females reported past-month use, followed by Native Hawaiian or Other Pacific Islander males (28.9 percent), males of multiple races (26.5 percent), Hispanic or Latino males (26.4 percent), American Indian or Alaska Native females (25.9 percent), females of multiple races (25.9 percent), American Indian or Alaska Native males (25.5 percent), Native Hawaiian or Other Pacific Islander females (23.7 percent), Hispanic or Latino females (22.9 percent), Black or African American males (19.8 percent), Black or African American females (18.2 percent), Asian males (17.6 percent), and Asian females (16.4 percent). As shown in Exhibit 2.9, among most races/ethnic groups, males and females reported similar rates of current alcohol use; however, among Whites, Blacks, Hawaiian or Other Pacific Islanders, and Hispanics, males ages 12 to 20 were more likely to report current use than females (SAMHSA, CBHSQ, NSDUH, Special Data Analysis, 2012). Although fewer Blacks report current

---

[19] To provide sample sizes sufficient to produce reliable estimates for each race/ethnic group, multiyear estimates of past-month alcohol use and binge drinking by race/ethnicity were calculated.

Exhibit 2.8: Rates of Binge Drinking in the Past 2 Weeks among Male and Female 8th, 10th, and 12th Graders, 1991–2011 (Johnston et al., 2012a)

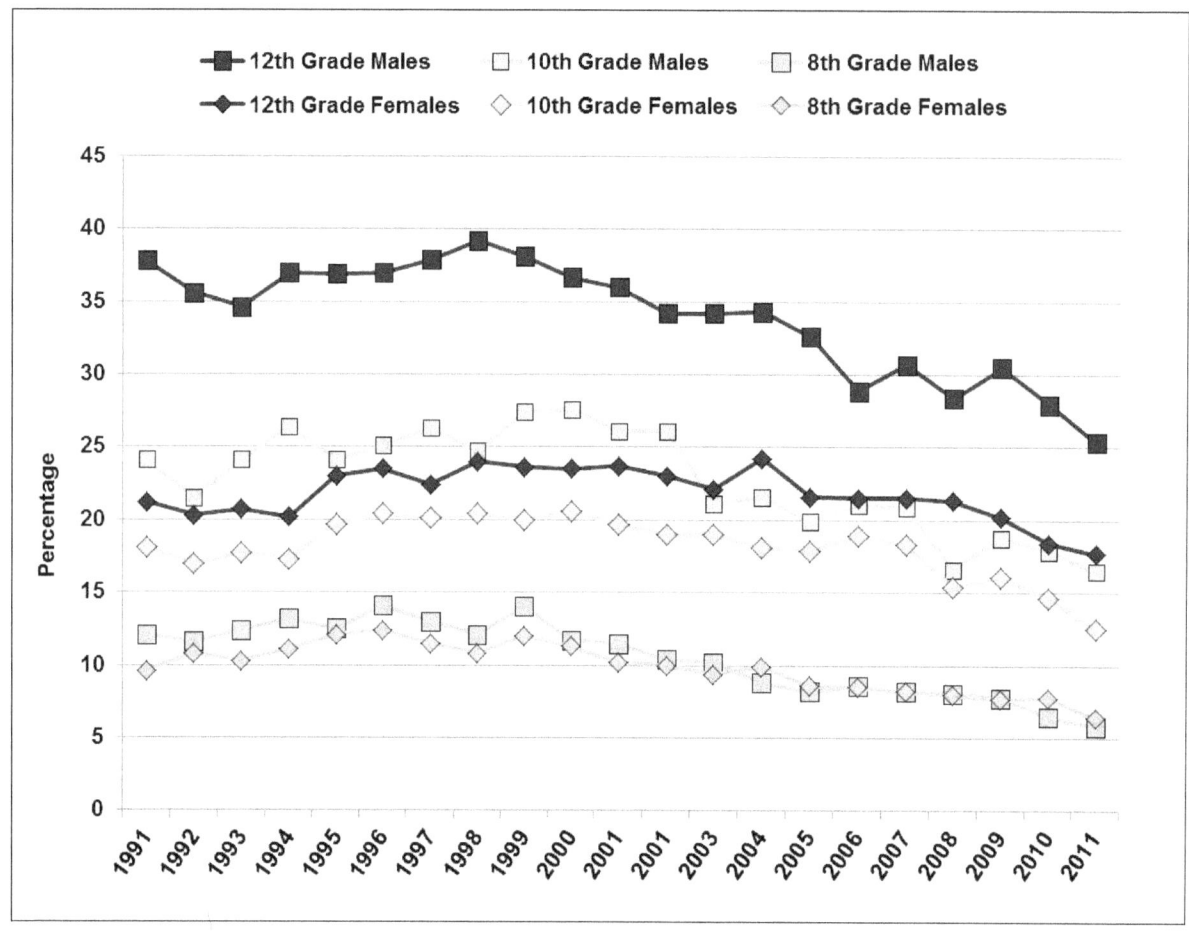

Exhibit 2.9: Alcohol Use and Binge Drinking in the Past Month among Persons Ages 12–20 by Race/Ethnicity and Gender, Annual Averages Based on 2002–2011 Data (SAMHSA, CBHSQ, NSDUH, Special Data Analysis, 2012)

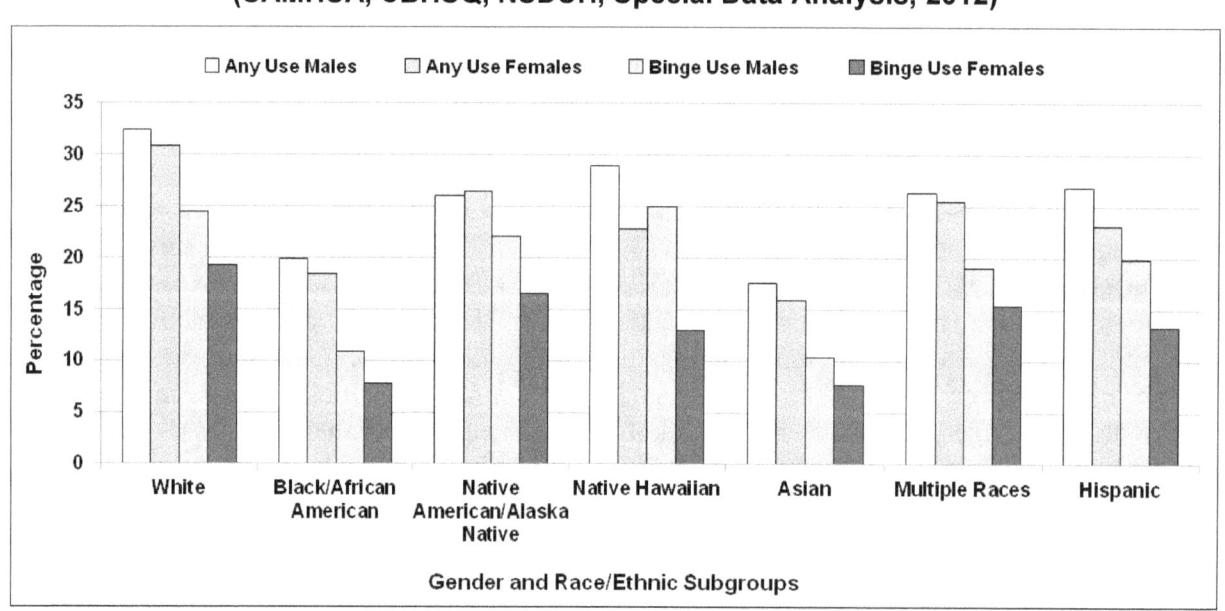

drinking, data from the 2011 YRBS suggest that prevalence of alcohol use before age 13 is greater among Black students (21.8 percent) and Hispanic students (25.2 percent) than among White students (18.1 percent) (CDC, 2012). Sample sizes from the MTF and the YRBS do not allow estimates of alcohol consumption by youth who are American Indian or Alaska Native, Native Hawaiian or Other Pacific Islander, or multiple races.

Multiyear NSDUH data (2002–2011) show that White, American Indian and Alaska Native, and Hawaiian and Other Pacific Islander males ages 12 to 20 were equally likely to report binge alcohol use in the past month. An estimated 24.9 percent of Native Hawaiians or Other Pacific Islander males reported having five or more drinks on the same occasion on at least 1 day within the past 30 days, followed closely by White males (24.1 percent) and American Indian or Alaska Native males (21.6 percent). Hispanic males (19.3 percent), White females (19.1 percent), males of multiple races (18.7 percent), and American Indian or Alaska Native females (16.9 percent) reported similar rates of binge drinking, followed by females of multiple races (15.5 percent), Hispanic females (13.5 percent), Native Hawaiian or Other Pacific Islander females (13.3 percent), Black males (10.8 percent), Asian males (10.3 percent), and Asian females (7.8 percent). As Exhibit 2.9 shows, rates of binge drinking were higher for males than females for each race/ethnic group, with the differences being greatest among Native Hawaiian or Other Pacific Islanders (males 24.9 percent vs. females 13.3 percent) and Hispanics (males 19.3 percent vs. females 13.5 percent) (SAMHSA, CBHSQ, NSDUH, Special Data Analysis, 2012).

These ethnic and racial differences must be viewed with some caution. As Caetano, Clark, and Tam (1998) note, there are important differences in alcohol use and related problems among ethnic and racial subgroups of Blacks, Hispanics, Asians, and Native Americans/Alaska Natives. Moreover, the patterns of consumption for any group or subgroup represent a complex interaction of psychological, historical, cultural, and social factors inadequately captured by a limited set of labels. With these cautions in mind, however, the data discussed thus far highlight the importance of considering race and ethnicity in underage drinking prevention measures.

Social Context of Alcohol Use

NSDUH began to collect data on the social context of last alcohol use in 2006. The following discussion combines data for 2010 and 2011. Most (81.2 percent) persons ages 12 to 20 who had consumed alcohol in the past month were with two or more people the last time they drank, 13.8 percent were with one other person the last time they drank, and 5.0 percent were alone. Underage persons who drank with two or more other people on the last occasion in the past month had more drinks on the last occasion on average (4.6 drinks) than those who drank with one other person (3.0 drinks) or drank alone (2.7 drinks) (SAMHSA, CBHSQ, NSDUH, Special Data Analysis, 2012; Pemberton, Colliver, Robbins, & Gfroerer, 2008).

The social context of drinking appears to differ across age groups. Among current drinkers, youths ages 12 to 14 were more likely to have been alone (12.3 percent) or with one other person (23.2 percent) the last time they drank compared with youths ages 15 to 17 (5.6 percent alone and 12.7 percent with one other person) or ages 18 to 20 (4.2 percent alone and 13.6 percent with one other person) (SAMHSA, CBHSQ, NSDUH, Special Data Analysis, 2012). In all age groups, underage current drinkers who drank with two or more other people averaged more drinks on the last occasion than those who drank with one other person or alone (Exhibit 2.10).

Exhibit 2.10: Average Number of Drinks Consumed on Last Occasion of Alcohol Use in the Past Month among Past-Month Alcohol Users Ages 12–20, by Social Context and Age Group: 2010–2011 (SAMHSA, CBHSQ, NSDUH, Special Data Analysis, 2012)

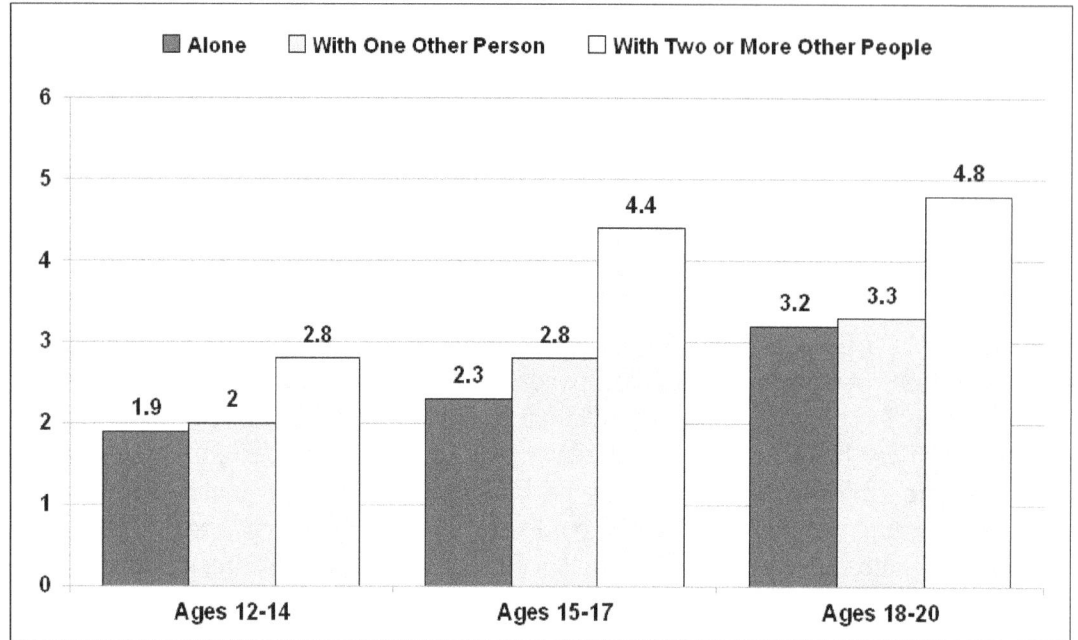

Gender, too, interacts with social context in determining alcohol use. Most male and female underage drinkers were with two or more other people on their last drinking occasion. However, female drinkers were more likely to be with two or more people the last time they drank (83.2 percent) than were male drinkers (79.5 percent); male drinkers were more likely to have been alone the last time they drank (6.4 percent) than female drinkers (3.3 percent).

Overall, underage persons who drank with two or more other people consumed more drinks on average (4.6) than those who drank alone (2.7) or with one other person (3.0). There were no significant differences in the mean number of drinks consumed between those who drank alone and those who drank with one other person. Males consumed more drinks than did females regardless of the social context; for example, when the last drinking occasion was with two or more other people, males averaged 5.4 drinks, compared with 3.8 drinks for females (SAMHSA, CBHSQ, NSDUH, Special Data Analysis, 2012).

Location of Alcohol Use

NSDUH began to collect data on location of last alcohol use in 2006. The following discussion combines data for 2010 and 2011. Most underage drinkers reported last using alcohol in someone else's home (56.1 percent, averaging 4.7 drinks) or their own home (28.9 percent, averaging 3.8 drinks). The next most popular drinking locations were at a restaurant, bar, or club (8.7 percent, averaging 4.8 drinks); in a car or other vehicle (4.3 percent, averaging 5.1 drinks); or at a park, on a beach, or in a parking lot (4.3 percent, averaging 4.9 drinks). Current drinkers ages 12 to 20 who last drank at a concert or sports game (1.7 percent of all underage drinkers) consumed an average of 5.8 drinks (SAMHSA, CBHSQ, NSDUH, Special Data Analysis, 2012).

Thus, most young people drink in social contexts that appear to promote heavy consumption and where people other than the drinker may be harmed by the drinker's behavior.

According to estimates based on 2010–2011 NSDUH data, drinking location varies substantially by age. For example, drinkers ages 12 to 14 were more likely to have been in their own homes the last time they drank (41.3 percent) than were older adolescents (25.4 percent for 15- to 17-year-olds and 29.5 percent for 18- to 20-year-olds). By contrast, 12- to 14-year-olds were less likely to report being in someone else's home the last time they drank (45.8 percent) than the older age groups (59.9 percent for 15- to 17-year-olds and 55.4 percent for 18- to 20-year-olds).

Drinkers ages 18 to 20 were more likely than those in younger age groups to have been in a restaurant, bar, or club on their last drinking occasion (11.5 percent for those ages 18 to 20 versus 1.1 percent for those ages 12 to 14 and 3.4 percent for those ages 15 to 17) (Exhibit 2.11) (SAMHSA, CBHSQ, NSDUH, Special Data Analysis, 2012). Female current alcohol users ages 12 to 20 were more likely than males to have had their last drink at a restaurant, bar, or club (10.8 percent versus 6.9 percent).

Taken together, these data suggest that underage drinking occurs primarily in a social context (three or more drinkers) at private residences. This conclusion is consistent with research that has found that underage drinking parties, where large groups of underage persons gather at

Exhibit 2.11: Location of Last Alcohol Use among Past-Month Alcohol Users Ages 12–20 by Age Group, 2010–2011 (SAMHSA, CBHSQ, NSDUH, Special Data Analysis, 2012)

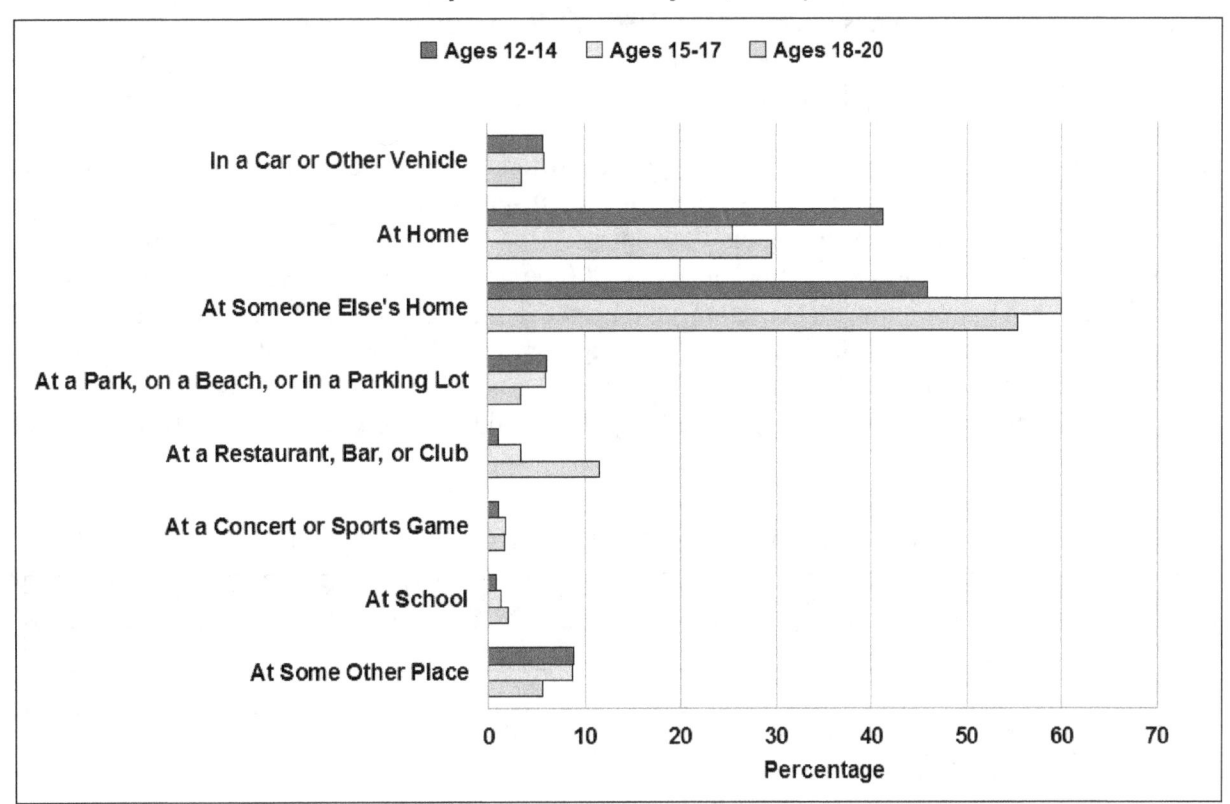

private residences, are high-risk settings for binge drinking and associated alcohol problems (Mayer, Forster, Murray, & Wagenaar, 1998). Similar findings exist for college student binge drinking (Clapp, Shillington, & Segars, 2000).

Types of Alcohol Consumed by Underage Drinkers

Different alcohol beverage types are likely associated with different patterns of underage consumption. Ease of concealment, palatability, alcohol content, marketing strategies, media portrayals, parent modeling, and economic and physical availability may all contribute to the quantity of and settings for consumption. Beverage preferences may also affect the policies and enforcement strategies most effective in reducing underage drinking (CDC, 2007). Tracking young people's beverage preferences is thus an important aspect of prevention policy.

Exhibit 2.12, based on 2011 MTF data, indicates the type of alcohol consumed by underage drinkers in the 8th, 10th, and 12th grades within the past 30 days. The five alcohol categories listed are beer, wine, wine coolers, spirits, and flavored alcoholic beverages (FABs), which are sometimes called "flavored malt beverages," "alcopops," or "malternatives." Alcopops are ready-to-drink, flavored alcoholic beverages that tend to be sweet and have between 4 and 6 percent alcohol by volume (similar to beer, which typically varies between 3 and 6 percent).

In some cases, the same adolescents reported drinking more than one type of alcohol. Thus, the percentage of adolescents for a given grade who have drunk alcohol may total more than 100 percent. For example, of 12th graders who drank alcohol in the 30 days before the survey, some percentage may have consumed both beer and wine. Distilled spirits have gained significantly in popularity among 12th graders over time. In 1988, 53.3 percent reported consuming beer in the past 30 days compared with 38.5 percent who reported distilled spirits consumption (Johnston et al., 2009c). By 2011, the gap in preferences had nearly disappeared, as shown in Exhibit 2.13.

Exhibit 2.13 shows that females, particularly, have shifted their beverage preference from beer to distilled spirits and FABs. In 1988, 46.3 percent of 12th-grade females reported consuming beer and 33.6 percent reported consuming distilled spirits. By 2011, the preference had shifted, with distilled spirits consumption remaining steady at 28.0 percent and beer consumption dropping to 22.4 percent. MTF data show that females have been more likely than males to prefer FABs since 2004 (Johnston et al., 2009a, 2012a). Beverage preferences vary by state. Data from eight states indicate that, among students in 9th through 12th grades who reported binge drinking, liquor was the most prevalent beverage type (Siegel, Naimi, Cremeens, & Nelson, 2011).

Exhibit 2.12: Past-Month Underage Alcohol Use by Category (Johnston et al., 2012a)

Grade	Beer	Wine	Wine Coolers	Spirits	Flavored Alcoholic Beverages
8	9.8%	n/c	n/c	n/c	8.6%
10	19.6%	n/c	n/c	n/c	15.8%
12	29.0%	10.2%	10.0%	29.8%	23.1%

Note: n/c indicates data not collected.

Exhibit 2.13: Trends in the Percentage of Male and Female 12th Graders Using Alcoholic Beverages by Beverage Type, 1988–2011 (Johnston et al., 2012a)

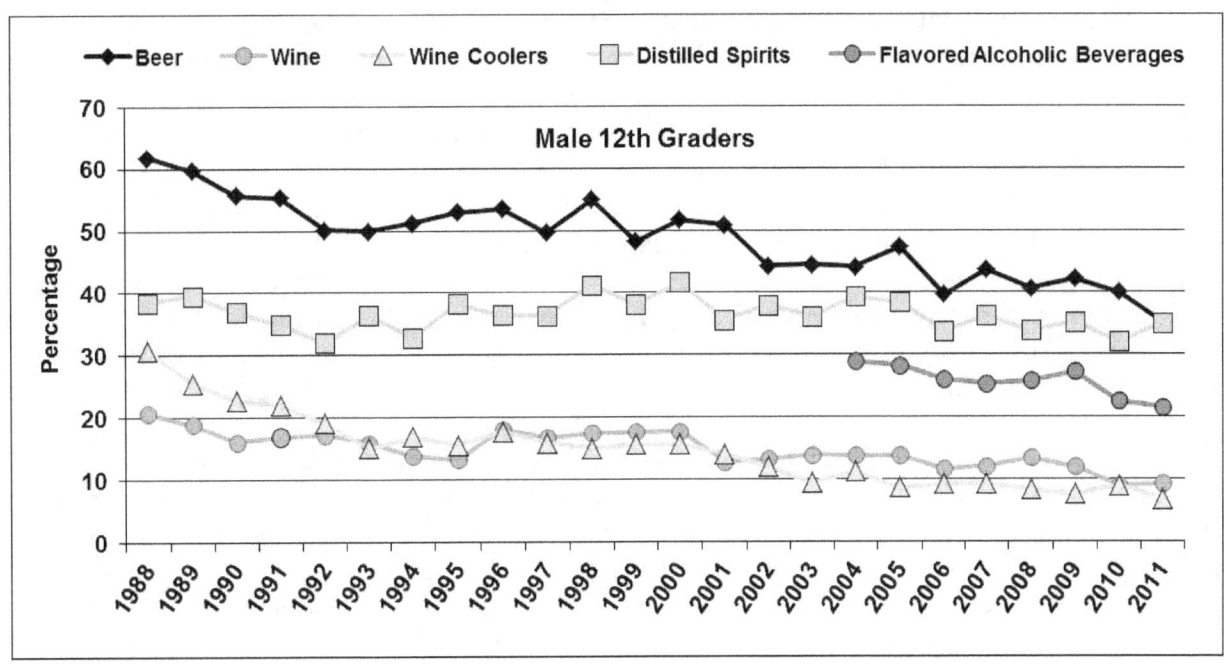

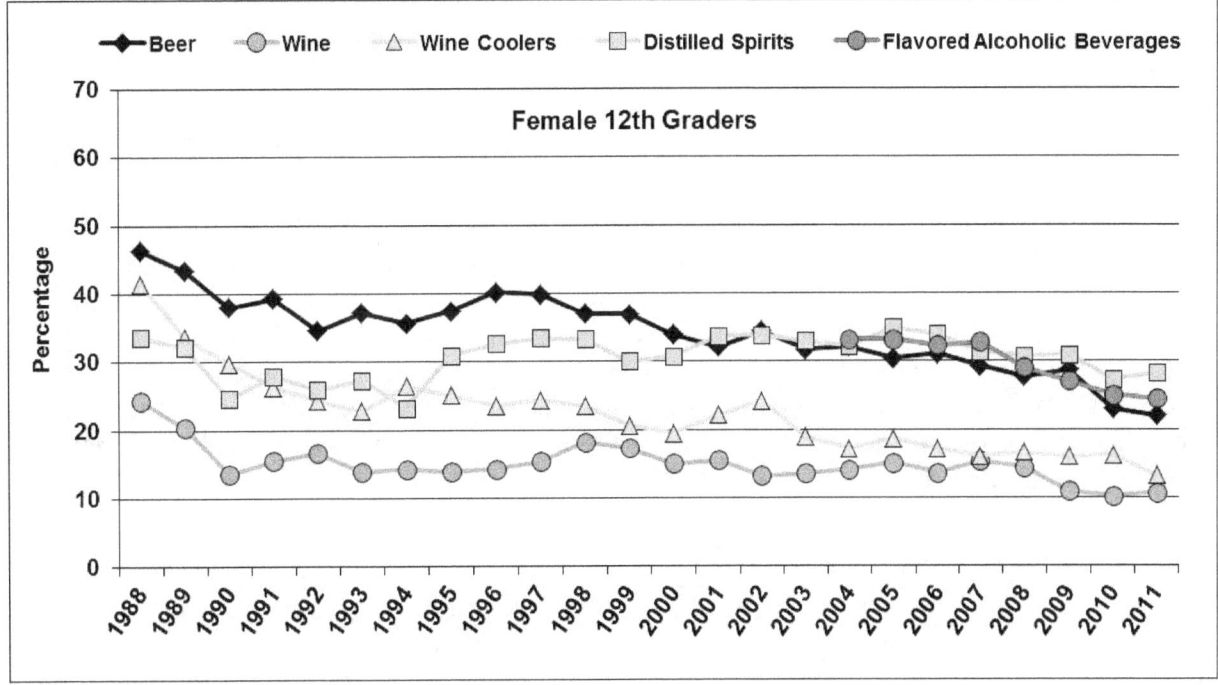

Alcohol Use in College Is Pervasive and Heavy

Although colleges and universities vary widely in their student binge-drinking rates, overall rates of college student drinking and binge drinking exceed those of age peers who do not attend college (Johnston et al., 2012b). Of college students, 80.5 percent drink and 36.1 percent report drinking five or more drinks on an occasion in the past 2 weeks. Unlike high school students and same-age peers not in college, binge-drinking rates among college students have shown little decline since 1993 (Johnston et al., 2012b). These differences are not easily attributable to differences between college attendees and nonattendees. Although college-bound 12th graders are consistently less likely than non-college-bound counterparts to report heavy drinking, college students report higher rates of binge drinking than college-age youth who are not attending college (Exhibit 2.14) (Johnston et al., 2012b). This finding suggests that college environments influence drinking practices (Hingson et al., 2002; Kuo, Wechsler, Greenberg, & Lee, 2003).

The consequences of underage drinking in college, discussed in detail in this chapter under "Adverse Consequences of College Drinking," are widespread and serious. About four out of five college students drink alcohol, about two in five engage in binge drinking (defined as five or more drinks in a row for men and four or more in a row for women within the past 2 weeks or 30 days, depending on the survey), and about one in five engages in frequent binging (three or more times in the past 2 weeks) (NIAAA, 2002a). Underage college students drink about 48 percent of the alcohol consumed by students at 4-year colleges (Wechsler et al., 2002). Some college students far exceed the binge criterion of five drinks per occasion (Wechsler et al., 1999; Wechsler & Nelson, 2008).

Alcohol Is Perceived as Readily Available by the Underage Population

Most teens see alcohol as readily available. In 2011, 59.0 percent of 8th graders, 77.9 percent of 10th graders, and 88.9 percent of 12th graders said alcohol would be "fairly easy" or "very easy" to get (Johnston et al., 2012a). Perceived availability, however, has declined in some groups. In 1992, 76.2 percent of 8th graders perceived alcohol as easily available, but by 2011 only 59.0 percent held that perception. For 10th graders, perception of availability peaked in 1996 at 90.4 percent, but by 2011 had declined to 77.9 percent. Data for 12th graders, first collected in 1999, show that 95.0 percent perceive alcohol to be readily available—a percentage that has remained relatively stable since then.

Alcohol Is Available from a Variety of Sources

Through the STOP Act, Congress required a report on measures of the availability of alcohol from commercial and noncommercial sources to underage populations. The STOP Act also calls for surveillance data on the means of underage access to alcohol. This emphasis reflects findings that alcohol availability and consumption are strongly correlated (Dent, Grube, & Biglan, 2005).

A few small studies show that the most frequent means of obtaining alcohol are parties, friends, and adult purchasers (Harrison, Fulkerson, & Park, 2000; Preusser, Ferguson, Williams, & Farmer, 1995; Wagenaar et al., 1996), and, for younger adolescents, family members (National Research Council [NRC], Institute of Medicine [IOM], 2004). The NRC and IOM report notes: "Use of friends under 21 and adult strangers as sources for alcohol appears to increase with age

Exhibit 2.14: Prevalence of Binge Drinking in the Past 2 Weeks by 12th Graders with and without College Plans, College Students, and Others 1 to 4 Years Past High School: 1991–2011 (Johnston et al., special runs, January 2010; 2011a,b; 2012a,b)

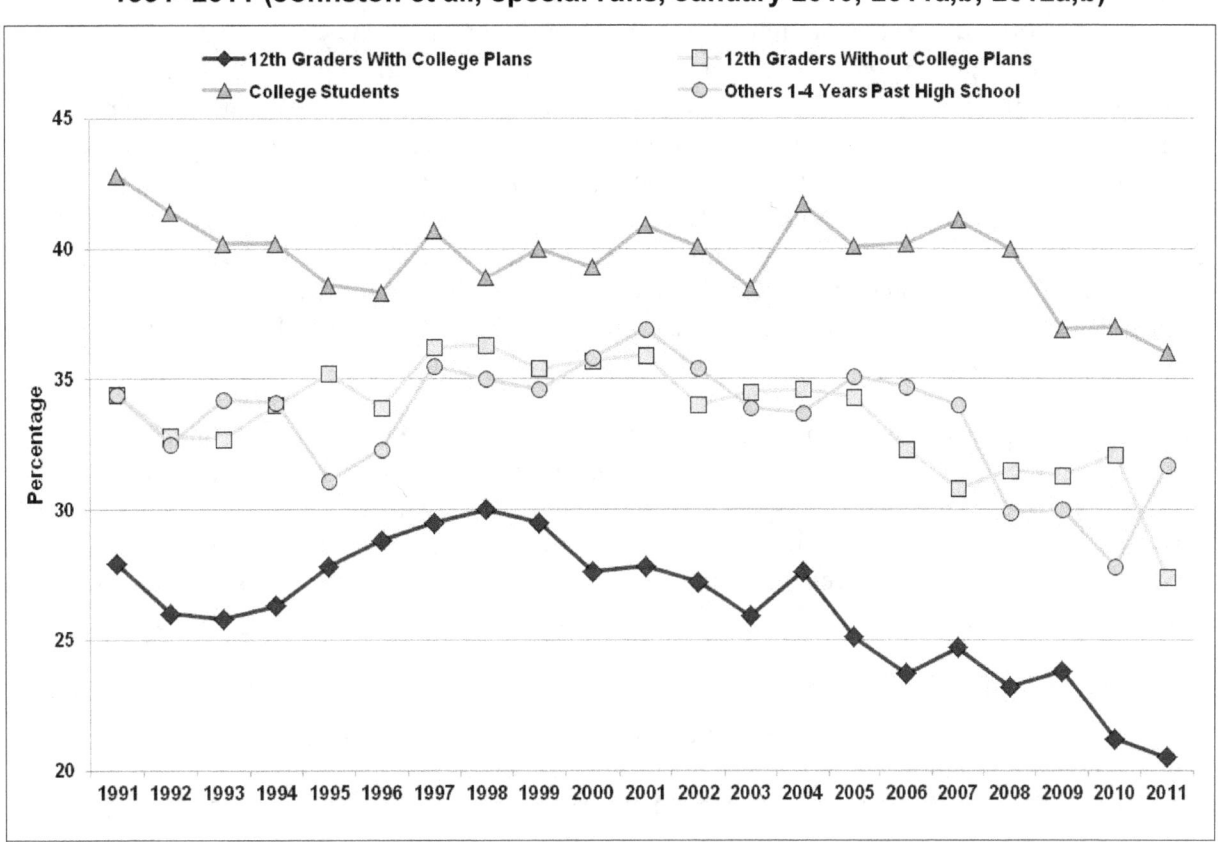

while reports of parents or other family members as sources decrease with age...use of commercial sources appears to be much higher among college students, in urban settings, and where possession and purchase laws are relatively weak or unenforced."

Before 2006, NSDUH collected data only on the *perception* of alcohol availability by those under 21. In 2006, new items were added to ascertain the *actual* source from which underage drinkers obtained their alcohol. NSDUH divides sources of last alcohol use into two categories: the underage drinker paid (he or she purchased it or gave someone else money to do so) or did not pay (he or she received it for free from someone or took it from his or her own home or someone else's home). Combined data from 2010 and 2011 show that among all underage current drinkers, 30.5 percent paid for alcohol the last time they drank (8.3 percent purchased the alcohol themselves; 22.0 percent gave money to someone else to do so). Those who paid for alcohol themselves consumed more drinks on their last drinking occasion (average of 5.6 drinks) than those who did not (average of 3.8 drinks). This difference is at least partially explained by the fact that older underage drinkers are more likely to pay for alcohol and to drink more.

Among all underage drinkers, 69.5 percent did not pay for the alcohol the last time they drank. A total of 27.5 percent were given alcohol for free by an unrelated individual age 21 or older,

6.5 percent got the alcohol from a parent or guardian, 9.1 percent got it from another family member age 21 or older, and 4.3 percent took it from their own home.

The most common sources of alcohol varied substantially by age. For youths ages 12 to 14, the most common sources were receiving it free from someone under age 21 (16.3 percent), receiving it from a parent or guardian (16.0 percent), or receiving it free from another family member age 21 or older (15.1 percent). For youths ages 15 to 17, the most common sources were receiving it free from an unrelated person age 21 or older (21.7 percent), receiving it free from someone under age 21 (19.7 percent), and giving somebody else money to purchase the alcohol (17.0 percent). As shown in Exhibit 2.15, among 18- to 20-year-olds, most current drinkers either received alcohol for free from an unrelated person age 21 or older (30.8 percent) or gave somebody else money to purchase the alcohol (25.4 percent) (SAMHSA, CBHSQ, NSDUH, Special Data Analysis, 2012).

Older underage persons were more likely to have paid for alcohol themselves (either by purchasing it themselves or by paying someone else to purchase it) on their last drinking occasion: 36.3 percent of 18- to 20-year-olds did so compared with 21.1 percent of 15- to 17-year-olds and 6.7 percent of 12- to 14-year-olds. Male underage drinkers were more likely to have paid for alcohol themselves on their last drinking occasion (36.5 percent) than their female counterparts (23.6 percent) (SAMHSA, CBHSQ, NSDUH, Special Data Analysis, 2012).[20]

Exposure of Underage Populations to Messages Regarding Alcohol in Advertising and Entertainment Media

The STOP Act requires the HHS Secretary to report to Congress on the extent of "the exposure of underage populations to messages regarding alcohol in advertising and the entertainment media as reported by the Federal Trade Commission (FTC)." To date, FTC has conducted three formal studies of the exposure of those under 21 to alcohol advertising, described below. FTC has not conducted any studies that measure alcohol depictions in entertainment media.

1999 Alcohol Report

In 1999, FTC reported that the voluntary codes of the alcohol industry permitted alcohol advertising in media where as little as 50 percent of the audience was of legal age. Only half the companies studied were able to show that nearly all of their ads reached a majority legal-age audience; the other half either provided data showing that a substantial portion of their ads did not comply with the 50 percent guideline or failed to obtain the data needed to evaluate their code compliance. Noting that the 50 percent standard permitted alcohol advertising to reach large numbers of underage consumers, FTC recommended that the industry raise the placement standard and measure compliance against reliable up-to-date audience composition data.[21]

---

[20] More detailed information can be found in the special report by Pemberton and colleagues entitled Underage Alcohol Use: Findings from the 2002-2006 National Surveys on Drug Use and Health. See http://www.oas.samhsa.gov/underage2k8/underage.pdf.

[21] For more information, see *Self-Regulation in the Alcohol Industry* (FTC, 1999), available at http://www.ftc.gov/reports/alcohol/alcoholreport.htm.

Exhibit 2.15: Source of Last Alcohol Used among Past-Month Alcohol Users Ages 12–20, by Age Group: 2010–2011 (SAMHSA, CBHSQ, NSDUH, Special Data Analysis, 2012)

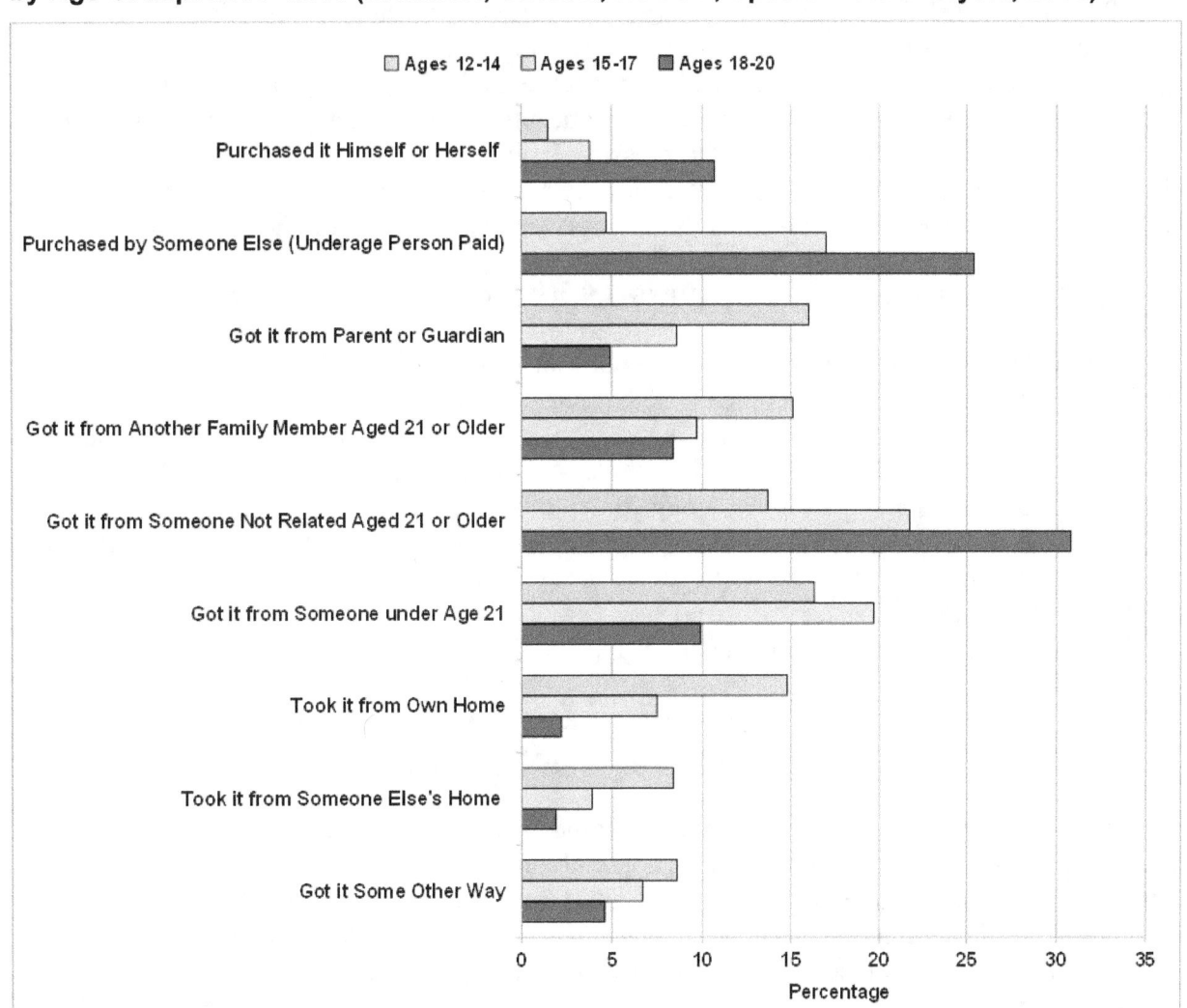

2003 Alcohol Report

FTC's 2003 review reported that over 99 percent of the radio, television, and magazine advertising budgets for alcohol brands whose target audience included 21-year-olds were expended in compliance with the 50 percent placement standard. FTC also announced that the alcohol industry had agreed to amend its voluntary codes to require that adults over 21 constitute at least 70 percent (thus reducing the permissible underage percentage to 30 percent) of the audience for TV, magazine, and radio ads, based on reliable data. To facilitate compliance, the revised codes of the beer and spirits industries required members to conduct periodic post-placement audits and promptly remedy any identified problems.[24]

---

[24] For more information, see *Alcohol Marketing and Advertising* (FTC, 2003), available at http://www.ftc.gov/os/2003/09/alcohol08report.pdf.

2008 Alcohol Report

In 2008, FTC published its third study of alcohol advertising, evaluating compliance with the 70 percent placement standard and other matters relating to underage exposure. Data showed that 92.5 percent of advertising placements complied with the 70 percent standard; furthermore, because placements that missed the target were concentrated in smaller media, more than 97 percent of total alcohol advertising "impressions" (individual exposures to advertising) met the standard. When advertising exposure data were aggregated across companies and measured media, about 86 percent of the alcohol advertising audience consisted of legal-age adults.[25]

Youth Drinking Is Correlated with Adult Drinking Practices

Generational transmission has been widely hypothesized as one factor shaping the alcohol consumption patterns of young people. Whether through genetics, social learning, or cultural values and community norms, researchers have repeatedly found a correlation between youth drinking practices and those of their adult relatives and other community adults (SAMHSA, 2008). Nelson and colleagues (2009) demonstrated this relationship at the population (state) level. State estimates of youth and adult current drinking and binge drinking from 1993 through 2005 were significantly correlated when pooled across years. These results suggest that some policies that primarily affect adult drinkers (e.g., pricing and taxation, hours of sale, on-premises drink promotions) may affect underage drinking.

Despite Meaningful Progress, Underage Drinking Remains Unacceptably High

Available data from 1975 to 2011 document that the prevalence of drinking among 12th graders peaked in 1978 for lifetime use and past-year use (Johnston et al., 2012a). Lifetime alcohol use among 12th graders in 2006 showed a statistically significant decline from 2005, dropping from 75.1 percent to 72.7 percent (Johnston, O'Malley, Bachman, & Schulenberg, 2007). Levels of lifetime alcohol use remained steady from 2007 to 2011 (Johnston et al., 2009a, 2012a). Past-month use among 12th graders increased from 1975 to 1978, decreased slightly from 1978 to 1988, decreased from 1988 to 1993, increased from 1993 to 1997, decreased from 1997 to 2002, remained steady from 2002 to 2005, and has decreased slightly since then (Johnston et al., 2009a,c; 2012a) (Exhibit 2.16).

Binge drinking in the past 2 weeks among 12th graders peaked in 1981, held steady in 1982, and then declined from 40.8 percent in 1983 to a low of 27.5 percent in 1993—a decrease of almost one third, and thus a significant improvement (Johnston et al., 2009a). From 1993 to 1998, binge drinking rose by about 4 percentage points among 12th graders. After increasing to 32 percent in 1998, the rate among 12th graders dropped to 25 percent by 2006, where it remained through 2009; it then declined significantly to 22 percent by 2011—a new low (Johnston et al., 2012a). An upward drift in binge drinking among 8th graders occurred from 1991 (10.9 percent) to 1996 (13.3 percent) and among 10th graders from 1991 (21.0 percent) to 2000 (24.1 percent). After those peaks, a slight decline in binge use occurred in all three grades until 2002, when rates fell

---

[25] For more information, see *Self-Regulation in the Alcohol Industry* (FTC, 2008), available at http://www.ftc.gov/os/2008/06/080626alcoholreport.pdf.

Exhibit 2.16: Trends in 30-Day Prevalence of Alcohol Use for 12th Graders, 1975–2011 (Johnston et al., 2012a)

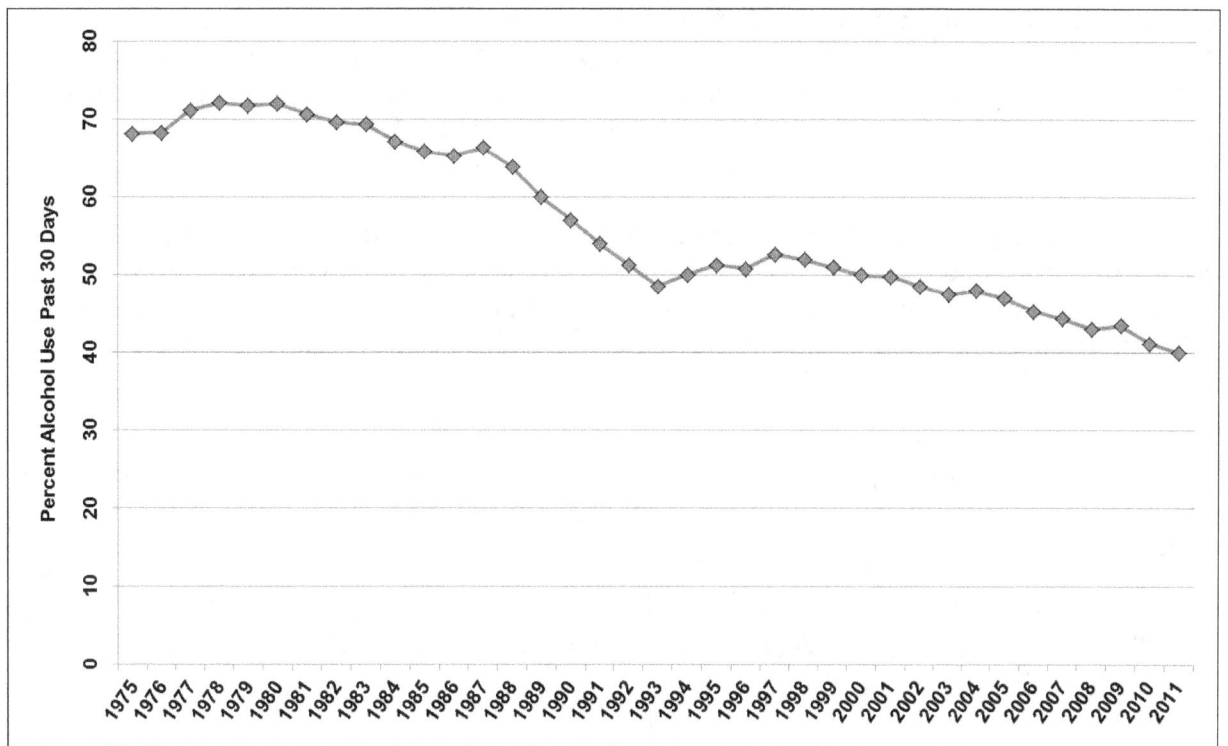

appreciably. Since 2002, there have been statistically significant declines in binging for all three grades (Johnston et al., 2012a). Faden and Fay (2004) examined similar underage drinking data from NSDUH, MTF, and YRBS from 1990 to 2002. Trend analyses "show a pattern of relative stability or decreases in the late 1990s and early 2000s for all groups on all measures with the exception of daily drinking by 10th graders in MTF and drinking five or more drinks in a row by 10th graders in YRBS" (Faden & Fay, 2004, p. 1393). These authors continue: "these results considered together offer stronger support for the finding of stability or decrease in youth drinking prevalence in the past 10 years or so than results from any one survey do by themselves." More recent analyses of the same data sources (Chen, Yi, & Faden, 2011) show continued declines in past-month and binge alcohol use through 2009.

These results are encouraging. Meaningful progress is being made. However, as the following sections demonstrate, the consequences of underage drinking remain a substantial threat to public health. From this perspective, the prevalence of alcohol use by persons under age 21 remains unacceptably high.

Consequences and Risks of Underage Drinking

Underage drinking is a problem for individuals and society. Underage drinking is a threat to public health and safety, with profound consequences for youth, their families, and their communities. According to the *Call to Action*, about 5,000 people under age 21 die annually from alcohol-related injuries involving underage drinking. Underage drinking also results in enormous economic costs. In 2006, almost $24.6 billion (about 11 percent) of the total $223.5

billion economic costs of excessive alcohol consumption were related to underage drinking. The costs largely resulted from losses in workplace productivity (58 percent of the total cost), law enforcement and other criminal justice expenses related to excessive alcohol consumption (19 percent of the total cost), health care expenses for problems caused by excessive drinking (15 percent of the total cost), and motor vehicle crash costs from impaired driving (6 percent of the total cost). Most productivity losses (28 percent) were due to deaths from alcohol-attributable conditions involving underage youth (Bouchery et al., 2011).

Underage drinking is a complex problem that results in a range of adverse short- and long-term consequences. The following sections describe some of these negative consequences, which include the negative effects of alcohol consumption on underage drinkers and consequences for those around them (referred to as secondary effects of underage alcohol use).

Alcohol-Related Motor Vehicle Traffic Crashes

The greatest mortality risk for underage drinkers is motor vehicle crashes. In 2010, of the 1,936 drivers ages 15 to 20 who were killed in motor vehicle traffic crashes:

- 587 (30 percent) had a BAC of 0.01 or higher.
- 97 (5 percent of all fatally injured drivers this age) had a BAC of 0.01 to 0.07 g/dL.
- 490 (25 percent of fatally injured drivers this age) had a BAC of 0.08 g/dL or higher (NHTSA FARS, 2010).

In 2010, of the 373 nonoccupants (pedestrians and pedal cyclists) in the 15- to 20-year-old age group killed in motor vehicle traffic crashes, 85 (23 percent) had a BAC of 0.01 g/dL or higher, 13 (3 percent of all nonoccupant fatalities this age) had a BAC of 0.01–0.07 g/dL, and 72 (19 percent of nonoccupant fatalities this age) had a BAC of 0.08 g/dL or higher (NHTSA FARS, 2010). Relative to adults, young people who drink and drive have an increased risk of alcohol-related crashes because of their increased impairment from a given amount of alcohol and, perhaps because of their relative inexperience behind the wheel. One study found that a BAC of 0.08 g/dL rendered adult drivers in all age and gender groups 11 times more likely than sober drivers to die in a single-vehicle crash. In a classic paper, Zador (1991) reported that in 16- to 20-year-olds, a BAC of 0.08 g/dL rendered male drivers 52 times more likely and female drivers 94 times more likely than sober gender-matched drivers the same age to die in a single-vehicle fatal crash.

The distribution of fatalities in motor vehicle traffic crashes involving a 15- to 20-year-old driver with a BAC of 0.08 g/dL or higher by person type in 2010 is shown in Exhibit 2.17.

According to 2011 NSDUH survey data, about 3.6 percent of 16-year-olds, 6.7 percent of 17-year-olds, 10.0 percent of 18-year-olds, 14.2 percent of 19-year-olds, and 16.5 percent of 20-year-olds reported driving under the influence of alcohol at least once in the past year (SAMHSA, detailed tables, 2012b). In general, the reported prevalence of driving under the influence of alcohol increases with age until about age 25, although there is some variation among survey years. For example, according to the 2010 NSDUH data, prevalence of driving under the influence of alcohol peaked at age 22, and then declined for older persons. Overall, 24.1 percent of high school students in the 2011 YRBS had, in the past 30 days, ridden with a driver who had been drinking; 27.7 percent of seniors had done so (CDC, 2012).

Exhibit 2.17: Distribution of Fatalities in Motor Vehicle Traffic Crashes Involving a 15- to 20- Year-Old Driver with a BAC of 0.08 or Higher by Person Type in 2010 (NHTSA FARS, 2010)

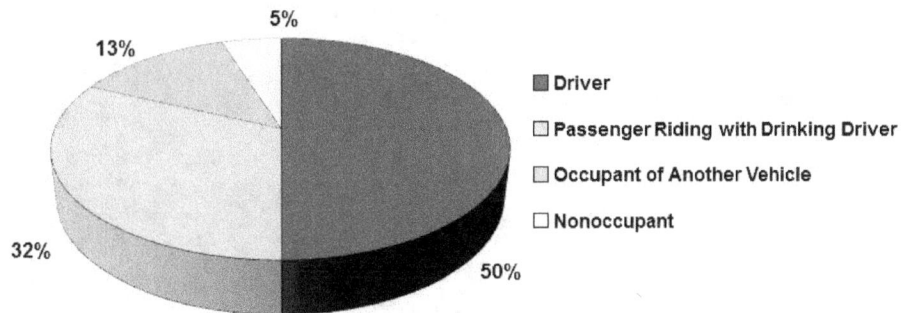

Other Unintentional Injuries such as Burns, Falls, and Drowning

Motor vehicle traffic crashes, homicide, and suicide are the three leading causes of death among youths ages 12 to 20 (Exhibit 2.18). In addition to motor vehicle crashes, underage drinking contributes to all major causes of fatal and nonfatal trauma experienced by young people. In 2009, 2,410 youths ages 12 to 20 died from unintentional injuries other than motor vehicle crashes, such as poisoning, drowning, falls, burns (CDC, 2011). Research suggests that about 40 percent of these deaths were attributable to alcohol (Smith, Branas, & Miller, 1999).

Suicide, Homicide, and Violence

Data from 17 states shows that among suicide decedents tested who were ages 10 to 19 (all of whom were under the legal drinking age in the United States), 12 percent had BACs >0.08 g/dL (Crosby et al., 2009). One study (Smith et al., 1999) estimated that, for the population as a whole, nearly a third (31.5 percent) of homicides and almost a quarter (22.7 percent) of suicides were attributable to alcohol (i.e., involved a decedent with a BAC of 0.10 g/dL or greater). Another study focused on youth suicide estimated that 9.1 percent of hospital-admitted suicide acts by those under 21 years old involved alcohol and that 72 percent of these cases were attributable to alcohol (Miller et al. 2006).

Police and child protective services records suggest that those under age 21 commit 30 percent of murders, 31 percent of rapes, 46 percent of robberies, and 27 percent of other assaults (Miller et al., 2006). As the authors note, relying on victim reports rather than agency records would yield higher estimates. For the population as a whole, an estimated 50 percent of violent crime is related to alcohol use by the perpetrator (Harwood, Fountain, & Livermore, 1998). The degree to which violent crimes committed by those under 21 are alcohol related is yet unknown.

Years of Potential Life Lost Due to Alcohol

Approximately 30 years of potential life are lost for persons with an alcohol-attributable death across all age groups (CDC, 2004). By comparison, each person who dies from cancer loses an average of 15 years of life, and each person who dies from heart disease loses an average of 11 years of life (Ries et al., 2003). Persons under age 21 who die as a result of alcohol use lose an average of 60 years of potential life (CDC, 2011).

Exhibit 2.18: Leading Causes of Death for Youth Ages 12–20: 2009 (CDC WISQARS, 2012)[26]

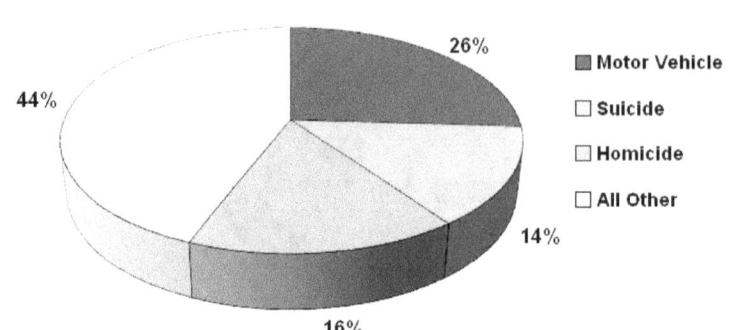

Risky Sexual Activity

According to the Surgeon General's *Call to Action*, underage drinking plays a significant role in risky sexual behavior, including unwanted, unintended, and unprotected sexual activity, as well as sex with multiple partners. Such behavior increases the risk for unplanned pregnancy and for contracting sexually transmitted diseases (STDs), including infection with HIV, the virus that causes AIDS (Cooper & Orcutt, 1997). When pregnancies occur, underage drinking may result in fetal alcohol spectrum disorders (FASDs), including fetal alcohol syndrome, which remains a leading cause of mental retardation (Warren & Bast, 1988; Stratton, Howe, & Battaglia, 1996; Jones, Smith, Ulleland, & Streissguth, 1973). A review article by Nolen-Hoeksema cites a number of studies suggesting that underage drinking by both victim and assailant increases the risk of physical and sexual assault (Nolen-Hoeksema, 2004; Abbey, 2011).

Adverse Consequences of College Drinking

One NIAAA-funded study (Abbey et al., 1996) reported that over half of college women respondents had experienced some form of sexual assault. Slightly less than one third of these assaults were characterized by respondents as attempted or completed rapes. However, the incidence of college sexual assaults is difficult to measure, and different studies report different rates. A review by Abbey (2011) of three relevant studies (Abbey et al, 2004; Seto and Barbaree, 1995; Testa, 2002) concludes that approximately half of all reported and unreported sexual assaults involve alcohol consumption by the perpetrator, victim, or both, Abbey further reports that, typically, if the victim consumes alcohol, the perpetrator does as well. Estimates of perpetrators' intoxication during the incident ranged from 30 percent to 75 percent.

Many other adverse social consequences are linked with college alcohol consumption. Hingson and colleagues (2009) estimated that annually more than 696,000 college students were assaulted or hit by another student who had been drinking; another 599,000 were unintentionally injured while under the influence of alcohol. Research suggests that roughly 474,000 students ages 18 to 24 have unprotected sex due to drinking, and each year more than 100,000 students ages 18 to 24 report having been too intoxicated to know if they consented to having sex (Exhibit 2.19). Approximately 25 percent of college students report academic consequences as a result of their

---

[26] CDC's web-based Injury Statistics Query and Reporting System (WISQARS) is an interactive database system that provides customized reports of injury-related data.

Exhibit 2.19: Prevalence of Alcohol-Related Morbidity and Mortality among College Students Ages 18–24 (calculated using methods presented in Hingson et al., 2005, 2009)

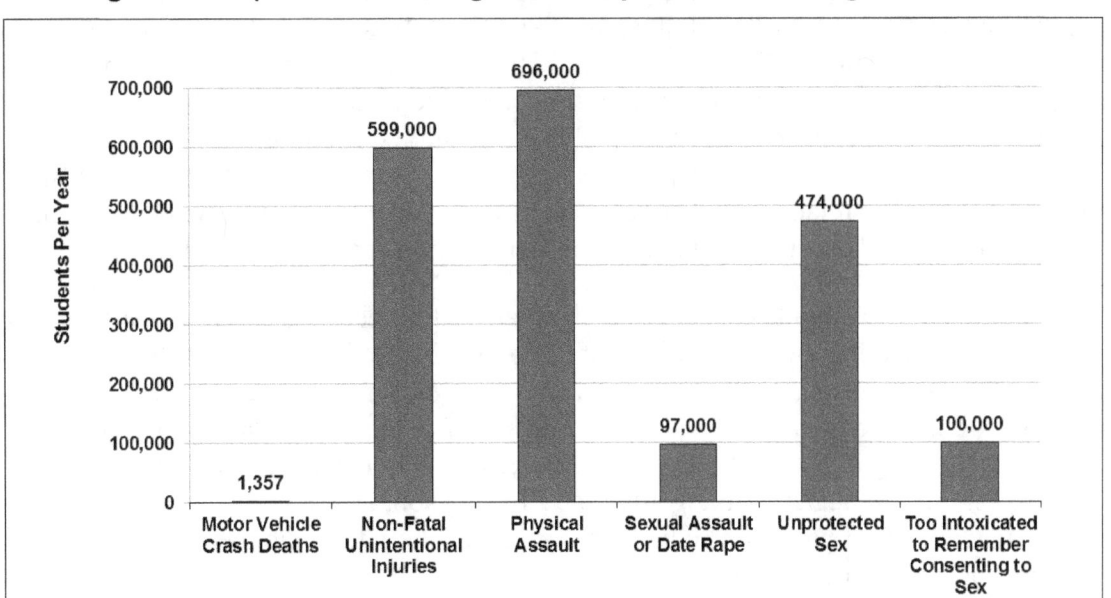

drinking, including missing class, falling behind, doing poorly on exams or papers, and receiving lower grades overall. About 11 percent of college student drinkers report having damaged property while under the influence of alcohol (Hingson et al., 2005).

Potential Brain Impairment

Adverse effects on normal brain development are a potential long-term risk of underage alcohol consumption. Neurobiological research suggests that adolescence may be a period of unique vulnerability to the effects of alcohol. For example, early heavy alcohol use may have negative effects on the actual physical development of the brain structure of adolescents (Brown & Tapert, 2004), as well as on brain functioning. Negative effects indicated by neuropsychological studies include decreased ability in planning, executive functioning, memory, spatial operations, and attention, all of which play important roles in academic performance and future levels of functioning (Giancola & Mezzich, 2000; Brown, Tapert, Granholm, & Dellis, 2000; Tapert & Brown, 1999; Tapert et al., 2001). As Brown and colleagues (2000) note, these deficits may put alcohol-dependent adolescents at risk for falling farther behind in school, putting them at an even greater disadvantage relative to nonusers. Some of these cross-sectional findings are supported by longitudinal analyses (Squeglia, Jacobus, & Tapert, 2009).

Impaired Academic Performance

Underage drinking including binge drinking affects academic performance. Students who reported binge drinking were three times more likely to report earning mostly Ds and Fs on their report cards compared with non–binge drinkers (Miller, Naimi, Brewer, & Jones, 2007).

Increased Risk of Developing an Alcohol Use Disorder Later in Life

Early-onset alcohol use (14 or younger), alone and in combination with escalated drinking in adolescence, has been noted in several studies as a risk factor for the development of alcohol-related problems in adulthood (Agrawal et al., 2009; Dawson et al., 2008; Grant & Dawson, 1997; Gruber, DiClemente, Anderson, & Lodico, 1996; Hawkins et al., 1997; Schulenburg, O'Malley, Bachman, Wadsworth, & Johnston, 1996; York, Welte, Hirsch, Hoffman, & Barnes, 2004). Grant and Dawson (1997) found that more than 40 percent of persons who initiated drinking before age 13 met diagnostic criteria for alcohol dependence at some time in their lives. By contrast, alcohol dependence rates among those who started drinking at ages 17 and 18 were 24.5 percent and 16.6 percent, respectively (Exhibit 2.20). Data from the 2009–2011 NSDUH survey suggest a similar relationship between age of initiation and development of alcohol-related problems. Only 10 to 11 percent of persons who started at age 21 or older met the criteria.

The onset of alcohol consumption in childhood or early adolescence is a marker for later alcohol-related problems, including heavier adolescent use of alcohol and other drugs (Robins & Przybeck, 1985; Hawkins et al., 1997). Adults who started drinking at age 14 were three times more likely to report driving after drinking too much ever in their lives than were those who began drinking after age 21. Crashes were four times as likely for those who began drinking at age 14 as for those who began drinking after age 21 (Hingson, Heeren, Levenson, Jamanka, & Voas, 2001). Children of parents who binge are twice as likely to binge themselves and to meet alcohol dependence criteria.

Underage Drinking: A Developmental Phenomenon

As the Acting Surgeon General wrote in the introduction to the *Call to Action*:

> …the latest research also offers hopeful new possibilities for prevention and intervention by furthering our understanding of underage alcohol use as a developmental phenomenon—as a behavior directly related to maturational processes in adolescence. New research explains why adolescents use alcohol differently from adults, why they react uniquely to it, and why alcohol can pose such a powerful attraction to adolescents, with unpredictable and potentially devastating outcomes.

This understanding of underage alcohol use as a developmental phenomenon is one of the major themes of the *Call to Action* and is an important concept in this report.

Exhibit 2.20: Ages of Initiation and Levels of DSM Diagnoses for Abuse and Dependence (Grant & Dawson, 1997)

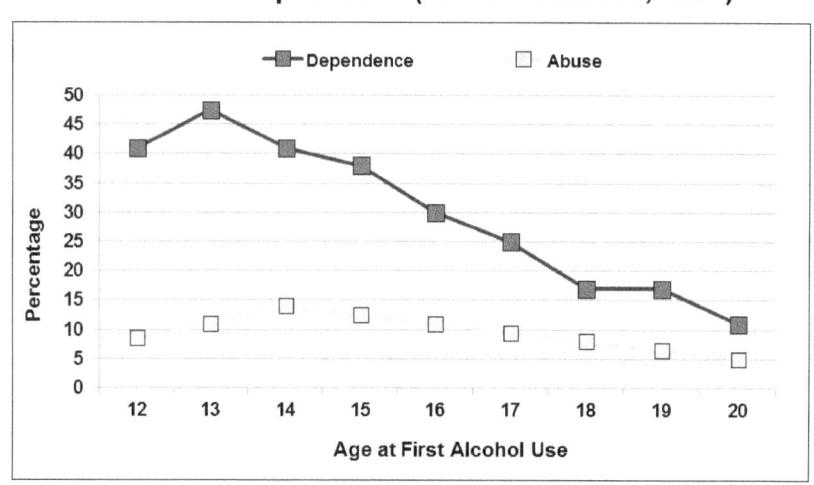

Adolescence is the period between the onset of puberty[27] and the assumption of adult roles. It is a time of particular vulnerability to alcohol use and its consequences for a variety of developmental reasons, some specific to the individual and others related to the biological and behavioral changes produced by adolescence itself. In addition, alcohol can present a special allure to some adolescents for social, genetic, psychological, and cultural reasons. Recent advances in the fields of epidemiology, developmental psychopathology, human brain development, and behavioral genetics have provided new insights into adolescent development and its relationship to underage alcohol use.

Adolescent alcohol consumption is a complex behavior influenced by multiple factors, including the normal maturational changes that all adolescents experience; the various social and cultural contexts in which adolescents live (e.g., family, peers, and school); genetic, psychological, and social factors specific to each adolescent; and environmental factors that influence the availability and appeal of alcohol (e.g., enforcement of underage alcohol policies, marketing practices, and media exposure). Biological factors internal to the adolescent, such as genes and hormones, interact with factors external to the adolescent, such as peers, school, and the overall culture, in determining whether and to what extent an adolescent will use alcohol. Internal and external factors influence each other in reciprocal ways as the adolescent's development unfolds over time. Youths are not uniformly at risk for alcohol consumption nor are they uniformly at risk over the span of their own adolescence.

An important aspect of understanding the adolescent attraction to alcohol, as well as the means by which its use can be prevented or reduced, is appreciating the significant influence of the many social systems in which adolescents operate. These different social systems both influence adolescents and are, in turn, influenced by adolescents (Bronfenbrenner, 1979). As shown in Exhibit 2.21, these systems include the adolescent's family, peers, school, extracurricular and

Exhibit 2.21: Systems That Influence Adolescent Behavior (HHS, 2007)

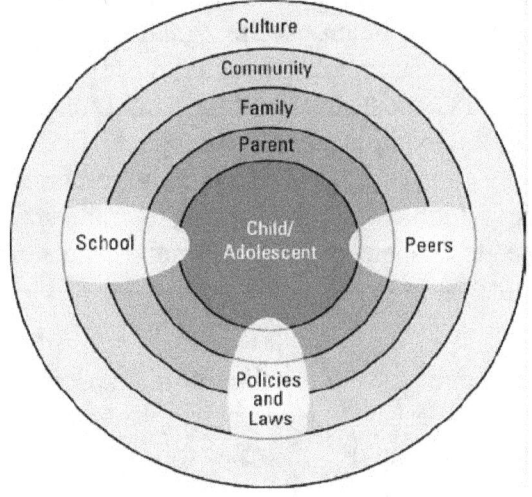

---

[27] For the purpose of this report, puberty is defined as a sequence of events by which a child becomes a young adult characterized by secretions of hormones, development of secondary sexual characteristics, reproductive functions, and growth spurts.

community activities, sports teams and clubs, religious institutions, other diverse organizations with which the adolescent interacts, part-time work, the community itself, the culture, and even influences from around the world accessed through the internet and other electronic resources. Each social system exposes the adolescent to both positive and negative influences, potentially increasing or decreasing the adolescent's risk of alcohol use. These multiple systems interact and may reinforce or counteract each other. Exhibit 2.21 represents the multiple systems in which adolescents are embedded. Their relative influences vary across development.

Each system may affect an adolescent's decision to use alcohol. To protect adolescents properly from alcohol use, parents and other adults must be involved in multiple social systems as individuals, citizens, and voters. By understanding the roles these systems play in the teen's life and by acting strategically on the basis of established and emerging research, parents, other adults, and the nation can reduce the risk and consequences of underage alcohol use.

An understanding of underage alcohol use as a developmental phenomenon sheds significant light on the particular vulnerabilities of adolescents to alcohol use, as well as protective measures likely to prevent and reduce underage drinking. Some of the most important developmental findings included in the *Call to Action* are discussed below.

The Developing Adolescent Brain

During adolescence, dramatic changes to the brain's structure, neuron connectivity ("wiring"), and physiology occur (Restak, 2001). These changes affect everything from emerging sexuality to emotionality and judgment. However, not all parts of the brain mature at the same time. Differences in maturational timing across the brain can result in impulsive decisions or actions, disregard for consequences, and emotional reactions that can lead to alcohol use or otherwise put teenagers at serious risk.

Stress and Adolescent Transitions

The physical effects of puberty create dramatic changes in the sexual and social experiences of maturing adolescents that require significant psychological and social adaptation, creating stress that may contribute to increased consumption of alcohol during the adolescent period (Tschann et al., 1994). In graduating from elementary to middle school, from middle to high school, and from high school to college or the workplace, adolescents face new stressors. Research shows a link between stress and alcohol consumption. For example, research on nonhuman primates shows that adolescent monkeys double their alcohol intake under stress and that excessive alcohol consumption is related to changes in stress hormones and serotonin (Barr et al., 2004).

Personality Traits

Studies of adolescent drinking have repeatedly failed to find specific sets of personality traits that uniquely predict alcohol use in adolescents. Nonetheless, research does show that adolescents who use alcohol heavily or have alcohol use disorders (AUDs) do exhibit certain shared personality traits (also shared by some adolescents who do not abuse alcohol). High levels of impulsiveness, aggression, conduct problems, novelty seeking (Gabel et al., 1999); low harm avoidance (Jones & Heaven, 1998); and other risky behaviors in childhood and early adolescence may be associated with future heavy alcohol use and AUDs (Soloff et al., 2000).

Mental Disorders

Depression and anxiety are risk factors for alcohol problems because some people drink to cope with internal distress. Adolescents with defined mental disorders have significantly elevated rates of alcohol and other drug use problems. Because many young people are involved not only with alcohol but also with other substances, and may also have a co-occurring mental disorder, interventions should be designed to address this complexity.

Adolescents from Families with a Family History of Alcohol Dependence

Children whose families include individuals who abuse alcohol are at increased risk for alcohol dependence throughout their lives. Genes account for over half of the risk for alcohol dependence; environmental factors account for the rest. However, no single gene accounts for the majority of risk. The development of a complex behavioral disorder such as alcohol dependence likely depends on specific genetic factors interacting with one another, multiple environmental factors, and the interaction between genetic and environmental factors. Research suggests that genes have a stronger influence on the development of problematic use, whereas environment seems to play a greater role in initiation of use (Rhee et al., 2003). The current college environment may increase the likelihood that persons with genetic predispositions to alcohol use disorders will have those predispositions expressed (Timberlake et al., 2007).

Sensitivity to Effects of Alcohol Use

Animal research indicates that adolescents in general are more sensitive than adults to the stimulating effects of alcohol and less sensitive to some of the aversive effects of acute alcohol intoxication, such as sedation, hangover, and ataxia (loss of muscular coordination) (Doremus et al., 2003; Little et al., 1996; Silveri & Spear, 1998; Varlinskaya & Spear, 2004; White et al., 2002; for review, see Spear, 2000, and Spear & Varlinskaya, 2005). This differing sensitivity may make adolescents more vulnerable to certain harmful effects of alcohol use. For example, adolescents are able to drink more than adults (who might pass out or be inclined to go to sleep) and therefore are more likely than adults to initiate activities when they are too impaired to perform them competently, such as driving. They are also more likely to drink to the point of coma. Furthermore, in the case of driving, each drink increases impairment more for adolescents than for adults (Hingson & Winter, 2003). Children whose parents abuse alcohol may be at even greater risk for excessive drinking resulting from a combination of genetic and developmental factors that lower their sensitivity to alcohol.

These issues are reviewed in detail in *Underage Drinking: Understanding and Reducing Risk in the Context of Human Development*, a special supplement of the journal *Pediatrics* (2008).

Intervening Amidst Complexity

Underage alcohol use is a highly complex phenomenon driven by a variety of interacting factors. A developmental approach to preventing and reducing underage alcohol use takes into account these complex forces and factors that determine an adolescent's decision to use or not use alcohol. Complex interactions among biological, social, cultural, and environmental factors evolve as maturation proceeds; thus, the same adolescent at age 13 and later at age 17 will have different developmental needs and require different protective structures and skills to avoid using alcohol. To further complicate matters, periods of rapid transition, reorganization, and growth spurts alternate with periods of quiet and consolidation—all within a changing social context. A developmental approach to the prevention and reduction of underage drinking recognizes the importance of all environmental and social systems that affect adolescents, as well as adolescents' maturational processes and individual characteristics.

An advantage of understanding underage alcohol use as a developmental phenomenon is the unique insight it provides into risk and protective factors. Although the problem of underage drinking is complex, it is not insurmountable. A developmental approach makes clear the need for a coordinated national effort to prevent and reduce underage drinking and for the active involvement of both public and private sectors as well as parents, other caregivers, and other adults. Success in solving a public health and safety problem as complex as underage drinking will require the engagement of every American, as the *Call to Action* puts it, "in a national effort to address underage drinking early, continuously, and in the context of human development. Underage alcohol use is everybody's problem—and its solution is everybody's responsibility."

Conclusion

As the data in this chapter demonstrate, characteristics of underage drinking such as age of initiation, current usage, and amounts consumed have fluctuated over the years. There is cause for some optimism, as the average age of first use has slowly risen, while binge-drinking rates show a gradual decline. Nevertheless, the overall rates of underage drinking remain unacceptably high, with the ability of youth to gain access to alcohol remaining relatively easy, particularly during the college years. The risks associated with this access are profound, resulting in traffic fatalities, injuries, suicides and homicides, and risky sexual behavior, as well as adverse effects on brain development and academic performance.

CHAPTER 3
A Coordinated Federal Approach to Preventing and Reducing Underage Drinking

The 2006 STOP Act records the sense of Congress that "a multi-faceted effort is needed to more successfully address the problem of underage drinking in the United States. A coordinated approach to prevention, intervention, treatment, enforcement, and research is key to making progress. This Act recognizes the need for a focused national effort, and addresses particulars of the federal portion of that effort as well as federal support for state activities."

A Coordinated Approach

The congressional mandate to develop a coordinated approach to prevent and reduce underage drinking and its adverse consequences recognizes that alcohol consumption by those under 21 is a serious, complex, and persistent societal problem with significant financial, social, and personal costs. Congress also recognizes that a long-term solution will require a broad, deep, and sustained national commitment to reducing the demand for, and access to, alcohol among young people. That solution will have to address not only the youth themselves but also the larger society that provides a context for that drinking and in which images of alcohol use are pervasive and drinking is seen as normative.

The national responsibility for preventing and reducing underage drinking involves government at every level: institutions and organizations in the private sector; colleges and universities; public health and consumer groups; the alcohol and entertainment industries; schools; businesses; parents and other caregivers; other adults; and adolescents themselves. This section of the present report, while equally inclusive, nonetheless focuses on the activities of the federal government and its unique role in preventing and reducing underage drinking. Through leadership and financial support, the federal government can influence public opinion and increase public knowledge about underage drinking; enact and enforce relevant laws; fund programs and research that increase understanding of the causes and consequences of underage alcohol use; monitor trends in underage drinking and the effectiveness of efforts designed to reduce demand, availability, and consumption; and lead the national effort.

All Interagency Coordinating Committee on Preventing Underage Drinking (ICCPUD) agencies and certain other federal partners will continue to contribute their leadership and vision to the national effort to prevent and reduce underage alcohol use. Each participating agency plays a role specific to its mission and mandate. For example, the National Institute on Alcohol Abuse and Alcoholism (NIAAA) supports biomedical and behavioral research on the prevalence and patterns of alcohol use across the lifespan and of alcohol-related consequences—including abuse and dependence injuries and effects on prenatal, child, and adolescent development. This body of research includes studies on alcohol epidemiology, metabolism, genetics, neuroscience, prevention, and treatment. NIAAA and the Centers for Disease Control and Prevention (CDC) provide the research to promote an understanding of the serious nature of underage drinking and its consequences. In general, the Substance Abuse and Mental Health Services Administration (SAMHSA), the National Highway Traffic Safety Administration (NHTSA), and the Department of Education (ED) conduct programs to reduce underage demand for alcohol, and the Department of Justice (DoJ), through its Office of Juvenile Justice and Delinquency Prevention (OJJDP), works to reduce underage consumption of and access to alcohol, as well as the availability of alcohol itself. SAMHSA, CDC, and NIAAA conduct surveillance that gathers the latest data on underage alcohol use and the effectiveness of programs designed to prevent and reduce it. NHTSA, CDC, SAMHSA, NIAAA, and the National Institute on Drug Abuse (NIDA) gather data on adverse consequences. As these agencies interact with one another, the activities and expertise of each inform and complement the others, creating a synergistic, integrated federal program for addressing underage drinking in all its complexity.

Federal Agencies Involved in Preventing and Reducing Underage Drinking

Multiple federal agencies are involved in preventing and reducing underage drinking. Each currently sponsors programs that address underage alcohol consumption, and each is a member of ICCPUD. The agencies and their primary roles related to underage drinking are as follows:

1. **U.S. Department of Health and Human Services (HHS)/Administration for Children and Families (ACF):** ACF is responsible for federal programs that promote the economic and social well-being of families, children, individuals, and communities. Many of these programs strengthen protective factors and reduce risk factors associated with underage drinking. Website: http://www.acf.hhs.gov

2. **HHS/Office of the Assistant Secretary for Planning and Evaluation (ASPE):** ASPE is the principal advisor to the HHS Secretary on policy development and is responsible for major activities in policy coordination, legislation development, strategic planning, policy research, evaluation, and economic analysis. Website: http://www.aspe.hhs.gov

3. **HHS/CDC:** CDC's mission is to promote health and quality of life by preventing and controlling disease, injury, and disability. Consistent with that mission, CDC is involved in strengthening the scientific foundation for the prevention of underage and binge drinking. This includes assessing the problem through public health surveillance and epidemiological studies of underage drinking and its consequences. CDC also evaluates the effectiveness of prevention policies and programs, and examines underage drinking as a risk factor through programs that address health problems such as injury and violence, sexually transmitted diseases, and fetal alcohol spectrum disorders (FASDs). CDC trains new researchers in alcohol epidemiology and builds state public health system capacity. CDC also conducts systematic reviews of what works to prevent alcohol-related injuries and harms. Website: http://www.cdc.gov

4. **HHS/Indian Health Service (IHS):** IHS is responsible for providing federal health services to American Indians and Alaska Natives. The IHS is the principal federal health care provider and health advocate for American Indians and Alaska Natives, and its goal is to raise their health status to the highest possible level. The IHS provides a comprehensive health service delivery system for approximately 2 million American Indians and Alaska Natives who belong to 566 federally recognized Tribes in 36 states. Website: http://www.ihs.gov

5. **HHS/National Institutes of Health (NIH) NIAAA:** NIAAA provides leadership in the effort to reduce alcohol-related problems by conducting and supporting alcohol-related research; collaborating with international, national, state, and local institutions, organizations, agencies, and programs; and translating and disseminating research findings to health care providers, researchers, policymakers, and the public. Website: http://www.niaaa.nih.gov

6. **HHS/NIH National Institute on Drug Abuse (NIDA):** NIDA's mission is to "lead the Nation in bringing the power of science to bear on drug abuse and addiction." NIDA supports most of the world's research on the health aspects of drug abuse and addiction, and carries out programs that ensure rapid dissemination of research to inform policy and improve practice. Website: http://www.nida.nih.gov

7. **HHS/Office of the Surgeon General (OSG):** The Surgeon General is America's chief health educator, giving Americans the best available scientific information on how to improve their health and reduce the risk of illness and injury. OSG oversees the 6,500-member Commissioned Corps of the U.S. Public Health Service and assists the Surgeon General with other duties as well. Website: http://www.surgeongeneral.gov

8. **HHS/SAMHSA:** SAMHSA's mission is to reduce the impact of substance abuse and mental illness on America's communities. SAMHSA works toward underage drinking prevention by supporting state and community efforts, promoting the use of evidence-based practices, educating the public, and collaborating with other agencies and interested parties. Website: http://www.samhsa.gov

9. **Department of Defense (DoD):** DoD coordinates and oversees government activities relating directly to national security and military affairs. Its alcohol-specific role involves preventing and reducing alcohol consumption by underage military personnel and improving the health of service members' families by strengthening protective factors and reducing risks factors in underage alcohol consumption. Website: http://www.defense.gov

10. **ED/Office of Safe and Healthy Students (OSHS):** OSHS administers, coordinates, and recommends policy to improve the effectiveness of programs providing financial assistance for drug and violence prevention activities and activities that promote student health and well-being in elementary and secondary schools and institutions of higher education. Activities may be carried out by state and local educational agencies or other public or private nonprofit organizations. OSHS supports programs that prevent violence in and around schools; prevent illegal use of alcohol, tobacco, and drugs; engage parents and communities; and coordinate with related federal, state, school, and community efforts to foster safe learning environments that support student academic achievement. Website: http://www2.ed.gov/about/offices/list/oese/index.html

11. **DoJ/OJJDP:** OJJDP provides national leadership, coordination, and resources to prevent and respond to juvenile delinquency and victimization. OJJDP supports states and communities in their efforts to develop and implement effective, coordinated prevention and intervention programs and to improve the juvenile justice system's ability to protect public safety, hold offenders accountable, and provide treatment and rehabilitation services tailored to the needs of juveniles and their families. OJJDP's central underage drinking prevention initiative, Enforcing the Underage Drinking Laws (EUDL), is a nationwide state- and community-based multidisciplinary effort that seeks to prevent access to and consumption of alcohol by those under age 21 with a special emphasis on enforcement of underage drinking laws and implementation programs that use best and most promising practices. Website: http://www.ojjdp.ncjrs.gov

12. **Department of the Treasury/Alcohol and Tobacco Tax and Trade Bureau (TTB):** TTB's mission is "to collect taxes owed, and to ensure that alcohol beverages are produced, labeled, advertised, and marketed in accordance with federal law." Website: http://www.ttb.gov

13. **Department of Transportation (DOT)/NHTSA:** NHTSA's mission is to save lives, prevent injuries, and reduce traffic-related health care and other economic costs. NHTSA develops, promotes, and implements effective educational, engineering, and enforcement programs to reduce traffic crashes and resulting injuries and fatalities, and reduce economic costs associated with traffic crashes, including underage drinking and driving crashes. Website: http://www.nhtsa.gov

14. **Federal Trade Commission (FTC):** FTC works to ensure that the nation's markets are vigorous, efficient, and free of restrictions that harm consumers. FTC has enforcement and administrative responsibilities under 46 laws relating to competition and consumer protection. As the enforcer of federal truth-in-advertising laws, the agency monitors alcohol advertising for unfair practices and deceptive claims and reports to Congress when appropriate. Website: http://www.ftc.gov

15. **Office of National Drug Control Policy (ONDCP):** The principal purpose of ONDCP is to establish policies, priorities, and objectives for the nation's drug control program. The goals of the program are to reduce illicit drug use, manufacturing, and trafficking; drug-related crime and violence; and drug-related health consequences. Part of ONDCP's efforts relate to underage alcohol use. Website: http://www.whitehousedrugpolicy.gov

The following section highlights current initiatives to prevent and reduce underage drinking and its consequences. Further details about departmental and agency programs to prevent and reduce underage drinking appear later in this chapter under "Inventory of Federal Programs by Agency."

How Federal Agencies and Programs Work Together

The STOP Act of 2006 requires the HHS Secretary, on behalf of ICCPUD, to submit an annual report to Congress summarizing "all programs and policies of federal agencies designed to prevent and reduce underage drinking." ICCPUD aims to increase coordination and collaboration in program development among member agencies so that the resulting programs and interventions are complementary and synergistic. For example, the Town Hall Meetings held in various parts of the country in 2006, 2008, 2010, and 2012 have been held in every state, the District of Columbia, and most of the Territories, and are an effective way to raise public awareness of underage drinking as a public health problem and mobilize communities to take action. At these meetings, communities have used NIAAA statistics, videos produced by NHTSA, and training materials developed by OJJDP through the EUDL program, and they have engaged governors' spouses as part of the Leadership To Keep Children Alcohol Free initiative. For the 2012 round of Town Hall Meetings, local communities were encouraged to make use of ICCPUD agency resources to create comprehensive action plans for community change.

A Commitment to Evidence-Based Practices

At the heart of any effective national effort to prevent and reduce underage drinking are reliable data on the effectiveness of specific prevention and reduction efforts. With limited resources available and human lives at stake, it is critical that professionals use the most time- and cost-effective approaches known to the field. Traditionally, efficacy has been ensured through practices that research has proven to be effective instead of those based on convention, tradition, folklore, personal experience, belief, intuition, or anecdotal evidence. The term for practices validated by documented scientific evidence is "evidence-based practices" (EBPs).

Despite broad agreement regarding the need for EBPs, there is currently no consensus on the precise definition of an EBP. Disagreement arises not from the need for evidence, but from the kind and amount of evidence required for validation. The gold standard of scientific evidence is the randomized controlled trial, but it is not always possible to conduct such trials. Many strong, widely used, quasi-experimental designs have and will continue to produce credible, valid, and reliable evidence—these should be relied upon when randomized controlled trials are not possible. Practitioner input is a crucial part of this process and should be carefully considered as evidence is compiled, summarized, and disseminated to the field for implementation.

The Institute of Medicine (IOM), for example, defines an EBP as one that combines the following three factors: best research evidence, best clinical experience, and consistency with patient values (IOM, 2001). The American Psychological Association (APA) adopted a slight variation of this definition for the field of psychology, as follows: EBP is "the integration of the best available research with clinical expertise in the context of patient characteristics, culture, and preferences" (APA, 2005).

The federal government does not provide a single, authoritative definition of EBPs, yet the general concept of an EBP is clear: some form of scientific evidence must support the proposed practice, the practice itself must be practical and appropriate given the circumstances under which it will be implemented and the population to which it will be applied, and the practice has a significant effect on the outcome(s) to be measured. For example, the Office of Safe and Healthy Students (OSHS) requires that its grantees use EBPs in the programs they fund, and NHTSA has produced a publication entitled "Countermeasures That Work" for use by State Highway Safety Offices (SHSOs) and encourages the SHSOs to select countermeasure strategies that have either been proven effective or shown promise.

National Registry of Evidence-Based Programs and Practices

SAMHSA developed the National Registry of Evidence-based Programs and Practices (NREPP) (http://www.nrepp.samhsa.gov), a searchable database of interventions for the prevention and treatment of mental and substance use disorders that have been reviewed and rated by independent reviewers. The purpose of this registry is to assist the public in identifying approaches to preventing and treating mental and/or substance use disorders that have been scientifically tested and that can be readily disseminated to the field. NREPP is one way that SAMHSA is working to improve access to information on tested interventions and thereby reduce the lag time between the creation of scientific knowledge and its practical application in the field. In addition to helping the public find evidence-based interventions, SAMHSA and other federal agencies use NREPP to inform grantees about EBPs and to encourage their use. The NREPP database is not an authoritative list; SAMHSA does not approve, recommend, or endorse the specific interventions listed therein. Policymakers, in particular, should avoid relying solely on NREPP ratings as a basis for funding or approving interventions. Nevertheless, NREPP provides useful information and ratings of interventions to assist individuals and organizations in identifying those practices that may address their particular needs and match their specific capacities and resources. As such, NREPP is best viewed as a starting point for further investigation regarding interventions that may work well and produce positive outcomes for a variety of stakeholders. As of fall 2012, more than 250 programs were evaluated by NREPP and posted on the NREPP website.

Guide to Community Preventive Services (Community Guide)

CDC supports the use of an evidence-informed approach for its broad range of recommendations, guidelines, and communications. This approach calls for transparency in reporting the evidence that was considered and requires that the path leading from the evidence to the recommendations or guidelines be clear and well described, regardless of the strength of the underlying evidence or the processes used in their development. The Community Guide provides the model for CDC's evidence-informed approach (http://www.thecommunityguide.org/index.html).

Under the auspices of the independent, nonfederal Community Preventive Services Task Force, the reviews found on the Community Guide website systematically assess all available scientific evidence to determine the effectiveness of population-based public health interventions and the economic benefit of all effective interventions. The Community Preventive Services Task Force reviews the combined evidence, makes recommendations for practice and policy, and identifies gaps in existing research to ensure that practice, policy, and research funding decisions are informed by the highest quality evidence.

CDC's Alcohol Program works with the Community Guide, SAMHSA, NIAAA, and other partner organizations on systematic reviews of population-based interventions to prevent excessive alcohol consumption, including underage and binge drinking and related harms. To date, the Community Preventive Services Task Force has reviewed the effectiveness of various community-based strategies for preventing underage and binge drinking, including limiting alcohol outlet density, increasing alcohol excise taxes, dram shop liability, limiting days and hours of alcohol sales, electronic screening and brief intervention for alcohol misuse, enhancing enforcement of minimum legal drinking age laws, lowering blood alcohol concentration (BAC) laws for younger drivers, and offering school-based instructional programs for preventing drinking and driving and for preventing riding with drunk drivers.

Strategies recommended by the Community Preventive Services Task Force for preventing excessive alcohol consumption include:

- **Promoting dram shop liability,** which allows the owner or server of a retail alcohol establishment where a customer recently consumed alcoholic beverages to be held legally responsible for the harms inflicted by that customer.
- **Increasing alcohol taxes,** which, by increasing the price of alcohol, is intended to reduce alcohol-related harms, raise revenue, or both. Alcohol taxes are implemented at the state and federal levels, and are beverage-specific (i.e., they differ for beer, wine, and spirits).
- **Maintaining limits on days of sale,** which is intended to prevent excessive alcohol consumption and related harms by regulating access to alcohol. Most policies limiting days of sale target weekend days (usually Sundays).
- **Maintaining limits on hours of sale,** which prevents excessive alcohol consumption and related harms by limiting the hours of the day during which alcohol can legally be sold.
- **Regulating alcohol outlet density** to limit the number of alcohol outlets in a given area.

- **Electronic screening and brief interventions (e-SBI)** to reduce excessive alcohol consumption and related harms, which use electronic devices (e.g., computers, telephones, or mobile devices) to facilitate delivery of key elements, including (1) screening individuals for excessive drinking and (2) delivering a brief intervention, which provides personalized feedback about the risks and consequences of excessive drinking.
- **Recommending against privatization of retail alcohol sales,** because privatization results in increased per capita alcohol consumption, a well-established proxy for excessive alcohol consumption. Further privatization of alcohol sales in settings with current government control of retail sales are recommended against.
- **Enhancing enforcement of laws prohibiting sales to minors,** by initiating or increasing the frequency of retailer compliance checks for laws against the sale of alcohol to minors in a community.

The Community Preventive Services Task Force also recommends the following interventions for preventing alcohol-impaired driving:

- **0.08 percent BAC and above laws,** making it illegal for a driver's BAC to equal or exceed 0.08 percent.
- **Lower BAC laws for young or inexperienced drivers,** which apply to all drivers under age 21. Between states, the illegal BAC level for young drivers ranges from any detectable BAC to 0.02 percent.
- **Maintain current minimum legal drinking age (MLDA) laws,** which specify an age below which the purchase or public consumption of alcoholic beverages is illegal. In the United States, the age in all states is 21 years.
- **Sobriety checkpoints,** where law enforcement officers stop drivers to assess their level of alcohol impairment.
- **Mass media campaigns,** intended to reduce alcohol-impaired driving and designed to persuade individuals to either avoid drinking and driving or prevent others from doing so.
- **Multicomponent interventions with community mobilization,** in which communities implement multiple programs and/or policies in multiple settings to influence the community environment to reduce alcohol-impaired driving.
- **Ignition interlocks,** devices that can be installed in motor vehicles to prevent operation of the vehicle by a driver who has a BAC above a specified level (usually 0.02 to 0.04 percent).
- **School-based instructional programs,** to reduce alcohol-impaired driving and riding with alcohol-impaired drivers.

More information on these recommended interventions for preventing alcohol-impaired driving can be found at http://www.thecommunityguide.org/index.html.

Underage Drinking–Related Goals

Healthy People 2020 provides science-based, national, 10-year objectives for improving health. It was developed by the Federal Interagency Workgroup (FIW), which includes representatives from numerous federal departments and agencies. SAMHSA and NIH served as co-leaders in developing Healthy People 2020 objectives for substance abuse, including underage drinking.[28]

A number of the programs listed below in "Inventory of Federal Programs for Underage Drinking by Agency" will advance the following Healthy People 2020 objectives related to underage drinking:

- Increase the number of adolescents who have never tried alcohol
- Increase the proportion of adolescents who disapprove of having one or two alcoholic drinks nearly every day and who perceive great risk in binge drinking
- Reduce the number of underage drinkers who engage in binge drinking
- Reduce the proportion of adolescents reporting use of alcohol or any illicit drugs during the past 30 days
- Reduce the proportion of adolescents who report that they rode, during the previous 30 days, with a driver who had been drinking alcohol

A smaller set of Healthy People 2020 objectives, called Leading Health Indicators, has been selected to communicate high-priority health issues and actions that can be taken to address them. These include the following indicator for underage drinking: "Adolescents using alcohol or any illicit drugs during the past 30 days." For more information on Healthy People 2020, please go to http://www.healthypeople.gov/2020/topicsobjectives2020.

Inventory of Federal Programs for Underage Drinking by Agency

As required by the STOP Act, this section of the report summarizes major initiatives under way throughout the federal government to prevent and reduce underage alcohol use in America.

Interagency Coordinating Committee on Preventing Underage Driving

Activities Specific to Underage Drinking

ICCPUD, established in 2004 at the request of the HHS Secretary and made permanent in 2006 by the STOP Act, guides policy and program development across the federal government with respect to underage drinking. The Committee is composed of representatives from DoD, ED/OSHS, FTC, HHS/OASH/OSG, HHS/ACF, HHS/ASPE, HHS/CDC, HHS/IHS, HHS/NIH/NIAAA, HHS/NIH/NIDA, HHS/SAMHSA, DoJ/OJJDP, ONDCP, DoT/NHTSA, and Treasury/TTB. (See Appendix D for a list of ICCPUD members.)

Town Hall Meetings: To engage communities nationwide in evidence-based efforts to prevent and reduce underage alcohol use, ICCPUD—with SAMHSA as the lead agency—supported Town Hall Meetings in 2006, 2008, 2010, and 2012. These meetings, which have been held in

---

[28] For details regarding these objectives, go to:

http://www.healthypeople.gov/2020/topicsobjectives2020/objectiveslist.aspx?topicId=40

every state, the District of Columbia, and some of the territories during each round, are an effective approach for raising public awareness of underage drinking as a public health problem and mobilizing communities to take preventive action. For example, a summary report by the Governor's Prevention Advisory Council (GPAC) Underage Drinking Prevention Workgroup on Town Hall Meetings held in California in 2010 found that 20 percent of these events resulted in plans to develop a social host ordinance or other alcohol-related legislation, 5 percent led to development of new prevention coalitions, and 17 percent recruited new members for existing coalitions. Iowa coordinates its Town Hall Meetings statewide to gather community feedback that can be used to assess progress in reducing and preventing underage alcohol use and its consequences. In 2012, 1,398 community-based organizations registered their intent to hold 1,546 events, despite decreasing budgets for many prevention organizations. During fiscal year (FY) 2012, one report was released on the results of the meetings: *2010 Town Hall Meetings: Mobilizing Communities to Prevent and Reduce Underage Alcohol Use, an Evaluation Report*. SAMHSA is developing a summary report on the 2012 Town Hall Meetings.

Messages: To strengthen the national commitment to preventing and reducing underage drinking, it is important that federal agencies convey the same messages at the same time. Therefore, the leadership of the ICCPUD agencies will continue to:

- Increase efforts to highlight in speeches and meetings across the country the need to prevent underage drinking and its negative consequences.
- Ensure that the Administration is speaking with a common voice on the issue.
- Reinforce the messages that ICCPUD has developed.
- Use a coordinated marketing plan to publicize programs, events, research results, and other activities and efforts that address underage drinking.

Support the Minimum Drinking Age: Agency leadership will continue to develop and use messaging that supports a 21-year-old drinking age and will promote this in speeches and message points.

Materials and Technical Assistance: ICCPUD has collected information on underage drinking prevention materials developed by participating agencies. This inventory is being used to strengthen each agency's efforts to provide high-quality and timely information and to help avoid unnecessary duplication of effort. In addition, ICCPUD has collected information on each agency's technical assistance activities, facilitating coordination of effort when possible.

Webinars: In fall 2012, ICCPUD launched a series of webinars on the prevention of underage drinking. Beginning with an overview from the Surgeon General and the SAMHSA Administrator and ICCPUD Chair Pamela Hyde, these webinars include presentations by CDC, ED, FTC, NHTSA, NIAAA, NIDA, OJJDP, ONDCP, SAMHSA, and TTB.

Web Portal: SAMHSA, on behalf of ICCPUD, maintains a web portal dedicated to the issue of underage drinking (http://www.stopalcoholabuse.gov) that consolidates comprehensive research and resources developed by the 15 federal ICCPUD agencies. The portal includes information on underage drinking statistics (i.e., prevalence, trends, and consequences), training events, evidence-based approaches, and other resources and materials that support prevention efforts. Direct links are provided to federally supported websites designed to prevent substance abuse, including alcohol. Information is intended to serve all stakeholders (e.g., community-based organizations involved in prevention, policymakers, parents, youth, and educators). The portal also includes a subsite for the Town Hall Meeting initiative and its supporting resources. SAMHSA, with input from ICCPUD, is currently restructuring the website to better serve the needs of diverse users. As of December 2012, the web portal was averaging 623 visits per day and the average time onsite was 10 minutes, 48 seconds.

Activities Related to Underage Drinking

None

Department of Defense

Activities Specific to Underage Drinking

Youth Program: As one of the core areas for Military Youth Programs, health and life skills develop young people's capacity to engage in positive behaviors that nurture their own well-being, set personal goals, and live successfully as self-sufficient adults. Through affiliation with the Boys & Girls Clubs of America, nationally recognized programs such as SMART Moves® (Skills Mastery and Resistance Training) helps young people resist alcohol, tobacco, drugs, and premature sexual activity. SMART Moves features engaging, interactive, small-group activities that increase participants' peer support, enhance their life skills, build resilience, and strengthen leadership skills. This year-round program, provided in Military Youth Programs worldwide, encourages collaboration among staff, youth, parents, and representatives from community organizations. The program's components are grouped to support youth ages 6–9, 10–12, and 13–15.

Department of Defense Education Activity (DoDEA):

1. *Adolescent Substance Abuse Counseling Service (ASACS):* The ASACS program is a partnership between DoDEA and the military services providing comprehensive community-based prevention and education, identification and referral, and outpatient substance abuse treatment services to U.S. forces identification card holders, including active duty, retired, nonappropriated and appropriated fund civilian government workers, and contractors and their families, throughout Europe and the Pacific Rim. Program services target adolescents (ages 12–18) and their families who have concerns/problems related to alcohol and other drugs. These programs are overseen with funding provided by each service depending on the location of the program.

   ASACS counselors, in conjunction with other community leaders, develop and implement community-based adolescent substance abuse prevention and treatment programs. They provide screening and assessment; individual, family, and group therapy; and aftercare services. Counselors provide a comprehensive community prevention education program using structured classroom lesson plans and group/individual experiential learning exercises. They facilitate parent support groups intended to improve parental communication skills, limit-setting skills, active listening, and discipline techniques. On request, ASACS counselors may provide professional consultation, training, and prevention materials to community officials and organizations that interact with adolescents. The ASACS program intends to enhance military readiness through increased family cohesiveness and support.

2. *Health Education Curriculum:* Health education develops essential health literacy skills along with health promotion and disease prevention concepts, to enable all students to obtain, interpret, and understand basic health information and services and to use such information and services in ways that enhance their health and the health of others. The content in the DoDEA health education standards is organized into seven strands. These standards teach essential and transferable skills that foster health efficacy. The standards in the Health Literacy Skills strand are consistent throughout all grade levels and matched at each grade level with content standards in the other strands as important similarities are identified. The standards in the remaining content strands—Personal and Community Health (HE1); Safety and Injury Prevention (HE2); Nutrition and Physical Activity (HE3); Mental Health (HE4); Alcohol, Tobacco, and Other Drugs (HE5); and Family Life and Human Sexuality (HE6) — progressively change through the grade levels. Strand HE5, Alcohol, Tobacco and other Drugs, specifically addresses alcohol abuse prevention starting in grade 5 and continues through to the grades 9–12 high school health course.

3. *Red Ribbon Week:* Sponsored by the National Family Partnership, Red Ribbon Week provides DoDEA schools and families a perfect opportunity to discuss the dangers of drug abuse and the benefits of a healthy and drug-free lifestyle. The Red Ribbon campaign is now the oldest and largest drug prevention program in the nation, reaching millions of young people each year. Red Ribbon celebration brings schools, commands, and communities together in DoDEA to raise awareness of the dangers of alcohol, tobacco, and other drugs and encourage prevention, early intervention, and treatment services.

4. *Substance Abuse and Violence Prevention (SAVP):* The goal of DoDEA's SAVP education is to provide all students with the knowledge and skills to resist illicit substance use and to build their capacity to make responsible decisions regarding use of legal substances. DoDEA is developing a 10-lesson digital SAVP curriculum for pilot testing in grade 5. This program will replace the DARE program, which is being phased out due to manpower constraints.

Law Enforcement: DoD ensures installation-level enforcement of underage drinking laws on all federal reservations. For underage active-duty members, serious consequences (such as productivity loss or negative career impact) are tracked via the Triennial Health-Related Behavior Survey.

Activities Related to Underage Drinking

Active Duty Health-Related Behaviors (HRB) Survey: DoD triennially conducts the HRB survey to measure more than 17 health-related behaviors for active-duty military personnel. The survey develops population estimates on health-related behaviors, which include alcohol and prescription drug use. Data are collected on the age of first substance use, prevalence, binge use, and heavy use. The measure chosen to validate "at risk use" is the well-researched Alcohol Use Identification Disorders Test. Results for the 2011 HRB Survey are due in December 2012.

Alcohol Abuse Countermarketing Campaign: DoD's TRICARE Management Activity launched "That Guy" in 2006 as an integrated marketing campaign targeting military enlisted personnel ages 18 to 24 across all branches of service. Based on research and behavior change marketing concepts, the campaign uses a multimedia, peer-to-peer approach to raise awareness of the negative short-term social consequences of excessive drinking. In doing so, "That Guy" promotes peer disapproval of excessive drinking and leads to reductions in binge drinking. This campaign includes an award-winning desktop and mobile website, http://www.thatguy.com, as well as social media channels including Facebook and YouTube; online and offline public service announcements; paid and pro bono billboard, print, and digital advertising; centrally funded promotional materials; central support of special events; online instructional videos; and a turnkey implementation plan and promotion schedule for installation project officers.

This campaign is funded by Defense Health Plan Program Objective Memorandum (POM) FY10-15, but depends on commanders to support and local program managers to implement the campaign and deliver its messages to the target audience. Successfully engaging with the target audience, "That Guy" is now actively deployed around the world. Cumulative achievements to date include:

- An average time of 11 minutes per user on the "That Guy" website.
- Over 28,500 "Likes" on Facebook.
- Over 3.5 million branded materials disseminated to all services.
- More than 5,650 points of contact (POCs) engaged across the globe.
- Forty-seven states and 23 different countries with a "That Guy" campaign presence, including: United States, Afghanistan, Australia, Belgium, Portugal, Qatar, Africa, Egypt, Bahrain, Greece, Japan, Germany, Italy, Spain, Turkey, Singapore, Cuba, Guam, South Korea, Saudi Arabia, Honduras, United Kingdom, and Iraq.
- Millions reached through video and radio public service announcements (PSAs) broadcast around the world pro bono through Armed Forces Radio and Television Service (AFRTS), Army and Air Force Exchange Service (AAFES), and community stations.
- More than 122 site visits to military installations around the world, adding up to more than 376 days on the road.
- Exhibits at 46 conferences for a total of 84 days spent exhibiting.
- A total of 218 briefings to leadership and at conferences for POCs.
- Sixty-five focus groups across all service branches, reaching a total of 465 members of the young enlisted target audience.

Awards: "That Guy" has received 19 awards for excellence in categories that include poster and web design, animation, gaming, marketing, and research. Recent awards include the PR Week Public Sector Campaign of the Year, PR Week Best Use of Research-Measurement, and Blue Pencil and Gold Screen Awards finalist in website category and winner in poster category.

Impact: According to Fleishman Hillard's analysis of the annual *Status of Forces Survey* performed by the Defense Manpower Data Center (DMDC), there has been a steady increase in campaign awareness within the target audience, rising from a "phantom awareness" of 3 percent in 2006 to 14 percent in 2007, 29 percent in 2008, 45 percent in 2009, and 58 percent in 2011 (the most recent figure based on a preliminary analysis of the January 2011 survey data). The campaign is active at more than 800 military locations including installations, aircraft carriers, ships, and submarines, and http://www.thatguy.com has received more than 1,465,291 cumulative visits since its launch in December 2006. Analysis of data by Fleishman Hillard also indicates that military personnel who are on installations actively implementing the "That Guy" campaign are less likely (only 21 percent) than personnel from nonengaged installations (29 percent) to agree that their peers believe it is acceptable to drink to the point of losing control. According to the Fleishman Hillard analysis of the 2008 HRB survey results (the most recent results currently available), binge drinking among enlisted service members ages 17 to 24 dropped from 51 percent in 2005 to only 46 percent in 2008 (across Army, Air Force, Navy, and Marines). More importantly, data suggest that binge-drinking rates are lower at installations actively implementing "That Guy":

- Army: 36 percent report binge drinking at installations actively implementing "That Guy" versus 56 percent at inactive installations.
- Air Force: 35 percent report binge drinking at installations actively implementing "That Guy" versus 45 percent at inactive installations.
- Navy: 45 percent report binge drinking at installations actively implementing "That Guy" versus 49 percent at inactive installations.
- Marines: The sample size was too small for analysis.

Note: The above data are from the Fleishman Hillard analysis of the "January 2011 DMDC Status of Forces" and the 2008 HRB survey reports.

Service-Level Prevention Programs

Marine Corps Substance Abuse Program: The Marine Corps substance abuse program provides plans, policy, and resources to support commanders in preventing problems that detract from unit performance and readiness, including substance abuse. Information about the risks of alcohol misuse, rules and regulations about drinking, and alternatives to drinking are provided. The program also highlights the negative impact of alcohol abuse.

1. The behavioral health branch is implementing an integrative universal training that will educate all Marines to the risks of alcohol use and misuse. This training will be offered in phases across a Marine's career designed to build on his or her education.

2. *Building Alcohol Skills Intervention Curriculum (B.A.S.I.C):* B.A.S.I.C. is a Train-the-Trainer program. This program is delivered by small unit leaders (squad/section) in two initial 90-minute sessions. The program is designed to help Marines assess and question their own drinking habits, decisions, and beliefs. Training topics include:
   - Extent and nature of alcohol problems.
   - Leading by example.
   - Alcohol's impact on performance.
   - Up-and-down effects of alcohol.
   - Risk reduction tips.
   - Encouraging alternative activities.
   - Recognizing and referring a problem.

   The USMC is exploring alternative evidence-based programming that will replace B.A.S.I.C.

3. *Prime for Life* is a 16-hour class utilized throughout the USMC for Marines who have been identified as having issues with the misuse or abuse of alcohol typically identified through an alcohol-related incident or who are in need of alcohol education. Prime for Life is conducted by alcohol abuse prevention specialists and alcohol and drug counselors who have received 24 hours of training to teach Prime for Life by the Prevention Research Institute.

4. *Adolescent Substance Abuse Counseling Service (ASACS (included under DoDEA)):* The ASACS program is a comprehensive community-based program that provides prevention and

education, identification and referral, and outpatient substance abuse treatment services to USMC, including active duty, retired, nonappropriated and appropriated fund civilian government workers, and contractors and their families, in Okinawa, Japan. The scope of care encompasses adolescents (ages 12–18) and their families who have concerns/problems related to alcohol and other drugs.

Navy Alcohol and Drug Abuse Prevention: The Navy's comprehensive substance abuse prevention program is designed to support fleet readiness by fighting alcohol and drug use. Our goal is to promote zero tolerance for drugs and responsible alcohol use, and prevent alcohol abuse. The Navy believes that preventing alcohol abuse and alcoholism greatly benefits the Navy by minimizing lost workdays and the need for costly treatment. As a result, Navy commanders are required to promote a "responsible use" and "zero tolerance" environment. In addition, our program includes educational programs, multimedia campaigns, and several all-hands events.

1. *Alcohol Aware Program:* This program is a command-level alcohol abuse prevention and deglamorization course designed for all hands. The goals of the program include:
   – Making participants aware of the effects of alcohol.
   – Pointing out the risks involved in using and abusing alcohol.
   – Providing the Navy's expectations, instructions, and core values.
   – Defining the responsible use of alcohol.

   Each participant is asked to anonymously evaluate his or her own pattern of drinking in an effort to determine whether it is appropriate and, where necessary, make adjustments.

2. *Alcohol Impact Program:* Alcohol Impact is the first intervention step in the treatment of alcohol abuse. It is an intensive, interactive educational experience designed for personnel who have had incidents with alcohol. The course is primarily an educational tool; however, objectives within the course could reveal the need for a higher level of treatment. This intervention program is normally given during off-duty hours.

3. Navy has launched several marketing campaign strategies that have been tested through focus groups, and has built a comprehensive communications campaign to reduce the prevalence of substance use among Navy personnel.

   – "Keep What You've Earned": Substance abuse prevention campaign developed using the National Cancer Institute's (NCI) Health Communications Model using media scans, surveys, interview, and focus groups that encourages thoughtful consideration of consequences and provides practical tools
   – "The Domino Strategy - How to Drink Responsibly": Social marketing that teaches sailors to pay attention to size, content, and amount of alcohol they consume
   – "Who Will Stand Your Watch?": Campaign that addresses the negative impact sailors' personal behavior has on their shipmates, families, and career

4. *Shot of Reality:* This 90-minute improvised show focuses on alcohol awareness and pitfalls of alcohol and drug abuse. The program is designed to help sailors make better decisions and take care of shipmates.

5. *Myth vs. Truth:* This program provides information about the range of social and professional problems and economic costs associated with underage drinking. The program

is also used to increase awareness that underage drinking is related to a host of serious problems, with the aim of informing policymakers about the importance of preventing underage drinking.

6. *Comedy is The Cure:* This 30-minute standup comedy show highlights the dangers and risks of alcohol and drug abuse and sexual assault and harassment. The program is designed to inspire military and civilian personnel to make smart, safe decisions and better prepare each unit for mission success.

Army Center for Substance Abuse Programs (ACSAP): The ACSAP Prevention and Training (P&T) Branch develops, establishes, administers, and evaluates all ACSAP substance abuse prevention, education certification, and training programs worldwide within the Active Component, National Guard, and Army Reserve. The goal of ACSAP is to provide commanders, Unit Prevention Leaders (UPLs), and Department of Army civilians, contractors, and family members with the education and training necessary to make informed decisions about alcohol and other drugs. The program also provides commanders with the necessary resources and tools to complete their annually required 4 hours of alcohol and other drug awareness training (requirement IAW AR 600-85) and provides them with prevention tools to deter substance abuse. ACSAP provides technical support for programs, acts as the lead agent for drug demand reduction issues, supports professional development, provides training for all nonmedical substance abuse prevention staff worldwide, and develops and distributes alcohol and drug abuse prevention training curricula, multimedia products, and other drug and alcohol resources to Army installations.

Air Force Innovative Prevention Program: The U.S. Air Force (USAF) 0-0-1-3 Program, which began at F.E. Warren Air Force Base (AFB), encourages healthy, controlled alcohol use (and nonuse for underage persons) as the normative lifestyle choice for young USAF personnel. The program establishes safe normative behaviors that move the DoD forward in addressing the health threats of both alcohol and tobacco. The 0-0-1-3 program was briefed to USAF senior leadership in 2005. As a result of this briefing, the USAF Assistant Vice Chief of Staff (CVA) instructed A1 (personnel) and the USAF Surgeon General (SG) to expand the 0-0-1-3 program to include a range of health-related behaviors that could negatively affect productivity, mission accomplishment, and readiness, and implement the program across the USAF. Consequently, working groups were formed and a Concept of Operations (CONOPS) was written to provide the theoretical underpinnings for a new program called the Culture of Responsible Choices (CoRC), which was designed to address a range of health-related behaviors such as underage drinking, alcohol misuse, illegal drug use, tobacco cessation, obesity, fitness levels, safety mishaps. It was also designed to produce a cultural shift within the USAF from "work hard/play hard" to "work hard/play smart." CoRC uses a comprehensive community-based approach with four levels:

- Strong leadership support (i.e., from top down and bottom up)
- Individual-level interventions (population screening, anonymous screening at primary care centers, education, short-term counseling with tailored feedback, etc.)
- Base-level interventions (media campaigns, alcohol-free activities, zero-tolerance policies for underage drinking and alcohol misuse, midnight basketball, cyber cafés, etc.)
- Community-level interventions (building coalitions between on-base and off-base groups, increased driving under the influence/driving while intoxicated [DUI/DWI] enforcement on and off base, etc.)

A variety of toolkits were generated, and implementation memoranda were signed by the CVA and A1. In 2006, CoRC materials including the CoRC CONOPS, toolkits, memoranda, best practices, and other elements were made available via the web (currently at vc.afms.mil/corc) and CoRC was launched across the USAF. Since the program's inception, the USAF has had a 6 percent reduction in alcohol-related misconduct incidents.

In addition to CoRC, the USAF partnered with DoJ and NIAAA to implement the EUDL program at five AFBs. EUDL uses evidence-based environmental strategies to reduce underage airmen's access to alcohol and decrease the prevalence of underage airmen drinking on base and in the surrounding local areas. In 2009, the EUDL program was expanded to two more AFBs and in 2013 two more will be added. NIAAA is supervising a 3-year evaluation of the EUDL program, which is described later in this report. Analysis of first-year EUDL data is promising. DoJ will support the evaluation's expansion to the additional AFBs.

Coast Guard (DHS) Substance Abuse Program: The United States Coast Guard (USCG) Substance Abuse Program provides USCG members substance abuse prevention plans, policy, and resources to support command in providing opportunities to prevent, screen, and diagnose problems that may inhibit unit performance, readiness, and worldwide deployment. Prevention training and education about the risks of alcohol and drug misuse, rules and regulations about drinking, and alternatives to drinking are provided. The program also describes the negative impact of alcohol abuse and offers preventive strategies to help counter negative peer influences.

Underage USCG members are mostly found in three major subgroups: USCG Academy, TRACEN Center Cape May (boot camp), and "A" Schools.

1. *USCG Academy:* The My Student Body curriculum used at the USCG Academy is a complete alcohol, drugs, and student wellness program for colleges and universities. It is used by leading public and private universities across the nation to manage institutional risks and positively impact student retention rates.
2. *TRACEN Center Cape May (boot camp) and "A" Schools:* Located in Petaluma, CA, and Yorktown, VA, all have substance abuse prevention specialists (SAPS) who hold frequent prevention trainings targeted to address underage drinking and emphasize the high-risk nature of their age group.

CG medical officers are now mandated to receive specialized training on how to conduct substance abuse screening. With its focus on "age of onset," "amount of times drunk in the past year," and other diagnostic criteria, the CG Medical Officer is uniquely qualified to detect "at-risk" drinking patterns in its members.

Department of Education

Activities Specific to Underage Drinking

Higher Education Center for Alcohol, Drug Abuse, and Violence Prevention (HEC): The HEC provided technical assistance and other resources to assist administrators and other prevention professionals at colleges and universities to prevent violence and substance abuse on their campuses and in surrounding communities through a variety of programs and services that support comprehensive prevention strategies. FY 11 was the last year of funding for the HEC, with technical assistance activities carried out in FY 12. The HEC publications and technical assistant activities were folded into a new and consolidated K-16 Safe and Supportive Learning TA center (http://safesupportiveschools.ed.gov).

Activities Related to Underage Drinking

Office of Safe and Healthy Students National Conference: In summer 2012, the Department of Education sponsored a national conference and listening session focused on special issues in the school climate at the K–12 level. There were five conference tracks, one of which focused on behavioral health issues in schools.

Federal Trade Commission

Activities Specific to Underage Drinking

Consumer Education: The FTC has continued its "We Don't Serve Teens" (WDST) program, promoting compliance with the legal drinking age of 21. Targeted to parents and other responsible adults, http://www.DontServeTeens.gov provides information about the rates and risks of teen drinking, relevant state laws, and things to say and do to reduce easy teen access to alcohol. In 2011, the FTC distributed thousands of two-sided adhesive WDST decals to state alcohol regulators, prevention organizations, police departments, school districts, and alcohol wholesalers and retailers nationwide. Decal messages included: "The legal drinking age is 21. Thanks for not providing alcohol to teens." and "Please don't provide alcohol to teens. It's unsafe. It's illegal. It's irresponsible." Also in 2011, the FTC worked with private partners to conduct PSA campaigns (including radio, transit ads, and billboards) promoting the WDST message in 11 cities.

Activities Related to Underage Drinking

Alcohol Advertising Program: In 2011, the FTC announced the initiation of a new study of alcohol marketing, publishing two *Federal Register* notices describing and soliciting comment on its proposed information collection orders to alcohol companies. The Office of Management and Budget approved the FTC's issuance of the orders in late 2011. In early 2012, the FTC issued orders requiring 14 alcohol companies to submit data and other information (including 2011 sales and marketing expenditure data, and legal age and underage audience composition data, for each ad placed in the first half of 2011, and information about digital marketing efforts). The FTC estimates that the study will be completed in late spring 2013.

Administration for Children and Families/HHS

Activities Specific to Underage Drinking

None

Activities Related to Underage Drinking

Runaway and Homeless Youth Program: The Family and Youth Services Bureau (FYSB) provides funding to local communities to support young people, particularly runaway and homeless youth and their families. Basic Center Program (BCP) grants offer assistance to at-risk youth (under age 18) in need of immediate temporary shelter. Shelters provide family and youth counseling and referrals to services such as substance abuse treatment. Through the Street Outreach Program (SOP), FYSB awards grants to public and private, nonprofit agencies to conduct outreach that builds relationships between grantee staff and street youth up to age 21 to help them leave the streets. The Transitional Living Program (TLP) supports projects that use trauma-informed services and the positive youth development (PYD) approach to provide longer term residential services to homeless youth ages 16 to 21 for up to 18 months. These services help successfully transition young people to independent living. TLPs enhance youths' abilities to make positive life choices through education, awareness programs, and support. They include services such as substance abuse education, life skills training, and counseling. Grantee sites are alcohol free, and it is expected that participation in these programs will prepare youth to make better choices regarding alcohol and drug use and other unhealthy behaviors.

Family Violence Prevention and Services: FYSB provides grants to state agencies, territories, state Domestic Violence Coalitions, and Indian Tribes for provision of immediate shelter and supportive services to victims of family violence, domestic violence, and dating violence, and their dependents. These grants fund more than 1,600 domestic violence shelters and 1,100 nonresidential service sites, which provide services such as crisis and mental health counseling, legal advocacy, emergency transportation, children's services, and other social services such as substance abuse counseling. In FY 2011, funded programs served more than 1.3 million victims and their children and responded to 2.8 million crisis calls. More than 14,000 youths under age 18 who were identified as victims of intimate partner violence were provided services. Programs provided over 94,000 educational presentations, reaching 2.3 million youths.

Abstinence Education Programs: FYSB provides support for abstinence education programs through the Competitive Abstinence Education Grant Program (CAEGP) and the Section 510 (Title V) State Abstinence Education Program. Programs focus on educating young people and creating an environment within communities that supports teen decisions to postpone sexual activity until marriage. Programs are encouraged to use evidence-based, medically accurate interventions to promote abstinence from risky behaviors that lead to poor health outcomes including substance abuse and underage drinking, unplanned pregnancy, and sexually transmitted diseases.

Personal Responsibility Education Programs (PREP): FYSB supports healthy decisionmaking through the PREP. As part of the Patient Protection and Affordable Care Act, Congress passed and the President signed the PREP into law. PREP funds are to be used to educate adolescents on both abstinence and contraception to prevent pregnancy and sexually transmitted infections and at least three of six congressionally mandated "adulthood preparation subjects" (APS). Several APS topics—adolescent development, healthy life skills, and healthy relationships— encompass substance abuse prevention messaging consistent with the *Surgeon General's Call to Action* (2007) and positive youth development (PYD).

Centers for Disease Control and Prevention/HHS

Activities Specific to Underage Drinking

Monitoring Youth Exposure to Alcohol Marketing: The CDC's Alcohol Program within the National Center for Chronic Disease Prevention and Health Promotion (NCCDPHP) funds the Center on Alcohol Marketing and Youth (CAMY) at the Johns Hopkins Bloomberg School of

Public Health to conduct ongoing, independent, company- and brand-specific monitoring of youth exposure to alcohol marketing; develop web-based tools to illustrate and compare youth and adult exposure to alcohol marketing; prepare translational resources on effective prevention strategies to reduce underage drinking; and train students, faculty, and public health professionals in methods for independent monitoring of youth exposure to alcohol marketing and in effective strategies to reduce this exposure. CAMY has extensive experience monitoring youth exposure to alcohol marketing, having previously received funds to do so on a pilot basis from the Robert Wood Johnson Foundation (RWJF) and the Pew Charitable Trust. For more information on CAMY, see http://www.camy.org.

Activities Related to Underage Drinking

Alcohol-Related Disease Impact (ARDI): ARDI is an online application that provides national and state estimates of average annual deaths and years of potential life lost (YPLL) due to excessive alcohol use. The application allows users to create custom data sets and generate local reports on these measures as well. Users can obtain estimates of deaths and YPLL attributed to excessive alcohol use among persons under age 21.

Behavioral Risk Factor Surveillance System (BRFSS): BRFSS is an annual random-digit-dial telephone survey of U.S. adults ages 18 years and older in all 50 states, the District of Columbia, Guam, Puerto Rico, the U.S. Virgin Islands, American Samoa, Palau, and the Federated States of Micronesia. It includes questions on current drinking, number of drinking days, average number of drinks per day, frequency of binge drinking (≥ 4 drinks per occasion for women; ≥ 5 per occasion for men), and the largest number of drinks consumed on a drinking occasion. The CDC's Alcohol Program has also developed an optional, seven-question binge-drinking module that can be used by states to obtain more detailed information on binge drinkers, including beverage-specific alcohol consumption and driving after binge drinking. CDC has also worked with national and international experts to develop an optional module to assess the delivery of screening and brief intervention for excessive alcohol use in clinical settings for the 2014 BRFSS. In 2011, BRFSS introduced changes to address the growing effects of cellphone-only households, resulting in higher estimates in many states for certain chronic disease indicators and risk behaviors, including binge drinking. For more information on BRFSS, see http://www.cdc.gov/brfss.

Youth Risk Behavior Surveillance System (YRBSS): The YRBSS monitors priority health-risk behaviors among youth and young adults. It includes a biennial, national school-based survey of 9th- through 12-grade students that is conducted by CDC, and state and local surveys of 9th- through 12th-grade students conducted by education and health agencies. These surveys include questions about the frequency of alcohol use, frequency of binge drinking, age of first drink of alcohol, and usual source of alcohol. States and cities that conduct their own survey have the option to include additional alcohol questions, such as type of beverage usually consumed and usual location of alcohol consumption. The YRBSS also assesses other health-risk behaviors, including sexual activity and interpersonal violence, that can be examined in relation to alcohol consumption. Additional information on the YRBSS is available at http://www.cdc.gov/yrbs.

School Health Policies and Practices Study (SHPPS): SHPPS is a national survey periodically conducted to assess school health policies and practices at the state, district, school, and classroom levels. It includes information about school health education on alcohol and drug use prevention, school health and mental health services related to alcohol and drug use prevention and treatment, and school policies prohibiting alcohol use. Additional information on SHPPS is available at http://www.cdc.gov/SHPPS.

Pregnancy Risk Assessment Monitoring System (PRAMS): PRAMS is a population-based mail and telephone survey of women who have delivered a live-born infant. It collects state-specific data on maternal attitudes and experiences before, during, and shortly after pregnancy. It also includes questions on alcohol consumption, including binge drinking during the preconception period and during pregnancy, along with other factors related to maternal and child health. For more information on PRAMS, see http://www.cdc.gov/prams.

National Violent Death Reporting System (NVDRS): NVDRS is a state-based active surveillance system that collects risk-factor data on all violence-related deaths, including homicides, suicides, and legal intervention deaths (i.e., deaths caused by police and other persons with legal authority to use deadly force, excluding legal executions), as well as unintentional firearm deaths and deaths of undetermined intent. For more information on NVDRS, see http://www.cdc.gov/ViolencePrevention/NVDRS.

Guide to Community Preventive Services: CDC's Community Guide Branch works with CDC programs and other partners to systematically review the scientific evidence on the effectiveness of population-based strategies for (1) preventing alcohol-impaired driving and (2) excessive alcohol use and related harms (see "Guide to Community Preventive Services" earlier in this chapter). In 2012, the Community Guide Branch, in collaboration with the National Center for Injury Prevention and Control (NCIPC), updated the 2001 sobriety checkpoints systematic review and, in collaboration with the CDC Alcohol Program, conducted a review of electronic delivery of screening and brief intervention for excessive alcohol use. The results of these reviews are summarized on the Community Guide website (http://www.thecommunityguide.org) and were published in the *American Journal of Preventive Medicine.*

Preventing Alcohol-Exposed Pregnancies: CDC's National Center on Birth Defects and Developmental Disabilities (NCBDDD) has a number of activities supporting the prevention of fetal alcohol spectrum disorders (FASD) among women of childbearing age (18–44 years). CDC continues to monitor alcohol consumption (any use and binge drinking) among women of childbearing age (18–44 years) in the United States using the Behavioral Risk Factor Surveillance System (BRFSS). These data are important to help reduce alcohol-exposed pregnancies by identifying groups of women at increased risk and designing prevention programs aimed at reducing risk behaviors and improving pregnancy outcomes. NCBDDD, in collaboration with NCHS, has added four additional alcohol questions to survey years 2011–2013 of the National Survey of Family Growth (NSFG). The NSFG data will provide useful information on alcohol consumption among women of reproductive age and their risk for alcohol-exposed pregnancy.

Five FASD Regional Training Centers provide training to medical and allied health students, residents, and professionals in alcohol use assessment and interventions for women of childbearing age. CDC supported the development of a K–12 curriculum that describes the consequences of drinking during pregnancy. This curriculum continues to be available from the National Organization on Fetal Alcohol Syndrome (NOFAS). The FAS Prevention Team has developed an evidence-based intervention (CHOICES) for nonpregnant women to reduce their risk for an alcohol-exposed pregnancy by reducing risky drinking, using effective contraception, or both. They are currently disseminating and evaluating integration of this intervention into selected sexually transmitted disease clinics, family planning clinics, and community health centers, and in American Indian communities.

In 2011, CDC published *CHOICES: A Program for Women about Choosing Healthy Behaviors*, a curriculum designed for use by professionals who will be conducting the CHOICES program and for trainers providing instruction on how to conduct the intervention, which is now available for order at http://www.cdc.gov/ncbddd/fasd/freematerials.html. SAMHSA uses the Project CHOICES model at alcohol and drug treatment centers in various states, and CHOICES has been accepted for review and possible inclusion in SAMHSA's National Registry of Effective Programs and Policies (NREPP). For more information on these and other program activities, see http://www.cdc.gov/ncbddd/fasd/index.html.

Alcohol Screening and Brief Intervention (aSBI) in Primary Care: NCBDDD has developed and is evaluating a guide to help primary care practices adapt and implement aSBI as a routine element of patient care. In addition, three CDC-funded FASD Regional Training Centers will implement and evaluate aSBI in primary care systems. In 2012, NCBDDD held a meeting with employers, insurers, health plans, and nonprofit groups to learn how to increase demand for aSBI from groups that influence primary care practice systems. NCBDDD is also collaborating with the CDC Alcohol Program to develop an optional module for the 2014 BRFSS survey to measure the delivery of aSBI-related services.

Indian Health Service/HHS

The IHS Division of Behavioral Health (DBH) is responsible for Alcohol and Substance Abuse Programming (ASAP) through funding of federal, urban, and tribally administered programs. Funding for Tribal programs is administered pursuant to P.L. 93-638 (codified as amended at 25 U.S.C. §§ 450a-450n (1975)). Nearly 85 percent of the ASAP budget is administered under 638 contracts or compacts made directly with tribally administered programs, which aim to provide community-based, holistic, and culturally appropriate alcohol and substance abuse prevention and treatment services. The ASAP is unique in that it is a nationally coordinated and integrated behavioral health system that includes Tribal and federal collaboration to prevent or otherwise minimize the effects of alcoholism and drug dependencies in American Indian/Alaska Native communities. The aim of the ASAP is to achieve optimum relevance and efficacy in delivery of alcohol and drug dependency prevention, treatment, and rehabilitation services, while respecting and incorporating the social, cultural, and spiritual values of Native American communities.

Activities Specific to Underage Drinking

None

Activities Related to Underage Drinking

Alcohol abuse in Native American communities is a problem that can begin prenatally and continue throughout the lifespan. Programs are therefore focused on family-oriented prevention activities rooted in the culture of the individual Tribes and communities in which they operate. In recognition of this shifting dynamic of local control and ownership of ASAP in Native

American communities, the IHS DBH has shifted focus from direct-care services to a technical assistance and supportive role.

Youth Regional Treatment Centers: The IHS currently provides recurring funding to 11 Tribal and federally operated Youth Regional Treatment Centers (YRTCs) to address the ongoing issues of substance abuse and co-occurring disorders among Native American youth. Through education and culture-based prevention initiatives, evidence- and practice-based models of treatment, family strengthening, and recreational activities, youths can overcome their challenges and recover their lives to become healthy, strong, and resilient leaders in their communities.

The YRTCs provide a range of clinical services rooted in a culturally relevant holistic model of care. These services include clinical evaluation; substance abuse education; group, individual, and family psychotherapy; art therapy; adventure-based counseling; life skills; medication management or monitoring; evidence-based/practice-based treatment; aftercare relapse prevention; and posttreatment followup services.

Methamphetamine and Suicide Prevention Initiative (MSPI): The DBH supports MSPI, which expands and strengthens current Tribal and urban responses to the methamphetamine and suicide crises and establishes new methamphetamine and suicide prevention and treatment programs. The goals of the MSPI are to:

- Prevent, reduce, or delay the use and/or spread of methamphetamine abuse.
- Build on the foundation of prior methamphetamine and suicide prevention and treatment efforts, in order to support the IHS, Tribes, and urban Indian health organizations in developing and implementing Tribal and/or culturally appropriate methamphetamine and suicide prevention and early intervention strategies.
- Increase access to methamphetamine and suicide prevention services.
- Improve services for behavioral health issues associated with methamphetamine use and suicide prevention.
- Promote the development of new and promising services that are culturally and community relevant.
- Demonstrate efficacy and impact.

This 3-year initiative supports 127 individual programs and/or communities in their efforts to develop their own focused programs. The MSPI consists of 112 Tribal and IHS awardees (MSPI-T), 12 urban grantees (MSPI-U), and 3 youth services grantees (MSPI-Y).

Addressing Fetal Alcohol Spectrum Disorder: DBH supports two projects that target FASD through the Northwest Portland Area Indian Health Board. First, the FASD training project with the University of Washington School of Medicine is a research-based project that focuses on FASD interventions within 10 Tribal sites throughout the State of Washington. Second, the Northwest Tribal FASD Project provides education and training on FASD and community readiness and assists communities in Idaho, Oregon, and Washington State to set up an all-systems-based response to FASD.

The DBH also funds the Indian Children's Program (ICP). The ICP provides services to meet the needs of American Indian and Alaska Native children, 0 to 18 years old, with special needs residing or attending school in the southwest region of the United States. The program provides

FASD services including assessment, intervention planning, and consultation with families. In addition, IHS participates in the Interagency Coordinating Committee on Fetal Alcohol Spectrum Disorders (ICCFASD), an interagency task force led by NIAAA that addresses multidisciplinary issues relevant to FASD.

Also, in 2010, the IHS Office of Clinical and Preventive Services and CDC's NCBDDD entered into a 3-year interagency agreement to implement and evaluate CHOICES within primary care settings serving the Oglala Sioux Tribe. CHOICES is an evidence-based program for nonpregnant women to reduce their risk for alcohol-exposed pregnancy by reducing risky drinking, using effective contraception, or both. This intervention supports IHS's Government Performance and Results Act (GPRA) performance measure for screening women of childbearing age for alcohol use to prevent FASD. The alcohol screening GPRA results have exceeded the targeted measure of 25 percent since FY 2006. Increases in performance results are due to increased provider awareness and an agency emphasis on behavioral health screening.

National Institute on Alcohol Abuse and Alcoholism/HHS

Activities Specific to Underage Drinking

Underage Drinking Research Initiative: This NIAAA initiative analyzes evidence related to underage drinking using a developmental approach. Converging evidence from multiple fields shows that underage drinking is best addressed and understood within a developmental framework because it relates directly to processes that occur during adolescence. Such a framework allows more effective prevention and reduction of underage alcohol use and its associated problems. This paradigm shift, along with recent advances in epidemiology, developmental psychopathology, and the understanding of human brain development and behavioral genetics, provided the scientific foundation for the Surgeon General's *Call to Action to Prevent and Reduce Underage Drinking*, continues to inform the work of ICCPUD and the related efforts of its member federal agencies and departments, the work of the Behavioral Health Coordinating Committee, and provides the theoretical framework for NIAAA's underage-drinking programs.

Developing Screening Guidelines for Children and Adolescents: Data from NIAAA's National Epidemiologic Survey on Alcohol and Related Conditions (NESARC) (see Appendix A) indicate that people between ages 18 and 24 have the highest prevalence of alcohol dependence in the U.S. population—meaning that, for most, drinking started in adolescence. These data, coupled with those from other national surveys (SAMHSA's National Survey on Drug Use and Health [NSDUH] [see Appendix A], Monitoring the Future [MTF], and CDC's Youth Risk Behavior Surveillance System [YRBSS] [see Appendix A]) showing the popularity of binge drinking among adolescents, prompted NIAAA to produce a guide for screening children and adolescents for risk for alcohol use, alcohol consumption, and alcohol use disorders.

The screening guide for children and adolescents, *Alcohol Screening and Brief Intervention for Youth: A Practitioner's Guide*, which became available in fall 2011, was developed by NIAAA in collaboration with a working group of experts. As part of a multiyear process, the working group heard from a number of research scientists, analyzed data from both cross-sectional national surveys and proprietary longitudinal studies, and worked with pediatricians from general pediatrics as well as pediatric substance abuse specialty practices. The process culminated in the development of an easy-to-use, age-specific, two-question screener for current and future alcohol use. The *Guide* also provides background information on underage drinking, and detailed supporting material on brief intervention, referral to treatment, and patient confidentiality. The screening process will enable pediatric and adolescent health practitioners to provide information to patients and their parents about the effects of alcohol on the developing body and brain in addition to identifying those who need any level of intervention.

In November 2011, NIAAA issued a Funding Opportunity Announcement (FOA) titled "Evaluation of NIAAA's Alcohol Screening Guide for Children and Adolescents" to solicit applications to evaluate the new NIAAA alcohol screener for youth. Although the questions were empirically developed, are based on a vast amount of data from national surveys as well as numerous prospective studies, and have high sensitivity and specificity in the sample studied, it is important that the precision of the screener be evaluated in practice. Applications were sought that would evaluate the two-question screener in youth ages 9 to 18 (a) as a predictor of alcohol risk, alcohol use, and alcohol problems including alcohol use disorders and (b) as an initial screen for other behavioral health problems, for example other drug use, smoking, or conduct disorder. Five projects have been funded to evaluate the guide in a variety of settings including primary care, a network of pediatric emergency rooms, juvenile justice, and the school system, and with youth who have a chronic health condition.

Research Studies: NIAAA supports a broad range of underage drinking research, including studies on the epidemiology and etiology of underage drinking, neurobiology, prevention of underage drinking, and treatment of alcohol use disorders among youth. Studies also assess short- and long-term consequences of underage drinking.

Research on the Effects of Adolescent Alcohol Abuse and Alcoholism on the Developing Brain: The powerful developmental forces of adolescence cause significant changes to the brain and nervous system, including increased myelination of neural cells and "pruning" of infrequently used synapses and neural pathways in specific regions of the brain. A key question is the extent to which adolescent drinking affects the developing human brain. A range of studies including research on rodents, studies of youth who are alcohol dependent, and recent longitudinal work beginning with youth before they begin drinking suggest that alcohol use during adolescence, particularly heavy use, can have deleterious short- and long-term effects. In December 2011, NIAAA followed the completion of initial human pilot studies with an FOA titled "Longitudinal Studies on the Impact of Adolescent Drinking on the Adolescent Brain (Phase II)" soliciting applications to more fully address the following issues: (1) what are the long-term and shorter term effects of child and adolescent alcohol exposure on the developing human brain; (2) what is the effect of timing, dose, and duration of alcohol exposure on brain development; (3) to what extent do these effects resolve or persist over time; (4) how do key covariates factor into alcohol's effects on the brain; and (5) the potential identification of early neural, cognitive, and affective markers that may predict alcohol abuse and dependence and onset or worsening of mental illness during adolescence and/or adulthood. A consortium of seven projects was funded in FY 2012. At the same time, ongoing animal studies funded in response to NIAAA's 2010 FOA titled "Neurobiology of Adolescent Drinking in Adulthood" seek to clearly define the persistent effects of adolescent alcohol exposure and begin to explore the neurobiological mechanisms underlying these effects.

College Drinking Prevention Initiative: The work of this initiative, which began more than a decade ago, continues to support and stimulate studies of the epidemiology and natural history of college-student drinking and related problems. Its ultimate goal is to design and test interventions that prevent or reduce alcohol-related problems among college students. NIAAA continues to have a sizable portfolio of projects that target college-age youth. Importantly, NIAAA recently convened a new College Presidents' Working Group to (1) provide input to the Institute on future research directions; (2) advise the Institute about what new NIAAA college materials would be most helpful to college administrators, and in what format; and (3) recommend strategies for communicating with college administrators. In response to the College Presidents' Working Group's request that NIAAA develop a "matrix" to help them and their staff navigate the many available interventions when making decisions about what to implement on their respective campuses, NIAAA commissioned a team of experts to develop such a matrix.

Simultaneously NIAAA is developing a computerized searchable tool and accompanying materials based on the matrix. The matrix will provide information about individual- and environmental-level strategies that have been or might be used to address alcohol use among college students. For each strategy, information is provided about the amount and quality of available research, estimated effectiveness, estimated cost and barriers related to implementation, and time to implement, factors that may be relevant to campus and community leaders as they evaluate their current approaches, and as they consider and select additional strategies to address college-student drinking using a comprehensive approach. The ultimate goal for NIAAA is to provide science-based information in accessible and practical ways in order to facilitate its use as a foundation for college drinking prevention and intervention activities.

Building Health Care System Responses to Underage Drinking: The overarching goal of this program is to stimulate primary care health-delivery systems in rural and small urban areas to address the critical public health issue of underage drinking. This is a two-phase initiative. In the first phase (now complete) systems were expected to evaluate and upgrade their capacity to become platforms for research assessing the extent of underage drinking in the areas they serve and to evaluate their ability to reduce it. In the second phase, they will prospectively study the development of youth alcohol use and alcohol-related problems in the areas they serve and implement and evaluate interventions that address underage drinking. Four Phase I awards were made at the end of FY 2006 and two 5-year Phase II awards were made at the end of FY 2007.

Brief Intervention Research: This research provides an evidence base for effective brief interventions targeting youth in emergency rooms following alcohol-related events. Health care providers capitalize on a "teachable moment" to deliver a brief intervention meant to reduce problem drinking and associated difficulties. This approach complements school-based primary prevention programs, which do not address cessation/reduction issues for adolescents who are already drinking, rarely address motivational issues related to use and abuse, and cannot target school dropouts.

Adolescent Treatment Research Program: NIAAA initiated an adolescent treatment research program in 1998. Since then, dozens of clinical projects have been funded, the majority of which are clinical trials. These include behavioral intervention trials, pharmacotherapy trials, and health services studies. The program's objective is to design and test innovative, developmentally tailored interventions that use evidence-based knowledge to improve alcohol treatment outcomes in adolescents. Results of many of these projects will yield a broad perspective on the potential efficacy of family-based, cognitive-behavioral, brief motivational, and guided self-change interventions in a range of settings.

Evaluation of EUDL: In 2006, OJJDP issued a solicitation for its EUDL Discretionary Program. Grants under this program sought to reduce the availability of alcoholic beverages to, and the consumption of alcoholic beverages by, persons under age 21 serving in the U.S. Air Force. The specific goals of the program are to decrease first-time alcohol-related incidents, incidence of unintentional injuries related to alcohol consumption, and alcohol-related traffic injuries or fatalities among underage USAF personnel. OJJDP awarded grants to four states in response to this solicitation: Arizona, California, Hawaii, and Montana. The AFBs that participated in this project, forming coalitions with their adjacent communities, are Davis-Monthan and Luke (AZ), Beale (CA), Hickam (HI), and Malmstrom (MT). NIAAA provided evaluation support for the project through a 48-month contract that included an evaluation of all activities developed at each AFB/community site.

Results published in the *Journal of Studies on Alcohol and Drugs* showed that the USAF-wide percentage of junior enlisted personnel reporting an AUDIT score of 8 or greater (indicating they are at elevated risk for problem drinking) fell from 20.4 percent in 2006 to 13.8 percent in 2008. On four of the five experimental bases, the percentage of junior enlisted airmen with AUDIT scores of 8 or higher fell significantly between baseline and 1 year after the intervention. It is important to note, however, that AUDIT scores across the USAF declined during the same period of time. Only two bases (Luke, AZ, and Malmstrom, MT) showed a significantly greater decline in the percentage of high AUDIT scores compared with their matched control bases.

Prevention for Multiethnic Urban Youth: As an outgrowth of Project Northland and Project Northland for Urban Youth, NIAAA continues to investigate how two programs with known efficacy in certain populations can be effectively implemented with multiethnic urban youth. The proposed project will examine trajectories, consequences, and multiple levels of influence on alcohol use among urban poor adolescents, explicitly comparing patterns of effects across ethnic and gender subgroups. This longitudinal study comparing patterns and trajectories of alcohol use and problems across these important subgroups will directly guide the development of further refined interventions of increased efficacy and effectiveness.

Multicomponent Community Interventions for Youth: NIAAA issued a request for applications titled "Multi-Component Youth/Young Adult Alcohol Prevention Trials," resulting in one award in 2011. The project will create, implement, and evaluate a community-level intervention to prevent underage drinking and negative consequences among American Indian and White youth in rural high-risk communities in northeastern Oklahoma. The study utilizes community environmental change and brief intervention and referral approaches that will be evaluated alone and in combination.

Publications: NIAAA issued a screening guide for children and adolescents for use by health care practitioners titled, *Alcohol Screening and Brief Intervention for Youth: A Practitioner's Guide.* NIAAA also disseminates information about the prevention of underage drinking through a variety of publications, including two new fact sheets, one on underage drinking (pubs.niaaa.nih.gov/publications/UnderageDrinking/Underage_Fact.pdf) and one on college drinking (pubs.niaaa.nih.gov/publications/CollegeFactSheet/CollegeFactSheet.pdf), an updated and expanded version of its booklet *Make a Difference—Talk to Your Child About Alcohol* (English and Spanish); two issues of *Alcohol Research and Health, Alcohol and Development in Youth: A Multidisciplinary Overview* (2004/2005) and *A Developmental Perspective on Underage Alcohol Use* (2009); several *Alcohol Alerts* including *Underage Drinking: Why Do Adolescents Drink, What Are the Risks, and How Can Underage Drinking Be Prevented?* (2006) and *A Developmental Perspective on Underage Alcohol Use* (2009); *Parenting to Prevent Childhood Alcohol Use* (2010); a number of seasonal fact sheets focusing on underage drinking issues surrounding high school graduation, the first weeks of college, and spring break; the widely cited report from NIAAA's college drinking task force, *A Call to Action: Changing the Culture of Drinking at U.S. Colleges* (2002a), and a brief update on college drinking, titled *What Colleges Need to Know Now: An Update on College Drinking Research* (2007).

NIAAA also sponsored and edited a special 2008 supplement to the journal *Pediatrics* titled *Underage Drinking: Understanding and Reducing Risk in the Context of Human Development.* Additional publications include a special July 2009 supplement to the *Journal of Studies on Alcohol and Drugs* on NIAAA's rapid response initiative to reduce college drinking and *Update on the Magnitude of the Problem*; a 2009 article in the journal *Alcohol Research and Health* titled "A Developmental Perspective on Underage Alcohol Use"; and the lead article in the December 2010 issue of the *American Journal of Preventive Medicine*, "Alcohol risk management in college settings: The Safer California Universities Randomized Trial."

In addition, recent issues of NIAAA's webzine, the *NIAAA Spectrum*, have highlighted underage and college drinking:
http://www.spectrum.niaaa.nih.gov/archives/v4i1Feb2012/media/pdf/
NIAAA_Spectrum_Newsletter_F eb2012.pdf and
http://www.spectrum.niaaa.nih.gov/media/pdf/NIAAA_Spectrum_Newsletter_Sept2012.pdf.

NIAAA Website: The NIAAA website, http://www.niaaa.nih.gov, provides adults with information about the science and prevention of underage drinking and includes links to NIAAA's college website (http://www.collegedrinkingprevention.gov) and its youth-targeted website (http://www.thecoolspot.gov).

- *College Drinking Prevention Website:* NIAAA's website addressing alcohol use among college students (http://www.collegedrinkingprevention.gov) was recently redesigned and updated to permit easier navigation by topic or by audience. Updated features include new statistics, recent research papers, and presentations from task force participants along with a new section on choosing the right college.
  - *Coolspot Website for Kids:* Targeted to youth ages 11 to 13 years old, http://www.thecoolspot.gov provides information on underage drinking, including effective refusal skills. Recent upgrades include a wide range of new sound effects and voiceovers throughout the site, a dedicated teacher and volunteer corner for use in middle-school classrooms or afterschool programs, and innovative ways to teach young people about peer pressure and resistance skills through a guided reading activity and two lesson plans that accompany the site's interactive features.

Leadership to Keep Children Alcohol Free: NIAAA was one of the founders of this nationwide organization, launched in 2000 and spearheaded by spouses of current and former governors. It is the oldest and largest organization of governors' spouses focused on a single issue. Now a 501c3 nonprofit foundation, it was previously supported by seven public and private funding organizations. The organization's goals are to:

- Make prevention of alcohol use among minors a national health priority.
- Focus state and national policymakers and opinion leaders on the seriousness of early-onset alcohol use.
- Educate the public about the incidence and impact of alcohol use by children ages 9 to 15.
- Mobilize the public to address these issues in a sustained manner and work for change within their families, schools, and communities.

In the past, members of Leadership to Keep Children Alcohol Free (Leadership) produced television PSAs directed at parents and other adults in their respective states and at supported youth-centered events. With support from NIAAA and SAMHSA, Leadership worked closely with the Office of the Surgeon General to ensure that the Surgeon General's *Call to Action to Prevent and Reduce Underage Drinking* was broadly disseminated. For example, governors' spouses who were members of Leadership worked with the Acting Surgeon General to "roll out" the *Call to Action* in various states. Leadership continues to collaborate with SAMHSA, NIAAA, and OSG in its work as an independent foundation.

Activities Related to Underage Drinking

Alcohol Policy Information System (APIS): APIS is an electronic resource that provides authoritative, detailed information comparable across states on alcohol-related policies in the United States at both state and federal levels. Designed primarily for researchers, APIS encourages and facilitates research on the effects and effectiveness of alcohol-related policies. Although not dedicated to underage drinking policies, APIS does provide information on policies relevant to underage drinking (e.g., retail alcohol outlet policies for preventing alcohol sales and service to those under age 21).

Longitudinal and Genetic Epidemiology Studies and the National Epidemiologic Survey on Alcohol and Related Conditions: A number of longitudinal studies following subjects first identified as adolescents (along with genetic epidemiology studies) are particularly pertinent to underage drinking, as is NESARC, which includes people ages 18 to 21. Such studies could potentially enhance understanding of the etiology, extent, and consequences of underage alcohol consumption. Analysis of NESARC data indicates that 18- to 24-year-olds have the highest prevalence of alcohol dependence of any age group in the general population, underscoring the need for enhanced early prevention efforts. In 2012, NIAAA launched the new nationally representative National Health and Alcohol Survey, which captures information on alcohol dependence and other related mental health conditions from over 46,000 individuals. DNA samples will also be collected. The NHAS will provide important prevalence data about alcohol use disorders, related disorders and problems, and overall health that can be used to inform advances in the prevention and treatment of alcohol use disorders, which affect millions of Americans of all ages every year.

National Institute on Drug Abuse/HHS

Activities Specific to Underage Drinking

None

Activities Related to Underage Drinking

Girl-Specific Intervention (GSI): Delivered via CD-ROM, GSI is a family-based intervention that targets mothers and their preadolescent and adolescent daughters to prevent substance use. GSI consists of 10 sessions targeting affective quality, coping, refusal skills, mood management, conflict resolution, problem solving, self-efficacy, body esteem, normative beliefs, social supports, and mother–daughter communication. In addition, the intervention targets family rituals, mothers' use of rules against substance use, child management, mother–daughter affective quality, and mothers' communication with their daughters. A previous test of the intervention with 202 pairs of predominantly White adolescent girls and mothers showed improvements in communication skills and conflict management. Compared with girls in the control condition, daughters who received the intervention reported improved alcohol use refusal skills, healthier normative beliefs about underage drinking, greater self-efficacy in avoiding underage drinking, less alcohol consumption (in the past 7 days, 30 days, and year), and lower intentions to drink as adults.

A recently completed randomized controlled trial tested the intervention with 11- to 13-year-old primarily Black and Hispanic girls and their mothers (*N*=546), delivered primarily within housing authority centers in New York (Schinke, Fang, Cole, & Cohen-Cutler, 2011). Girls in the intervention condition reported significant improvements in the quality of their communications with their mothers, perceptions of family rules against their substance use, perceptions of parental monitoring, and normative beliefs about substance use, compared with girls in the control condition. Rates of 30-day alcohol consumption were lower for girls in the intervention condition compared with girls in the control condition. The intervention also had a significant impact on girls' reports of depression, self-efficacy to avoid drugs, and intentions to drink, smoke, and use drugs in adulthood. Outcomes for mothers also favored GSI, with mothers in the intervention condition reporting significantly more rules against the use of drugs, and higher levels of parental monitoring at posttest, than mothers in the control condition.

Strong African-American Families (SAAF) Program: SAAF is a family-centered risk behavior prevention program that enhances protective caregiving practices and youth self-regulatory competence. SAAF consists of separate parent and youth skill-building curricula and a family curriculum. Evaluations have confirmed SAAF's efficacy for 11-year-olds in preventing, across several years, the initiation of risk behaviors, including alcohol use; enhancing protective parenting practices; and increasing youth self-regulatory capabilities. The program was effective when primary caregivers had clinical-level depressive symptoms and when families reported economic hardship; it can also ameliorate genetic risk for involvement in health-compromising risk behaviors across preadolescence. A recently completed randomized controlled trial of SAAF targeted African American adolescents in high school (*N*=505). This study found that 22 months after baseline the intervention had a significant impact on substance use and substance use problems (including alcohol), conduct problems, and depression symptoms for youth in the intervention condition compared with youth in the control condition (Brody et al., 2012).

After Deployment: Adaptive Parenting Tools (ADAPT): Adapted from an evidence-based Parent Management Training-Oregon (PMTO) model intervention, Parenting through Change, the ADAPT program is designed for military families with a parent reintegrating from the conflicts in Afghanistan and Iraq (OEF/OIF). ADAPT is a modified version of PMTO that is enhanced with web-based supports, and is specific to military families and culture. ADAPT utilizes small-group parenting sessions that provide support and skills for positive parent–child interactions, emotion regulation, and effective parenting practices. Previous research on PMTO interventions for families from universal and high-risk populations (e.g., divorcing families, low-income families, and youth with early-onset conduct problems) have demonstrated that the program is effective in reducing coercive parenting and increasing positive parenting. Longitudinal followup studies have shown positive effects of PMTO on a broad array of outcomes, including child and parent adjustment, youth substance use and related behavior problems, as well as other areas of family functioning. Currently, a study of the ADAPT model is being conducted with 400 reintegrating Army National Guard families with 6- to 12-year-old children to test the effectiveness of the intervention for improving parenting and reducing child risk for substance use and related behavior problems, and satisfaction with the program. A recent article describes the need for programs such as ADAPT, the PMTO evidence base supporting the program, and recommendations for providers, for supporting parenting among military families as a way to reduce youth risk factors and promote well-being (Gewirtz, Erbes, Polusny, Forgatch, & Degarmo, 2011).

Coping Power: Coping Power is a multicomponent child and parent preventive intervention directed at preadolescent children at high risk for aggressiveness and later substance abuse and delinquency. The child component is derived from an anger coping program primarily tested with highly aggressive boys and shown to reduce substance use. The Coping Power Child Component is a 16-month program for children in the 5th and 6th grades. Group sessions usually occur before or after school or during nonacademic periods. Training focuses on teaching children how to identify and cope with anxiety and anger; control impulsiveness; and develop social, academic, and problem-solving skills at school and home. Parents are also trained throughout the program. Efficacy and effectiveness studies show Coping Power to have preventive effects on youths' aggression, delinquency, and substance use (including alcohol use). In a study of the intensity of training provided to practitioners, greater reductions in children's externalizing behaviors and improvements in children's social behaviors and academic skills occurred for those whose counselors received more intensive Coping Power training than for those in the basic Coping Power training or control conditions. A currently funded study of Coping Power is comparing the child component delivered in the usual small-group format with a newly developed individual format to determine whether the latter will produce greater reductions in substance use, children's externalizing behavior problems, and delinquency at a 1-year followup assessment.

EcoFIT (previously, Adolescent Transitions Program): This tiered intervention, targeted to children, adolescents, and their parents, recognizes the multiple environments of youth (e.g, family, caregivers, peers, school, and neighborhood). EcoFIT in schools uses a tiered approach to provide prevention services to students in middle and junior high school and their parents. The universal intervention level, directed to parents of all students in a school, establishes a Family Resource Room to engage parents, establish parenting practice norms, and disseminate information about risks for problem behavior and substance use. The selective intervention level uses the Family Check-Up, which offers family assessment and professional support to identify families at risk for problem behavior and development of youth substance use and mental health problems. The indicated level, the Parent Focused curriculum, provides direct professional support to parents to make the changes indicated by the Family Check-Up. Services may include behavioral family therapy, parenting groups, or case management services. Findings showed that the EcoFIT model reduced substance use in high-risk students 11 to 14 years old (grades 6–9), with an average of 6 hours of contact time with the parents. Adolescents whose parents engaged in the Family Check-Up had less growth in alcohol, tobacco, and marijuana use and problem behavior from ages 11 through 17, along with decreased risk for substance use disorder diagnoses and arrests by age 18. The National Institute on Child Health and Human Development funded a study in 2012, with co-funding from NIDA, which will examine the role of parent–youth relationships in late adolescence on substance use and abuse during the transition to adulthood. This study will also evaluate the preliminary efficacy of a late adolescence version of the Family Check-up for preventing escalation of substance use during this developmental period, and promoting positive behavioral health outcomes in early adulthood.

Strengthening Families Program for Parents and Youth 10–14 (SFP 10–14): SFP is a seven-session skill-building program for parents, youth, and families to strengthen parenting and family functioning and to reduce risk for substance abuse and related problem behaviors among youth. Program implementation and evaluation have been conducted through partnerships that include state university researchers, cooperative extension system staff, local schools, and community implementers. Longitudinal comparisons with control group families showed positive effects on parents' child management practices (e.g., setting standards, monitoring children, and applying consistent discipline) and on parent–child affective quality. In addition, an evaluation of this program found delayed initiation of substance use at the 6-year followup. Other findings showed improved youth resistance to peer pressure to use alcohol, reduced affiliation with antisocial peers, and reduced levels of problem behaviors. Importantly, conservative benefit–cost calculations indicate returns of $9.60 per dollar invested in SFP 10–14. A longitudinal study of SFP 10-14 and Life Skills Training (LST) together and LST alone found that 5.5 years after baseline (end of grade 12) both interventions together and LST alone reduced growth in substance initiation. Both interventions also prevented more serious substance use outcomes among youth at high risk (use of at least two substances) at baseline. A currently funded study is supporting a long-term followup of a randomized trial of the multicomponent SFP 10–14 plus LST compared with LST alone, or a minimal contact control condition, following youth during late adolescence emerging adulthood to understand the long-term public health impact of universal prevention.

Good Behavior Game (GBG): GBG is a universal preventive intervention that provides teachers with a method of classroom behavior management. It was tested in randomized prevention trials in 1st- and 2nd-grade classrooms in 19 Baltimore City public schools beginning in the 1985–1986 school year and was replicated in the 1986–1987 school year with a second cohort. The intervention was aimed at socializing children to the student role and reducing early antecedents of substance abuse and dependence, smoking, and antisocial personality disorder—specifically, early aggressive or disruptive behavior problems. Analyses of long-term effects in the first-generation sample (1985–1986) at ages 19 to 21 show that, for males displaying more aggressive and disruptive behaviors in 1st grade, GBG significantly reduced drug and alcohol abuse and dependence disorders, regular smoking, and antisocial personality disorder. Currently, NIDA is supporting a long-term second-generation (1986–1987) followup through age 25, including DNA collection for gene x environment analyses. NIDA supported a trial of GBG delivery in a whole-school-day context that emphasizes reading achievement, along with pilot research on models for implementing GBG in entire school districts. In addition, NIDA supported a pilot study for formative research on the large-scale implementation of GBG within a school district that could inform a system-level randomized trial on scaling up GBG. The pilot research focused on developing district partnerships, determining community-level factors that influence program implementation, and ensuring the acceptance, applicability, and relevance of measures and intervention design requirements for a large-scale trial. The conceptual framework guiding the development of the partnership and lessons learned are described in an article (Poduska, Gomez, Capo, & Holmes, 2012) that also addresses the implications for implementing evidence-based universal prevention programs such as GBG through research and practice partnerships.

Life Skills Training (LST): LST addresses a wide range of risk and protective factors by teaching general personal and social skills, along with drug resistance skills and normative education. This universal program consists of a 3-year prevention curriculum for students in middle or junior high school, with 15 sessions during the first year, 10 booster sessions during the second year, and 5 sessions during the third year. The program can be taught in grades 6, 7, and 8 (for middle school) or grades 7, 8, and 9 (for junior high schools). LST covers three major content areas: drug resistance skills and information, self-management skills, and general social skills. The program has been extensively tested and found to reduce the prevalence of tobacco, alcohol, and illicit drug use relative to controls by 50 to 87 percent. NIDA currently funds a study examining the dissemination, adoption, implementation, and sustainability of LST.

Media Detective: Media Detective is a media literacy education program for elementary schools to increase children's critical thinking skills about substance use media messages and reduce their intent to use tobacco and alcohol products. The program is a 10-lesson curriculum that was developed through NIDA's Small Business Innovation Research (SBIR) program. A short-term, randomized controlled trial was conducted to evaluate the effectiveness of Media Detective, through a comparison of outcomes among students (ages 7–13) in schools randomly assigned to receive the intervention and schools assigned to a wait-list control condition. Findings from this trial revealed that students in the Media Detective group who reported using alcohol or tobacco in the past reported significantly less intention to use and more self-efficacy to refuse substances than students in the control condition who reported prior use of alcohol or tobacco (Kupersmidt, Scull, & Austin, 2010). Also, boys in the Media Detective group reported significantly less interest in alcohol-branded merchandise than boys in the control group. This was an evaluation of the short-term effects (pretest/posttest) of a relatively brief intervention designed to improve students' media literacy related to alcohol and tobacco use. These early results suggest that the program is having both universal and targeted influence on school children's intentions to use substances. Currently, a similar methodology is being used to develop a media literacy prevention intervention for high school teachers and students. The intervention uses active learning methods and is designed to be implemented in public, private, and home school settings as well as community-based settings.

Project Towards No Drug Abuse (Project TND): This intervention targets youth in alternative or traditional high schools to prevent their transition from drug use to drug abuse. It considers the developmental issues faced by older teens, particularly those at risk for drug abuse. The core of Project TND is 12 in-class sessions that provide motivation and cognitive misperception correction and social and self-control skills, along with decisionmaking materials that target the use of cigarettes, alcohol, marijuana, and hard drugs as well as participation in violence-related behavior, such as carrying a weapon. The classroom program has been found effective at 1-year followup in three experimental field trials. Although promising classroom program effects have been obtained in previous trials, only main effects on hard drug use and cigarette smoking have been maintained past 1-year followup, but not a main effect for marijuana or alcohol use.

A recently completed randomized controlled trial on the dissemination and implementation of Project TND in traditional high schools, in which schools were randomly assigned to one of three conditions (comprehensive implementation support for teachers, regular workshop training only, or standard care control) found that comprehensive training approaches may improve implementation fidelity, but improvements in fidelity may not result in strong program outcomes of Project TND (Rohrbach, Gunning, Sun, & Sussman, 2010). Results indicated that, relative to the controls, both intervention conditions produced effects on hypothesized program mediators, such as greater gains in program-related knowledge, greater reductions in substance use intentions (cigarette, marijuana, and hard drugs), and more positive changes in drug-related beliefs. In addition, there were stronger effects on implementation fidelity in the comprehensive training condition, than in the regular training condition. However, despite these effects, 7 of the 10 immediate student outcome measures showed no significant differences between conditions. A current study of Project TND is examining the role of brief telephone booster sessions based on motivational interviewing and delivered over multiple years—from late adolescence into emerging adulthood—to sustain and possibly enhance long-term outcomes (Barnett et al., 2012).

Community-Level Studies: Community-level studies address questions related to the dissemination and implementation of evidence-based substance abuse prevention programs. Examples include the following.

- *Communities That Care (CTC):* An operating system for quality implementation of evidence-based preventive interventions targeted to specific risk and protective factors within the community, CTC provides a framework for assessing and monitoring community-level risk and protective factors, training, technical assistance, and planning and action tools for implementing science-based prevention interventions through community service settings and systems. The Community Youth Development Study (CYDS) is testing CTC in 7 states with 12 matched pairs of communities randomized to receive the CTC system or serve as controls. CYDS targets youth in grades 6 through 12. Participating communities selected and implemented evidence-based prevention interventions based on their community profile of risk and protective factors. A panel of 4,407 5th graders were recruited and followed annually to assess impact of the CTC system on substance use and related outcomes. Annual surveys of youth in grades 6, 8, 10, and 12 were also conducted. Initial results from the longitudinal panel demonstrated that mean levels of risk exposure were significantly lower for youth in the CTC condition than youth in the control condition (Hawkins et al., 2008). From grades 5 through 8, youth in the intervention condition had lower incidences of alcohol, cigarette, and smokeless tobacco initiation, and significantly lower delinquent behavior than those in the control condition.

In grade 8, the prevalence of alcohol and smokeless tobacco use in the last 30 days, binge drinking in the last 2 weeks, and delinquency behaviors in the past year were significantly lower for youth in CTC communities than for youth in control communities (Hawkins et al., 2009). At grade 10, the prevalence of current cigarette use and past-year delinquent and violent behavior were lower in CTC communities than in control communities (Hawkins et al., 2012). Also, the odds of initiating alcohol use by grade 10 were significantly lower (38 percent lower) in CTC communities than in the control communities. Arthur and colleagues (2010) examined the implementation of core intervention elements by coalitions in CYDS and found that, compared with control coalitions, CYDS coalitions implemented significantly more of the CTC core elements (e.g., using community-level data on risk and protective factors to guide selection of effective prevention programs) and also implemented significantly higher numbers of tested, effective prevention programs. In addition, CTC communities had greater sustainability of tested and effective programs and delivered the programs to more children and parents than control communities (Fagan, Arthur, Hanson, Briney & Hawkins, 2011). A recent economic analysis of CTC found a benefit–cost ratio of $5.30 per $1 invested (Kuklinski, Briney, Hawkins, & Catalano, 2012).

- *PROmoting School/Community-University Partnerships To Enhance Resilience (PROSPER):* An innovative partnership model for the diffusion of evidence-based preventive interventions that reduce youth substance use and other problem behaviors, the PROmoting School/ Community-University Partnerships to Enhance Resilience (PROSPER) partnership model links land-grant university researchers, the cooperative extension system, the public school system, and community stakeholders. A randomized trial of PROSPER was conducted in 28 school districts in rural and semiurban communities in Iowa and Pennsylvania, blocked on size, and randomly assigned to the PROSPER partnership model or to a usual programming control condition. Approximately 10,000 6th graders recruited across two cohorts were enrolled in the study along with approximately 1,200 students and their parents. In the PROSPER condition, communities received training and support to implement evidence-based prevention through the partnership and selected interventions from a menu of efficacious and effective universal prevention programs. Analyses 18 months after baseline revealed significant intervention effects compared with the control condition, particularly reduced new-user rates of marijuana, methamphetamine, ecstasy, and inhalant use; lower rates of initiation of gateway and illicit substance use; and lower rates of past-year marijuana and inhalant use and drunkenness (Spoth et al., 2007).

In a study of 10th-grade findings, 4.5 years past baseline, youth in the PROSPER condition reported significantly lower lifetime/new-user rates of marijuana, cigarettes, inhalants, methamphetamine, ecstasy, alcohol use, and drunkenness compared with the control condition (Spoth et al., 2011). Among youth at higher risk for substance use at baseline, those in the intervention condition showed significantly slower growth in substance use between 6th grade and 10th grade relative to controls. Sustainability of implementation quality was examined 6 years after initiating the PROSPER model (Spoth, Guyll, Redmond, Greenberg, & Feinberg, 2011). Adherence to the school-based and family-based intervention models was high, averaging near 90 percent across multiple implementation cohorts (five school-based cohorts; six family-based cohorts). A continuation study was funded in 2012 to understand effects of PROSPER in emerging adulthood, for participants who received evidence-based interventions in middle school. Reductions in substance abuse, antisocial behaviors, sexual risk behaviors, and improvements in healthy adult functioning will be examined.

- *Building Infrastructure and Capacity to Support Sustained, Quality Implementation of Evidence-Based Interventions:* NIDA supported a large-scale grant to address the lack of well-integrated infrastructure across public education systems to support quality delivery of evidence-based interventions. The project was based on the PROSPER model—a partnership model for implementation of evidence-based prevention interventions targeting alcohol, tobacco, and other drug use and abuse and related problems. Activities included in-depth capacity and resource assessments at state (Cooperative Extension Service; Departments of Education, Health, and Juvenile Justice) and community levels and capacity building, including awareness building, organizational and leadership networking, resource generation, and introductory training on the PROSPER model. Another feature included developing a web-based process and outcome evaluation system. A goal of this grant was to develop research-based approaches to build the nation's capacity to reduce youth substance use, including alcohol use and abuse, and create rapid advances in the prevention science field from research to practice.

- *Creating the Scientific Infrastructure for the Promise Neighborhood Initiative:* NIDA supported a large-scale infrastructure grant focused on the implementation of comprehensive preventive interventions in the nation's highest poverty neighborhoods. This project coordinated with the Promise Neighborhood initiative that is being led by the U.S. Department of Education. The grant supported the Promise Neighborhood Consortium (PNC), which provided an infrastructure through which the scientific community could assist America's high-poverty neighborhoods in translating existing knowledge into widespread improvements in well-being, including the prevention of substance abuse, antisocial behavior, risky sexual behavior, depression, and academic failure, and the promotion of diverse forms of prosocial behavior and academic achievement. The goals of the grant were to (1) establish the infrastructure for the PNC; (2) create a state-of-the-art website system to enable the research and neighborhood members of the PNC to communicate and collaborate; (3) specify measures of neighborhood well-being and the risk and protective factors that influence multiple problems; (4) define a menu of evidence-based policies, programs, and practices for use across a neighborhood or community to reduce the prevalence of substance abuse and related social, emotional, behavioral, and health problems; and (5) create at least eight intervention research teams to design intervention research in high-poverty neighborhoods. The prevention plan focused on the promotion of nurturing environments and emphasizes impact on children, youth, and families. One of the products from the consortium was a framework for the promotion of child health and development in high-poverty neighborhoods, including risk and protective factors that could be impacted by evidence-based interventions (Komro, Flay, Biglan, & PNC, 2011).

- *Community Monitoring Systems—Tracking and Improving the Well-Being of America's Children and Adolescents:* Community Monitoring Systems is a monograph that describes federal, state, and local monitoring systems that provide estimates of problem prevalence; risk and protective factors; and profiles regarding mobility, economic status, and public safety indicators. Data for these systems come from surveys of adolescents and archival records. Monitoring the well-being of children and adolescents is a critical component of efforts to prevent psychological, behavioral, and health problems and to promote successful adolescent development. Research during the past 40 years has helped identify aspects of child and adolescent functioning that are important to monitor. These aspects, which encompass family, peer, school, and neighborhood influences, have been associated with both positive and negative outcomes for youth. As systems for monitoring well-being become more available, communities will become better able to support prevention efforts and select prevention practices that meet community-specific needs.

Preventing Drug Use among Children and Adolescents: A Research-Based Guide for Parents, Educators, and Community Leaders, 2nd Edition: This booklet is based on a literature review of all NIDA prevention research from 1997 through 2002. Before publication, it was reviewed for accuracy of content and interpretation by a scientific advisory committee and reviewed for readability and applicability by a Community Anti-Drug Coalitions of America (CADCA) focus group. The publication presents the principles of prevention; information on identifying and using risk and protective factors in prevention planning; applying principles in family, school, and community settings; and summaries of effective prevention programs.

National Drug Facts Week (NDFW): NDFW is a health observance week for teens that aims to provide accurate information about alcohol, tobacco, and other drug abuse. During this week, NIDA also holds a Drug Facts Chat Day, where NIDA scientific staff and colleagues from NIMH and NIAAA respond to questions and concerns from students on substance abuse and mental health topics. A companion NIDA publication, titled *Drug Facts: Shatter the Myths* is also a resource for NDFW. This publication answers teens' most frequently asked questions about alcohol, tobacco, and other drug use. Information on NDFW can be found at: http://drugfactsweek.drugabuse.gov/index.php. The most recent NDFW was scheduled for January 28–February 3, 2013, and the Drug Facts Chat Day was scheduled for January 31, 2013.

Monitoring the Future (MTF): MTF is an ongoing study of substance abuse (including alcohol) behaviors and related attitudes of secondary school students, college students, and young adults. Students in grades 8, 10, and 12 participate in annual surveys (8th and 10th graders since 1991, and 12th graders since 1975). Within the past 5 years, 45,000 to 47,000 students have participated in the survey each year. Followup questionnaires are mailed to a subsample of each graduating class every 2 years until age 35 and then every 5 years thereafter. Information on current findings from MTF can be found on the NIDA website: http://www.drugabuse.gov/related-topics/trends-statistics/monitoring-future.

Substance Abuse and Mental Health Services Administration/HHS

Activities Specific to Underage Drinking

Development of an Underage Drinking Prevention National Media Campaign: SAMHSA's Center for Substance Abuse Prevention (CSAP) is creating a new, research-based national media campaign that will motivate parents of children ages 9 to 15 to take action to prevent underage drinking. CSAP conducted a literature review, convened an expert panel, held stakeholder interviews, and conducted a series of focus groups with parents and interviews with children in the target age range. CSAP engaged five pilot sites across the United States to test campaign materials before the national launch of the campaign in February 2013. Campaign messages have been developed and tested in the pilot sites for television, radio, and print.

Leadership to Keep Children Alcohol Free: Leadership to Keep Children Alcohol Free (Leadership) is a nationwide organization of current and former governors' spouses who focus on preventing alcohol use by youth ages 9 to 15 (also see NIAAA entry on this organization). SAMHSA works with Leadership to link the agency's Substance Abuse Prevention and Treatment Block Grant prevention programs, other SAMHSA-supported programs such as town hall meetings, and the agency's public service announcements with Leadership's initiatives. In addition, SAMHSA supported Leadership in its efforts to disseminate the Surgeon General's *Call to Action.* Leadership is also represented on the expert panel advising the SAMHSA underage drinking prevention national media campaign.

Underage Drinking Prevention Education Initiatives: This SAMHSA/CSAP effort provides resources, message development, public outreach and education, and partnership development for preventing underage alcohol use among youth up to age 21. The initiative provides ongoing support for the ICCPUD web portal and town hall meetings, Too Smart To Start, Building Blocks for a Healthy Future (Building Blocks), the state/Territory Video Initiative (all detailed below), and other national and community-based prevention initiatives conducted by SAMHSA and CSAP.

- *ICCPUD Web Portal:* SAMHSA, on behalf of ICCPUD, maintains a web portal (http://www.stopalcoholabuse.gov) dedicated to the issue of underage drinking and consolidates comprehensive research and resources developed by the 15 federal agencies of ICCPUD. The portal includes information on underage drinking statistics (i.e., prevalence, trends, and consequences), training events, evidence-based approaches, and other resources and materials that support prevention efforts. Direct links are provided to federally supported websites designed to prevent substance abuse, including alcohol. Information is intended to serve all stakeholders (e.g., community-based organizations involved in prevention, policymakers, parents, youth, and educators). The portal also includes a subsite for the town hall meeting initiative and its supporting resources. SAMHSA, with input from ICCPUD, is currently restructuring the website to better serve the needs of diverse users. As of December 2012, the web portal was averaging 623 visits per day and the average time onsite at 10 minutes, 48 seconds.

- *Town Hall Meetings:* To engage communities nationwide in evidence-based efforts to prevent and reduce underage alcohol use, ICCPUD—with SAMHSA as the lead agency— has supported town hall meetings in 2006, 2008, 2010, and 2012. These meetings, held in every state, the District of Columbia, and some of the territories during each round, are an effective approach for raising public awareness of underage drinking as a public health problem and mobilizing communities to take preventive action. For example, a summary report by the Governor's Prevention Advisory Council (GPAC) Underage Drinking Prevention Workgroup on town hall meetings held in California in 2010 found that 20 percent of these events resulted in plans to develop a social host ordinance or other alcohol-related legislation, 5 percent led to development of new prevention coalitions, and 17 percent recruited new members for existing coalitions. Iowa coordinates its town hall meetings statewide to gather community feedback that can be used to assess progress in reducing and preventing underage alcohol use and its consequences. In 2012, nearly 1,400 community-based organizations registered their intent to hold more than 1,500 events, despite decreasing budgets for many prevention organizations. During FY 2012, one report was released on the results of the meetings: *2010 Town Hall Meetings: Mobilizing Communities to Prevent and*

Reduce Underage Alcohol Use, an Evaluation Report. SAMHSA is developing a summary report on the 2012 town hall meetings.

- *Webcasts:* SAMHSA hosted two live national webcasts in support of the 2012 Town Hall Meeting initiative: Making the Grade on College Drinking Prevention (February 6, 2012) and Getting to Outcomes Through Town Hall Meetings (May 21, 2012). Both webcasts featured national experts and prevention specialists who were achieving notable progress in reducing underage drinking prevention in their communities. Both webcasts attracted a broad audience: 542 individuals attended the first webcast in person or online; 350 attended the second webcast online. These national webcasts are achieved and available for viewing at: http://www.stopalcoholabuse.gov/TownHallMeetings/resources/training.aspx. In addition, page views of the ICCPUD website at http://www.stopalcoholabuse.gov soared during the 2 months in which the webcasts were broadcast: 1,849,224 during February and 1,044,193 during May. The average number of page views for all other months from September 2011 to August 2012 was 288,158/month. These events were promoted through social media, stakeholder e-mail lists, and national and community partner organizations.

- *Too Smart To Start (TSTS):* TSTS is a national community education program targeting youth and teens as well as their parents, other caregivers, and educators. TSTS provides professionals, volunteers, and parents with tools and materials that help shape healthy behaviors and prevent alcohol use for a lifetime. TSTS includes an interactive website (http://www.toosmarttostart.samhsa.gov), technical assistance, and a community action kit. The program actively involves entire communities in sending clear, consistent messages about why children should reject underage drinking, and includes materials and strategies that are flexible enough to be used in communities of all sizes.

- *Building Blocks for a Healthy Future*: Building Blocks is an early childhood substance abuse prevention program that educates parents and caregivers of children 3 to 6 years old about ways to reduce basic risk factors and enhance protective factors related to the behavioral health of their children. This evidence-based program is based on six protective steps identified by NIDA and SAMHSA that adults can take to help children avoid later drug use, such as establish and maintain good communication with their children and make clear rules and enforce them consistently. Building Blocks materials are available in both English and Spanish. SAMHSA holds training workshops on the use of Building Blocks materials at semiannual meetings held by the National Head Start Association and the conferences of other child-serving organizations. The website (http://www.bblocks.samhsa.gov) offers several lessons plans each year for early childhood educators, and pairs them with materials for parents so they can reinforce classroom activities at home. During FY 2012, SAMHSA established a relationship with regional Head Start programs as the groundwork for an evaluation of program outcomes.

- *State/Territory Video Initiative*: SAMHSA initiated this project in 2006 to explore the potential benefits of developing a series of short videos (each 7 to 10 minutes long) showcasing underage alcohol use prevention efforts in the states. The videos are intended to:
  - Build awareness of current prevention efforts.
  - Promote resources available to community organizations.
  - Empower parents, youth, and organizations through opportunities to join these efforts.

- Report on the measurable results of state/territory and community activities and initiatives (e.g., holding of town hall meetings and implementation of evidence-based approaches).

Following a positive response to videos developed in direct collaboration with and pilot-tested by four states (Arizona, Louisiana, Mississippi, and Texas), SAMHSA expanded the video initiative to include all states and territories. SAMHSA aims to produce videos for all 50 states, 8 territories, and the District of Columbia before 2014. During FY 2012, SAMHSA provided video production support to 17 states (Alabama, Arizona, Idaho, Illinois, Indiana, Kansas, Maine, Maryland, Massachusetts, Michigan, New Hampshire, North Carolina, New Jersey, Ohio, South Carolina, Tennessee, and Wisconsin), the District of Columbia, and Puerto Rico. The number of videos produced to date is 37 (some states and territories produced more than one). Completed videos can be viewed on the SAMHSA YouTube page at http://www.youtube.com/user/SAMHSA#g/c/6F25AC126268A2B3, where they have been viewed more than 27,000 times to date. This initiative incorporates continuous evaluation of the process and the outcomes of the videos. A full report is expected in 2014.

- *American Indian Underage Drinking Prevention Video*: In late 2010, SAMHSA began collaborating with its Native American Center for Excellence and its Expert Panel to plan a video supporting efforts by American Indian communities to keep their youth alcohol free. Interviews with 21 youth and 3 elders, based on the concept that "culture is prevention," were recorded in June 2012 during a national meeting of Native American youth. A first cut of this video is being produced.

- *Regional Meetings with States/Territories/Tribes/Communities*: SAMHSA conducted a series of five HHS regional meetings during summer 2011 with the goals of producing (1) a summary of effective regional underage drinking prevention efforts and (2) recommendations for stronger prevention approaches and resources needed by community-level prevention organizations to support their implementation. SAMHSA held these meetings with state prevention stakeholders recommended by National Prevention Network representatives and the National Association of State Alcohol and Drug Abuse Directors. In addition, SAMHSA has solicited input from key national groups, including those targeted to youth and those at the college level such as Students Against Destructive Decisions and the Network Addressing Collegiate Alcohol and Other Drug Issues. SAMHSA presented a summary report of its findings on successful prevention efforts, barriers to implementing strategic plans, policy concerns, and recommendations to its federal ICCPUD partners, who are working collaboratively on developing a unified national strategy

Strategic Prevention Framework State Incentive Grant (SPF SIG) Program: SPF SIG is one of CSAP's infrastructure grant programs. SPF SIGs provide funding for up to 5 years to states, territories, and Tribes that wish to implement the SPF to prevent the onset and reduce the progression of substance abuse, including childhood and underage drinking; reduce problems related to substance abuse in communities; and build prevention capacity and infrastructure at the state/Tribal/territory and community levels. The SPF itself is a five-step planning process that uses a public health approach to guide state/Tribal and community prevention activities. SPF SIGs require grantees to assess their prevention needs based on epidemiological data; build their prevention capacity; develop a strategic plan; implement effective evidence-based community prevention programs, policies, and practices; and evaluate outcomes.

Each SPF SIG is guided by a governor or Tribal advisory committee that includes state/Tribe/territory, community, and private-sector representation. Grantees are required to develop epidemiological workgroups at the state/Tribal/territory level to identify state-level priority substance abuse problems. Grantees must then allocate a minimum of 85 percent of the total grant award directly to communities to address those problems.

CSAP has awarded SPF SIGs to 49 states, the District of Columbia, 8 U.S. territories, and 19 Tribes. Cohort I grants were awarded in FY 2004; Cohort II in FY 2005; Cohort III in FY 2006; Cohort IV in FY 2009; and Cohort V in FY 2010. All SPF SIGs support the goals of the underage drinking initiative because all grant tasks, including needs assessment, capacity building, planning, implementation, and evaluation, must be carried out with consideration for the issue of underage drinking. As of 2010, 64 of the 78 grantees funded in Cohorts I through V had approved SPF SIG plans and had disseminated funds to communities to address identified priority substance abuse problems. By the end of FY 2009, more than 70 percent of SPF SIG states had reduced past-30-day underage drinking. In 2004, 33 percent of SPF SIG states reported improvement in perceived risk of alcohol use among youth ages 12 to 20. By 2008, that number had increased to more than 59 percent. Additionally, 48 percent of communities targeting underage binge drinking showed improvement and 62 percent of communities targeting underage 30-day use also showed improvement. An interim report on state and community outcomes data was published in September 2011.

Treatment of Adolescent Alcohol Abuse and Alcoholism/Replication of Effective Alcohol Treatment Interventions for Youth: The Assertive Adolescent and Family Treatment Program, which builds on effective interventions for youths with alcohol or other drug problems, is a program of SAMHSA's Center for Substance Abuse Treatment (CSAT). Participating sites receive funds to provide training and certification on using the Adolescent Community Reinforcement Approach and Assertive Continuing Care, both of which are proven youth interventions. This program increases the availability and effectiveness of treatment for youths with alcohol and drug problems and targets youths ages 12 to 20.

Sober Truth on Preventing Underage Drinking (STOP) Grant Program: In December 2006, the STOP Act was signed into public law establishing the STOP Act grant program. The program requires SAMHSA's CSAP to provide $50,000 per year for 4 years to current or previously funded Drug-Free Communities Program (DFC) grantees to enhance the implementation of evidence-based practices that are effective in preventing underage drinking. It was created to strengthen collaboration among communities, the federal government, and state, local, and Tribal governments; enhance intergovernmental cooperation and coordination on the issue of alcohol use among youth; and serve as a catalyst for increased citizen participation and greater collaboration among all sectors and organizations of a community that have demonstrated a long-term commitment to reducing alcohol use among youth.

STOP Act grant recipients are required to develop strategic plans using SAMHSA's Strategic Prevention Framework process, which includes a community needs assessment, an implementation plan, a method to collect data, and the evaluation, monitoring, and improvement of strategies being implemented to create measurable outcomes. Grantees are required to report every 2 years on four core Government Performance and Results Act (GPRA) measures: age of onset, frequency of use (past 30 days), perception of risk or harm, and perception of parental disapproval across at least three grades from grades 6 through 12. SAMHSA's CSAP currently funds 103 community coalitions in 34 states across the United States. CSAP awarded 22 grants in Cohort II (which extends from FY 2009 to FY 2013) and 81 grants in Cohort III (which extends from FY 2012 to FY 2016).

Activities Related to Underage Drinking

Substance Abuse Prevention and Treatment (SAPT) Block Grant: The SAPT Block Grant is a major funding source for substance abuse prevention and treatment in the United States. States can and do use it to prevent and treat alcohol use disorders among adolescents. The SAPT Block Grant contains a primary substance abuse prevention set-aside that reserves a minimum of 20 percent of each state's Block Grant allocation for primary prevention activities. Although most primary prevention programs supported by these funds address substance abuse in general, many have an impact on underage drinking. The Block Grant application encourages states to report voluntarily on underage drinking strategies, such as implementation of public education and/or media campaigns; environmental strategies that focus on social marketing; laws against alcohol consumption on college campuses; policies or enforcement of laws that reduce access to alcohol by those under age 21, including event restrictions, product price increases, and penalties for sales to the underage population; data for estimated age of drinking onset; and statutes restricting alcohol promotion to underage audiences.

Partnership for Success: State and Community Prevention Performance Grant (PFS): The PFS is designed to provide states with up to 5 years of funding to achieve quantifiable decline in statewide substance abuse rates, incorporating a strong incentive to grantees that have met or exceeded their prevention performance targets by the end of the third year of funding. Grant awards were made to states with the infrastructure and demonstrated capacity to reduce substance abuse problems and achieve specific program outcomes. The overall goals of the PFS are to reduce substance abuse–related problems; prevent the onset and reduce the progression of substance abuse, including childhood and underage drinking; strengthen capacity and infrastructure at the state and community levels in support of prevention; and leverage, redirect, and realign statewide funding streams for prevention. Four states were funded in cohort I and one state funded in cohort II of the grant.

Strategic Prevention Framework, Partnership for Success (SPF-PFS II): Over a 3-year period, the SPF-PFS II is designed to address two of the nation's top substance abuse prevention priorities: (1) underage drinking among persons ages 12 to 20 and (2) prescription drug misuse and abuse among persons ages 12 to 25. PFS II grantees are permitted to choose a subset of these respective age ranges for the two prevention priorities based on their data findings. The SPF-PFS II is also intended to bring SAMHSA's Strategic Prevention Framework to a national scale. These awards provide an opportunity for recipients of the Substance Abuse Block Grant (SABG) that have completed an SPF SIG and are not currently funded through SAMHSA's Partnership for Success grants to acquire additional resources to implement the SPF process at the state and community levels. Equally important, the SPF-PFS II program promotes alignment and leveraging of prevention resources and priorities at the federal, state, and community levels. SPF-PFS II grantees are expected to meet several key requirements: (1) States must use a data-driven approach to identify which of the substance abuse prevention priorities they propose to address using the SPF-PFS II funds. States must use SPF-PFS II funds to address one or both of these priorities. At their discretion, states may also use SPF-PFS II funds to target an additional, data-driven prevention priority in their state. (2) States must develop an approach to funding communities of high need (i.e., subrecipients) that ensures that all funded communities receive ongoing guidance and support from the state, including technical assistance and training. Of the 15 states awarded funding, 11 have chosen to target underage drinking. Three of the 11 have chosen underage drinking as their sole priority.

National Helpline (1-800-662-HELP): Individuals with alcohol or illicit drug problems or their family members can call the SAMHSA National Helpline for referral to local treatment facilities, support groups, and community-based organizations. The Helpline is a confidential, free, 24-hour-a-day, 365-days-a-year information service available in English and Spanish. Information can be obtained by calling the toll-free number or visiting the online treatment locator at http://www.samhsa.gov/treatment.

Targeted Capacity Expansion (TCE) Program: TCE in SAMHSA's CSAT addresses emerging substance abuse trends and the disparity between demand for and availability of appropriate treatment in some areas. The program supports rapid, strategic responses to unmet demand for alcohol and drug treatment services in communities with serious, emerging substance abuse problems and in communities with innovative solutions to these unmet needs. Adolescents are one of the target populations served by TCE grants.

Screening, Brief Intervention, Referral, and Treatment (SBIRT) Grants: SBIRT involves implementation of a system in community and specialist settings that screens for and identifies individuals with substance use–related problems. Depending on the level of problems identified, the system either provides for a brief intervention in a generalist setting or motivates and refers individuals with high-level problems and probable substance dependence disorder diagnoses to a specialist setting for assessment, diagnosis, and brief or long-term treatment. This includes training in self-management and involvement in mutual help groups, as appropriate. SBIRT grants are administered by CSAT. Several SBIRT grantees have developed programs that are available to individuals under age 21. Additional SBIRT information, including related publications, is available at http://www.sbirt.samhsa.gov.

Offender Reentry Program (ORP): This CSAT program addresses the needs of juvenile and adult offenders who use substances and are returning to their families and communities from incarceration in prisons, jails, or juvenile detention centers. ORP forms partnerships to plan, develop, and provide community-based substance abuse treatment and related re-entry services for target populations. The juvenile ORP targets youths ages 14 to 18, and the adult ORP includes adults ages 19 to 20.

Program To Provide Treatment Services for Family, Juvenile, and Adult Treatment Drug Courts: By combining the sanctioning power of courts with effective treatment services, drug courts break cycles of child abuse and neglect, criminal behavior, alcohol and/or drug use, and incarceration or other penalties. Motivational strategies are developed and used to help adolescents deal with the often-powerful negative influences of peers, gangs, and family members. SAMHSA/CSAT funds Juvenile Treatment Drug Court grants to provide services to support substance abuse treatment, assessment, case management, and program coordination for those in need of treatment drug court services.

Programs for Improving Addiction Treatment: SAMHSA/CSAT supports a variety of programs to advance the integration of new research into service delivery and improve addiction treatment nationally. For example, the Addiction Technology Transfer Center (ATTC) Network identifies and advances opportunities for improving addiction treatment. It assists practitioners and other health professionals in developing their skills and disseminates the latest science to the treatment community, providing academic instruction to those beginning their careers as well as continuing education opportunities and technical assistance to people already working in the addictions field. For more information on the ATTC Network, including related publications and resources, see http://www.ATTCNetwork.org.

In addition, CSAT has produced several Treatment Improvement Protocols (TIPs) that address a wide array of concerns. These TIPs include *TIP 16: Alcohol and Drug Screening of Hospitalized Trauma Patients*; *TIP 24: A Guide to Substance Abuse Services for Primary Care*; *TIP 26: Substance Abuse Among Older Adults*; *TIP 31: Screening and Assessing Adolescents for Substance Use Disorders*; *TIP 32: Treatment of Adolescents with Substance Use Disorders*; and *TIP 34: Brief Interventions and Brief Therapies for Substance Abuse.*

Fetal Alcohol Spectrum Disorders: SAMHSA's FASD Center for Excellence (CFE) is SAMHSA's largest alcohol prevention initiative, addressing innovative techniques and effective strategies for preventing alcohol use among women of childbearing age and providing assistance to persons and families affected by FASD. States, communities, juvenile justice systems, and academic institutions are in the process of improving their service delivery systems and policies and procedures to screen at intake for FASD among children, youth, and adults and refer individuals for interventions or for diagnosis, if necessary. These systems also participate in surveillance to create sustainable evidence-based responses to FASD. This initiative does not specifically target underage drinkers, but it is expected that through the current FASD CFE's collaboration with SAMHSA/CSAP underage drinking programs, more children, youth, and adults will be reached, educated, and trained on co-occurring issues (substance use/abuse) across the lifespans of individuals with FASD. The FASD CFE website, http://www.fasdcenter.samhsa.gov, reported 187,467 unique visitors and 493,276 total visits from January to December 2011, and 160,364 unique visitors and 429,991 total visits from January to September 2012. SAMHSA is also a member of the Interagency Coordinating Committee on FASD (ICCFASD), comprising federal partners such as NIAAA, the National Center for Birth Defects and Disabilities (NCBDD) of the Centers for Disease Control and Prevention, the Health Resources Services Administration (HRSA), and the Indian Health Service.

Access to Recovery (ATR): SAMHSA/CSAT ATR grants allow state and Tribal organizations the flexibility of designing and implementing a voucher program that meets the treatment and recovery support needs of consumers in their community. In doing so, ATR provides consumers with choices among substance abuse clinical treatment and recovery support service providers, expands access to comprehensive clinical treatment and recovery support options (including faith-based options), and increases substance abuse treatment capacity. Grantees are encouraged to support any mix of traditional clinical treatment and recovery support services that is expected to yield successful outcomes for the most people at the lowest possible cost. In addition, states and Tribal grantees may implement the program statewide or target geographic areas of greatest need, specific populations in need, or areas with a high degree of readiness to implement a voucher program. More information on ATR, including related publications, can be accessed at http://www.atr.samhsa.gov.

Native American Center for Excellence (NACE): NACE was established by SAMHSA in 2007 as a national training and technical assistance resource on issues related to American Indian and Alaska Native (AI/AN) substance abuse prevention and behavioral health. NACE serves tribal health systems, community-based organizations, regional health boards, and others. NACE supports community-driven initiatives and solutions and brings cultural attention and sensitivity to all of its interactions and relationships with AI/AN communities. A 15-member panel of experts guides NACE services on a wide range of topics including AI/AN behavioral health assessment, capacity building, program planning, evidence-based practice implementation, evaluation, youth issues, and traditional healing. Culturally competent expert consultants and trainers representing a broad range of disciplines and approaches to wellness add to the rich pool of service providers that NACE offers. NACE also builds and supports strong collaborative initiatives as well as learning communities: virtual meetings of interested stakeholders on special topics where participants can talk, teach, share materials, and inspire each other. NACE contributes to AI/AN engagement and youth prevention throughout Indian Country in supporting the development of multimedia projects prevention video and culturally appropriate youth healing modalities.

Safe Schools/Healthy Students (SS/HS) Initiative: SS/HS seeks to create healthy learning environments that help students thrive, succeed in school, and build healthy relationships. A central goal of the initiative is to prevent children from consuming alcohol and other drugs, and the implementation of evidence-based programs such as Class Action, Family Matters, and Project Alert helps achieve this goal. The initiative also supports a variety of prevention activities involving families and communities such as "Safe Home Pledges" that ask parents to commit to maintaining a safe and alcohol-free environment (e.g., not serve alcohol to minors) and public forums and town hall meetings on drug and alcohol abuse. The results demonstrate the initiative has been successful in reducing alcohol consumption among students at participating SS/HS school districts. Between Year 1 and Year 3 of the grant, the percentage of students who reported drinking declined from 25.4 percent to 22.4 percent (according to GPRA data). This represents a decrease from 27,521 students drinking in Year 1 to 24,270 students drinking in Year 3. Furthermore, more than 80 percent of school staff reported the SS/HS grant helped reduce alcohol and other drug use among students. Reported 30-day alcohol use decreased nearly 12 percent from year 1 to year 3 of the grant (25.4 percent to 22.4 percent) for the 2005–2007 cohorts. This correlates to approximately 3,250 fewer students drinking in year 3, enough to fill 130 classrooms.

Implementing Evidence-Based Prevention Practices in Schools (Prevention Practices in Schools): This grant program provides funding to schools to implement the Good Behavior Game (GBG), a universal classroom preventive evidence-based practice provided to school-aged children. It has been proven to reduce antisocial behavior, alcohol and tobacco addiction, and suicidal ideation in young adults. Disruptive and aggressive behavior in classrooms, as early as the 1st grade, has been identified as a risk factor for the development of substance abuse, antisocial behavior, and violent criminal behavior. GBG was rigorously tested in clinical trials in Baltimore City public schools. Prevention Practices in Schools is a pilot grant program in its third year of a 5-year grant and has reached 16,019 of students so far.

Community Resilience and Recovery Initiative (CRRI): CRRI is a place-based initiative to improve behavioral health outcomes through enhanced coordination and evidence-based health promotion, illness prevention, treatment, and recovery support services in communities affected by the economic downturn. CRRI grants direct resources toward preventing or intervening early in behavioral health problems. They also aim to prevent a downward cycle that leads to chronic declines in community resilience and long-term behavioral health issues and unemployment among their residents. Through coordinated services, the CRRI grants work in funded communities to: reduce excessive drinking (and other substance use if the community chooses); reduce child maltreatment and family violence; enable communities to better identify and respond to suicide risk; build a sense of cohesiveness and connectedness; enable coordination across service systems and community organizations; and improve community resilience and reduce the impact of the economic downturn on behavioral health problems. CRRI grants are positively affecting client outcomes in their programs. These outcomes chart the progress of clients for whom both intake and 6-month followup data were available. These outcomes include increases in abstinence from alcohol/drugs, employment and education, stability in housing, and social connectedness and decreases in arrests and the negative social consequences of alcohol and drug use.

National Survey on Drug Use and Health (NSDUH): Conducted by SAMHSA, NSDUH (formerly the National Household Survey on Drug Abuse) is a primary source of national and state-level data on the prevalence and patterns of alcohol, tobacco, and illegal drug use, abuse, and dependence in the noninstitutionalized U.S. civilian population (ages 12 and older). The survey collects data through face-to-face interviews with approximately 68,000 respondents each year. NSDUH tracks information on underage alcohol use and provides a database for studies on alcohol use and related disorders.

Behavioral Health Services Information System (BHSIS): BHSIS, conducted by SAMHSA's Center for Behavioral Health Statistics and Quality (CBHSQ), is the primary source of national data on substance abuse treatment services. Although not specific to youth, BHSIS offers information on treatment facilities with special programs for adolescents as well as demographic and substance abuse characteristics of adolescent treatment admissions. It has four components:

- *Inventory of Behavioral Health Services (I-BHS)* is a list of all known public and private substance abuse and mental health treatment facilities in the United States and its territories.
- *National Survey of Substance Abuse Treatment Services (N-SSATS)* is an annual survey of all substance abuse treatment facilities in the I-BHS. It collects data on location, characteristics, services offered, and utilization, and is used to update the National Directory of Drug and Alcohol Abuse Treatment Programs and the online Substance Abuse Treatment Facility Locator.
- *National Mental Health Services Survey (N-MHSS)* is an annual survey of all mental health treatment facilities in the I-BHS. It collects data on location, characteristics, services offered, and utilization and is used to update the Mental Health Treatment Facility Locator.
- *Treatment Episode Data Set (TEDS)* is a compilation of data on the demographic and substance abuse characteristics of admissions to and discharges from substance abuse treatment, primarily at publicly funded facilities. State administrative systems routinely collect treatment admission information and submit it to SAMHSA in a standard format.

Drug Abuse Warning Network (DAWN): Conducted by SAMHSA, DAWN was a nationally representative public health surveillance system that continuously monitored drug-related visits to hospital emergency departments (EDs). Using a stratified two-stage cluster sampling design, SAMHSA collected data from a sample of approximately 250 nonfederal, short-stay, general hospitals with 24-hour EDs in the first stage, and a large fraction of the ED visits within those hospitals at the second stage. For each sampled ED visit caused by or related to drugs, DAWN collected up to 22 drugs involved in the visit, along with demographic information including patient's age and gender. In 2012, SAMHSA and the National Center for Health Statistics (NCHS), CDC, began work to incorporate DAWN's ED survey into the redesigned ED component of the new National Hospital Care Survey conducted by NCHS. DAWN data showed that in 2011, patients aged 20 or younger made nearly 440,000 drug-abuse-related ED visits, almost half of which (188,706 visits, or 43.2 percent) involved alcohol.

National Registry of Evidence-Based Programs and Practices: NREPP is a searchable online registry of mental health and substance abuse interventions that have been reviewed and rated by independent reviewers. It identifies scientifically tested approaches to preventing and treating mental and/or substance use disorders that can be readily disseminated to the field. NREPP exemplifies SAMHSA's work toward improving access to information on tested interventions and thereby reducing lag between the creation of scientific knowledge and its practical application in the field. For every intervention NREPP reviews, it publishes an intervention summary on its website that describes the intervention and its targeted outcomes and provides expert ratings of the quality of the research and its readiness for dissemination. This information helps individuals and organizations determine whether a particular intervention may meet their needs. SAMHSA advises having direct conversations with intervention developers and other contacts listed in the summary before selecting and/or implementing an intervention. As of fall 2012, more than 250 programs were evaluated by NREPP and posted on the NREPP website. For more information on NREPP, visit http://www.nrepp.samhsa.gov.

Center for the Application of Prevention Technologies (CAPT): SAMHSA's CAPT is a national training and technical assistance (T/TA) system committed to strengthening substance abuse prevention efforts at the regional, state, and local levels and building the nation's prevention workforce. SAMHSA's CAPT provides face-to-face and electronic T/TA services to 75 entities (52 states, 14 Tribes, and 9 jurisdictions) receiving funding through any of the following SAMHSA grant programs: Strategic Prevention Framework State Incentive Grants (SPF SIGs), Partnerships for Success I and II, the Substance Abuse Block Grant, and the State Epidemiological Outcomes Workgroups.

The CAPT provides a range of services focusing on underage drinking prevention. For example, from April to June 2012, the CAPT's West Resource Team facilitated a series of four webinars to introduce local prevention workers to specific underage drinking evaluation strategies, such as social host ordinances, responsible beverage service training, taxation and licensing, and social norms. The CAPT's Central Resource Team conducted a literature review on the risk factors for underage binge drinking and corresponding evidence-based prevention strategies—states in the CAPT's Central service area then used this information to inform community-level prevention planning processes. In January the CAPT provided assistance to Vermont on revising a draft set of performance and outcome measures for school-based prevention activities. In addition, in FY2012 the CAPT delivered more than 30 trainings to states, Tribes, and jurisdictions on using the SPF to prevent underage drinking. In June, for example, CAPT T/TA providers conducted a 2-day onsite training for community-level prevention providers in the Federated States of Micronesia on underage drinking risk and protective factors and developing logic models.

Service to Science Initiative: Administered through CAPT (see above), SAMHSA/CSAP's Service to Science initiative helps innovative programs addressing critical substance abuse prevention to enhance their evaluation capacity. Since the initiative's inception in 2004, over 500 programs serving diverse populations in various settings have received direct TA. After their year of participation, programs are eligible to apply for 1-year subcontract awards to further enhance their evaluation capacity. In FY2012, 52 programs participated in the initiative. On behalf of SAMHSA, the CAPT also awarded subcontracts in FY2012 to 22 programs that had participated in FY2011. Of these funded programs, 10 addressed prevention or deterrence of underage drinking and 3 of these 10 addressed underage drinking prevention exclusively.

Office of the Surgeon General/HHS

Activities Specific to Underage Drinking

Dissemination of the* Call to Action *and the* Guides*: The ICCPUD agencies continue to promote the 2007 *Call to Action* and the accompanying *Guides to Action* as a key source of information on addressing the national health problem of underage drinking. The *Call to Action* and the *Guides* are available at http://www.surgeongeneral.gov and http://www.stopalcoholabuse.gov.

Activities Related to Underage Drinking

National Prevention Strategy: America's Plan for Better Health and Wellness: On June 16, 2011, the National Prevention, Health Promotion, and Public Health Council announced the release of the National Prevention Strategy, a comprehensive plan that will help increase the number of Americans who are healthy at every stage of life. Included in the Prevention Strategy is the section "Preventing Drug Abuse and Excessive Alcohol Use," which specifically addresses the need to prevent excessive alcohol use, including underage drinking. The recommendations made in this section of the strategy identify the need for more stringent alcohol control policies, advocate for the creation of environments that empower young people not to drink, and promote the use of SBIRT to screen for abuse.

Office of Juvenile Justice and Delinquency Prevention/DoJ

Activities Specific to Underage Drinking

Enforcing Underage Drinking Laws (EUDL): The EUDL program provides national leadership in ensuring that states, territories, and communities have the information, training, and resources needed to enforce underage drinking laws. Through EUDL, the OJJDP supports and enhances efforts by states and local jurisdictions to prohibit the sale of alcoholic beverages to minors and the purchase and consumption of alcoholic beverages by minors. (Minors are defined as individuals under 21 years old.) A governor-designated agency, through its EUDL coordinator, implements the EUDL initiative. State and territory agencies that implement OJJDP-supported EUDL programs include justice agencies, highway safety offices, alcohol beverage control agencies, health and human services agencies, youth services agencies, and offices of the governor. Agency contacts are listed on the Underage Drinking Enforcement Training Center (UDETC) website (http://www.udetc.org).

The EUDL block grant program supports task forces of state, territory, and local law enforcement, and judicial and prosecutorial agencies; encourages innovative programming; and conducts public advertising programs that inform and educate alcohol retailers about underage drinking and its consequences. The EUDL program encourages and supports partnerships between law enforcement and underage drinking prevention advocates. EUDL requires that all discretionary programs include multidisciplinary coalitions that use environmental, enforcement-oriented local approaches. EUDL grantees routinely partner with a number of other private and public organizations. For example, 54 states/territories and the District of Columbia have worked and continue to work closely with state/territory alcohol beverage control agencies or other state/territory-level enforcement agencies that specialize in alcohol enforcement. A total of 49 states/territories and the District of Columbia have incorporated and continue to incorporate college communities into EUDL funding priorities; 37 states/territories have engaged and many continue to engage members of the Leadership to Keep Children Alcohol Free initiative in their state and territory EUDL programs; and 15 states/territories have linked and many continue to link with U.S. military bases to address underage and hazardous drinking behavior by troops. During the 2012 EUDL Coordinator Symposium, OJJDP highlighted, through a panel discussion, effective EUDL/federal partnerships established during the program. In 2012, EUDL experienced a significant funding reduction (from $25 million to $5 million). Therefore, the EUDL block grant was not supported that year.

Standard local EUDL discretionary programming can also include the development and use of youth leadership to plan and implement community programs. Designated youth assist law enforcement with compliance checks, use the media to promote underage drinking prevention, hold alcohol-free events, and participate in training to learn about underage drinking issues.

Underage Drinking Enforcement Training Center (UDETC): A major component of the EUDL program, UDETC provides training and technical assistance to adults and youth. UDETC identifies science-based strategies, publishes supporting documents, delivers training, and provides technical assistance to support the enforcement of underage drinking laws. Since 1999, UDETC has been working with EUDL Coordinators in all 50 states, the District of Columbia, and 5 territories to coordinate training and technical assistance for prevention and reduction of underage drinking. UDETC accomplishes its mission by providing onsite trainings, expert technical assistance by UDETC staff, monthly audio teleconferences, publications, a toll-free technical assistance hotline, a website, distance-learning opportunities, and an annual national conference and/or symposium on underage drinking prevention and enforcement. As a national program, UDETC has responded to more than 11,000 technical assistance requests each year, completed 126 national audio calls/webinars reaching more than 19,000 individuals, conducted 595 onsite trainings reaching 32,193 participants, developed more than 270 documents (guides, toolkits, case studies, and resource reports), and has had more than 24 million website hits.

UDETC has published the following documents to help states and local communities enforce retail establishment compliance with underage drinking laws:

- *Guide to Responsible Alcohol Sales: Off Premise Clerk, Licensee and Manager Training*— Offers sales personnel training tools that support management policies to prevent sales of alcohol to those under age 21.

- *Preventing Sales of Alcohol to Minors: What You Should Know About Merchant Education Programs*—Describes such programs and their role in comprehensive community strategies to reduce underage drinking. It also identifies necessary components and resources for more information.

- *Reducing Alcohol Sales to Underage Purchasers: A Practical Guide to Compliance Check Investigations*—Indicates the importance of enforcement in retail establishments as the cornerstone of enforcing underage drinking laws, and provides the essential elements of carrying out compliance checks using minors or young-looking adults.

- *Strategies for Reducing Third-Party Transactions of Alcohol to Underage Youth*—Dissuades adults from providing alcohol to underage persons. The publication discusses the problem of nonretail sources of alcohol for underage drinkers and describes the essential elements of shoulder-tap operations, along with other techniques, to deter adults from buying or providing alcohol to underage drinkers.

UDETC also publishes the following documents about the costs of underage alcohol use and effective policies and procedures for reducing underage alcohol use:

- *Strategies to Reduce Underage Alcohol Use: Typology and Brief Overview*—Available in both English and Spanish, it summarizes common strategies to reduce underage drinking and their effectiveness based on research and evaluation.

- *Cost sheets* for each of the 50 states and the District of Columbia highlighting the costs incurred by each state and the District of Columbia because of underage drinking. Using the most current data available, these sheets give state-specific costs for a host of serious problems, including alcohol poisoning and treatment for alcohol abuse and dependence.

Additional publications to support enforcement and prevention work, including over 140 success stories that feature measurable outcomes, are available from the UDETC website (http://www.udetc.org).

UDETC maintains a small library of radio and TV public service announcements aimed at increasing awareness among parents and other adults of underage drinking and its consequences. EUDL state coordinators and EUDL-funded communities voluntarily forward PSAs to UDETC, which shares the collection with state coordinators and others seeking guidance or assistance with their own PSAs.

National Leadership Conferences: Through UDETC, OJJDP has conducted 12 annual National Leadership Conferences, which provide training opportunities and promote cooperation, coordination, and collaboration among such partners as highway safety offices, health agencies, justice agencies, law enforcement, schools, youth advocacy groups, health care professionals, and alcohol prevention service providers. In August 2011, more than 1,400 partners attended the conference. In August 2012, OJJDP conducted an invitation-only EUDL Coordinators Symposium designed to engage state EUDL coordinators and selected invitees in strategizing ways to enhance EUDL outcomes in states and local communities. More than 130 attendees participated in focused discussions, workshops, and collaborative meetings.

In December 2010, with an interest in making their resources accessible, UDETC developed distance-learning curriculums. UDETC's distance-learning opportunities featured courses that presented best practices and strategies for enforcement of underage drinking laws and efforts to reduce underage drinking. The web-based, online courses are free to participants and designed to provide basic information as a foundation for onsite followup training provided by the UDETC. Participants can receive a certificate after completion of each course. Currently, more than 1,000 individuals have completed the two online courses (Conducting Compliance Check Operations and Environmental Strategies). Future courses include Party Prevention and Controlled Party Dispersal and Techniques for Managing Special Events. UDETC also began a weekly internet radio program titled "A National Conversation on Protecting Our Youth— Enforcing Underage Drinking Laws" developed to serve less mobile audiences. The weekly programs are also available after show times by request through the UDETC website.

Judicial Project: EUDL's UDETC tackled the Judicial Project, an innovative initiative offering resources to the judiciary and probation fields on the broad and encompassing problems related to underage alcohol use. With judges assuming a leadership role within a community and having the ability to influence community norms around underage drinking, the objective of the project is to collect the most up-to-date science, research, and court practices on the myriad of health-related issues that impact youth who appear before the courts on alcohol-related offenses. The project delivers information in a variety of ways to judges, court professionals, and community members who are concerned about the societal impact of underage drinking. The project does not attempt to influence the impartiality of judges but serves to provide information and resources to judges who request information on relevant topics and learn how other courts are responding to these types of cases.

EUDL Discretionary Program:

- *NIAAA Studies, Through the Prevention Research Center, of EUDL Discretionary Programming in Rural Sites:* In FYs 2004 and 2005, the EUDL Discretionary Program partnered with NIAAA to address underage drinking in rural communities. In 2009, OJJDP-supported program activity had been completed in all seven of the states (CA, IL, NV, NM, OR, PA, WA) attempting to conduct best and most promising EUDL activities in up to five rural sites in their jurisdictions. Currently, NIAAA is funding and managing site evaluation by the Prevention Research Center. The effort established community coalitions to reduce/prevent underage drinking in rural areas.

- *OJJDP EUDL Partnership with the United States Air Force (USAF) and NIAAA:* In 2006, OJJDP issued a solicitation for the EUDL Discretionary Program that sought to reduce the availability of alcoholic beverages to—and the consumption of alcoholic beverages by—persons serving in the USAF who are under 21. Specific goals were to reduce the number of first-time alcohol-related incidents, incidence of unintentional injuries related to alcohol consumption, and number of alcohol-related traffic injuries or fatalities among underage USAF personnel. OJJDP awarded grants to four states that identified AFBs to participate and form coalitions with adjacent communities. The participating AFBs were Davis-Monthan and Luke (AZ), Beale (CA), Hickam (HI), and Malmstrom (MT). NIAAA provided evaluation support for the project through a 48-month contract that included evaluation of all activities developed at each AFB/community site. In 2011, OJJDP produced a bulletin to highlight the evaluation findings (see http://www.udetc.org, within the Research/Evaluation/Military Discretionary Program Evaluation tab).

In FY 2009, OJJDP issued another solicitation for discretionary EUDL work that sought to build on the EUDL/USAF partnerships by providing grant funding to two additional states (MO and WY). The decision was made to expand the EUDL/USAF program when preliminary evaluation findings suggested the program produced positive outcomes worth replicating. Programs are being implemented, in concert with adjacent communities, on Whiteman AFB in Missouri and F.E. Warren AFB in Wyoming. The expanded OJJDP-supported evaluation includes these states and bases.

In FY 2012, OJJDP issued a third solicitation for discretionary EUDL work, to build on the EUDL/USAF partnerships to include the U.S. Marine Corps by providing grant funding to two additional states. Programs will be implemented, in concert with adjacent communities.

- *NIAAA Studies, Through ICF International, of EUDL Discretionary Programming in Selected Communities and AFBs:* As mentioned above, in FY 2006, the EUDL discretionary program partnered with NIAAA to address underage drinking among underage USAF personnel. OJJDP-supported program activity in partnership with USAF implemented in select communities and five AFBs in four states (AZ, CA, HI, MT). NIAAA funded and managed ICF International's evaluation of the EUDL/USAF partnerships and their design and implementation of a set of interventions to reduce underage drinking among airmen at grantee sites. In FY 2009, the evaluation was expanded to two added AFBs in two new states (MO, WY). In FY 2012, the evaluation will be expanded once again to include two added AFBs in two new states. OJJDP is funding and managing ICF International's evaluation of the sites funded in FY 2009 and FY 2012 as well.

- *OJJDP FY 2008 EUDL Discretionary Program To Address Underage Drinking on College/University Campuses:* In FY 2008, OJJDP focused its EUDL discretionary funding on addressing underage drinking by university/college students. The program is being implemented in Illinois, Nevada, and South Carolina. Participating college/university sites are Eastern Illinois University; University of Illinois at Champaign/Urbana; University of Nevada Reno; and—in South Carolina—Furman University, University of South Carolina, Clemson University, and College of Charleston. This effort is committed to establishing university- and college-based programs in partnership with adjacent communities to implement research-based and promising practices that will reduce underage drinking among university/college students younger than 21, with emphasis on environmental strategies.

  Six core areas of implementation revolve around these best and most promising practices: (1) develop and strengthen coalitions that include campus and community leaders, (2) enhance policies and procedures related to underage drinking, (3) conduct compliance checks on and off college campuses, (4) conduct DWI enforcement operations focused on underage persons, (5) conduct enforcement operations aimed at reducing social availability of alcohol to underage youth, and (6) implement other environmental strategies for reducing underage alcohol consumption. Illinois has completed its implementation of the program, South Carolina is about to conclude its program efforts, and Nevada will finish its program implementation by June 2013.

- *OJJDP FY 2010 EUDL Assessment, Strategic Planning, and Implementation Initiative (SASPII):* In FY 2010, OJJDP focused its EUDL discretionary funding on reducing the availability of alcoholic beverages to and the consumption of alcoholic beverages by persons younger than 21 through assessment, strategic planning, and program implementation. Maine, Nevada, and Washington were grant recipients of the 2010 EUDL SASPII discretionary demonstration project awards. The selected states and communities conducted an independent assessment of both state and local underage drinking in the first year of the program, developing a long-range strategic plan based on the independent assessment as part of first-year program activities, and implementing selected elements of the strategic plan during the rest of the grant period. The unique feature of the FY 2010 discretionary program is the independent assessment process that culminates in a report to the state that provides recommended action steps for reducing underage access to and consumption of alcohol.

Office of National Drug Control Policy

Activities Specific to Underage Drinking

None

Activities Related to Underage Drinking

National Youth Anti-Drug Media Campaign: Through its teen brand "Above the Influence" (ATI), the National Youth Anti-Drug Media Campaign provides ongoing messaging and tools to support underage drinking prevention. In FY 2012, new ATI advertising featured teens sharing their stories of rising above drugs and drinking, broadcast nationally on television and in digital media. As a call-to-action, teens were encouraged to tell their own stories and post them on the ATI Facebook page. Among the thousands of responses were many video submissions focused on challenges related to underage drinking and growing up with alcoholic parents. The ATI Facebook page has surpassed 1.8 million "likes." ONDCP regularly provides posts related to underage drinking to stimulate discussion on the page. The ongoing editorial calendar ensures this issue remains prominent throughout the year.

Teens regularly turn to the internet to access credible information related to alcohol and underage drinking. The ATI website's (http://www.abovetheinfluence.com) most frequented section is Drug Facts, which includes a downloadable Alcohol Facts page. To ensure that teens seeking this information click to the ATI page, ONDCP engaged heavily in "Paid Search," purchasing keywords from search engine companies. The Campaign had more than 1,000 keywords directly related to alcohol abuse.

An important element of the Media Campaign is grassroots outreach for ATI, as part of ONDCP's primary objective to localize ATI – making it more relevant, usable, and customizable to teens and youth-serving organizations in local communities. Thus the Campaign has partnered with 100 youth-serving organizations in over 62 communities across the country and provided technical assistance and training on the ATI Activity Toolkit to more than 8,000 community organizations through conference workshops and webinars since 2010. Specifically, the Campaign has worked closely with youth-serving partner organizations, including Students Against Destructive Decisions chapters, Boys and Girls Clubs of America, Y's (formerly the YMCA), ONDCP's Drug Free Communities grantees, and others.

Drug-Free Communities (DFC) Support Program: The DFC program, created by the Drug-Free Communities Act of 1997, is the nation's leading effort to mobilize communities to prevent youth substance use. Directed by ONDCP in partnership with SAMHSA, the DFC Program provides grants to community coalitions to strengthen the infrastructure among local partners to create and sustain a reduction in local youth substance use. Recognizing the fundamental concept that local problems need local solutions, the program requires funded coalitions to implement environmental strategies—broad initiatives aimed at addressing the entire community through the adaptation of policies and practices related to youth substance use. Currently, the program has funded more than 2,000 community coalitions and mobilized nearly 9,000 community coalition members throughout the United States, Puerto Rico, American Samoa, Palau, and Micronesia. DFC grantees collect data every 2 years on four substances—alcohol, tobacco, marijuana, and prescription drugs—for at least three grade levels between 6th and 12th grades. Grantees collect data on the following four measures: past 30-day use, perception of risk or harm of use, perception of parental disapproval of use, and perception of peer disapproval of use. Grantees consistently report that alcohol is the most significant youth substance use problem in their communities, with 92 percent rating it as the drug of greatest concern for middle school youth, and 95 percent for high school youth. In the past 8 years of program evaluation, DFC-funded communities have achieved significant reductions in youth substance use. For additional information, visit the DFC website at http://www.whitehouse.gov/ondcp/Drug-Free-Communities-Support-Program.

Demand Reduction Interagency Working Group (IWG): In 2009, ONDCP reinstituted the IWG, comprising 35 federal agencies whose missions involve some connection to substance abuse. Agency leaders identified four major cross-cutting issues: prevention and education, prescription drugs, electronic health records, and data. These committees have helped shape the 2010, 2011, 2012, and 2013 National Drug Control Strategies. Underage drinking is an issue receiving great attention in several of these IWG committees. In 2012, ONDCP along with its federal partners participated in several events with associations and institutions of higher education on underage drinking to encourage implementation of evidence-based practices that are motivational and empowering along with the development of strategies that foster ongoing collaboration and communication on policy, curriculum development, programs, and resources on college and university campuses

National Highway Traffic Safety Administration/DOT

Activities Specific to Underage Drinking

Programs Encouraging States To Enact Minimum Drinking Age and Zero Tolerance Laws:
NHTSA implemented congressionally mandated programs to encourage states to enact minimum drinking age and zero tolerance laws. Zero tolerance laws make it unlawful for persons under age 21 to drive with any detectable amount of alcohol in their systems. Minimum drinking age laws make it unlawful for persons under age 21 to purchase or publicly possess alcohol. All 50 states and the District of Columbia have enacted both laws. NHTSA continues to monitor state compliance with these federal mandates. Failure to comply results in financial sanctions to the states.

Youth Traffic Safety Media Campaign Development: NHTSA has initiated a three-prong strategy to address youth traffic safety concerns. This strategy is the basis of a developing national media campaign with an overarching focus primarily on adults/parents of youth, which incorporates all three NHTSA youth traffic safety priority areas: teen belt use, graduated driver licensing (GDL), and youth access to alcohol. To emphasize this, NHTSA has created the Teen Driver and Teens & Parents web pages to highlight the importance of parents talking to their teens (http://www.nhtsa.gov/Teen-Drivers). The Traffic Safety Marketing website provides template materials such as talking points, earned media tools, collateral materials, and other marketing materials designed to help maximize local outreach efforts to various key audiences (http://www.trafficsafetymarketing.gov). The program strategy that supports the media includes:

- Reducing youth access to alcohol through high-visibility enforcement of underage purchase, possession, and provision laws to create a significant deterrent for violation of youth access laws, reduce underage drinking, and decrease youth alcohol-related crashes. Parental responsibility is crucial to educating and protecting teens, so a key program component reminds parents to obey the law and help keep their teens safe.
- Increasing safety belt use among teens through primary seat belt laws, high-visibility enforcement of seat belt laws, and education to complement the laws and enforcement.
- Enforcement of GDL laws, including enactment of three-stage GDL legislation, high-visibility enforcement of GDL laws, and increased parental responsibility for monitoring compliance. This effort targets youth ages 15 to 18, parents, and other adults.

High-Visibility Enforcement of Underage Drinking Laws/Youth Access to Alcohol and Social Marketing Campaign to Parents: High-visibility enforcement of traffic laws has been proven to be effective in reducing impaired driving, increasing seat belt use, and otherwise improving traffic safety. NHTSA is conducting a demonstration project to apply this principle to reduce underage access to alcohol and underage drinking and driving in four locations. This project will demonstrate, in particular, the use of high-visibility enforcement, coupled with communication strategies that publicize the enforcement, and source investigations, which seek to identify the persons from whom the underage drinkers obtained alcoholic beverages and hold those persons accountable. Enforcement strategies include traffic enforcement, party patrols, compliance checks, as well as source investigations. Communications include paid, earned, and social media. Strategies vary depending on the characteristics of the participating communities.

SMASHED: Toxic Tales of Teens and Alcohol: NHTSA, SAMHSA, and ED's Office of Safe and Healthy Students (OSHS) collaborated with Recording Artists, Actors and Athletes Against Drunk Driving (RADD) and its partner, HBO Family, to develop and disseminate *SMASHED*, an educational package including a documentary on underage drinking and alcohol-related driving, to thousands of schools and communities across the country. HBO licensed RADD and federal partners to use *SMASHED*. In Phase II, NHTSA is funding an independent evaluator to determine how tools like *SMASHED* can be used most effectively to stimulate community action and promote or initiate evidence-based programs and practices to address issues like underage drinking. Targets for this effort are youth, their families, and community/school leaders.

Project YOUTH-Turn: Under a cooperative agreement with NHTSA, the National Organizations for Youth Safety (NOYS) has developed the first component of an online program titled "Project YOUTH-Turn," which enhances protective factors that help change attitudes toward underage drinking and driving. NOYS also trains national youth leaders to teach their peers strategies for preventing underage drinking and driving. They also offer leadership materials on their website (http://www.noys.org). Current funding supports the marketing of the tools on this website to youth organizations. This effort targets youth ages 8 to 24.

Activities Related to Underage Drinking

State Highway Safety Funding: NHTSA provides federal funding to states and local communities through state Highway Safety Offices. Funds may be used for activities related to underage drinking and driving under the following programs: 402 (state and community programs); 410 (impaired driving incentive grants); 154 (open container transfers); 157 (occupant protection incentive grants); and 164 (repeat offender transfer).

Under YOUR Influence: NHTSA has worked with NOYS to create a new website (http://www.underYOURinfluence.org) focused on helping parents teach their teens how to drive safely. The site helps parents set house rules so that teens learn to "Drive by the Rules, Keep the Privilege," a messaging campaign created by NHTSA that includes a PSA and posters empowering parents in their role as the primary educators of their teens. The website includes a youth/community toolkit; a message board; links to internet resources for parents; talking tips for parents; information about state laws regarding underage drinking, seat belt use, and GDL; creative ideas for talking to teens about the importance of safe driving; and more. Parents can subscribe to an online monthly newsletter covering the three NHTSA priority youth traffic safety issues: underage drinking, teen belt use, and GDL.

National Roadside Survey of Impaired Driving: In 2007, NHTSA's Office of Behavioral Safety Research conducted this survey, which produced groundbreaking research data on the incidence of alcohol- and drug-positive drivers on weekend nights (including much-needed data on over-the-counter, prescription, and illegal drug use). The survey was conducted at 60 sites across the country, and involved approximately 7,500 drivers. This study also obtained oral fluid and blood samples from many drivers to determine incidence of drug use by drivers on the road. Previous roadside surveys conducted in 1973, 1986, and 1996 that obtained blood alcohol concentrations, provided an opportunity for comparison over four decades. The next National Roadside Survey of Impaired Driving will be conducted in 2013.

Exhibit 3.1: Expenditures by Select Interagency Coordinating Committee on Preventing Underage Drinking (ICCPUD) Agencies for Programs Specific to Underage Drinking

ICCPUD Agency	Underage Drinking Amount			
	FY 2009 Actual	FY 2010 Actual	FY 2011 Actual	FY 2012 Actual
Department of Education[1]	$42,519,506	$40,580,995	$8,782,000	
Centers for Disease Control and Prevention	$800,000	$1,200,000	$1,041,730	$1,081,200
National Institute on Alcohol Abuse and Alcoholism	$46,418,745[2] $6,671,773[3]	$56,000,000[4] $2,000,000[5]	$57,000,000[6]	$62,000,000
Substance Abuse and Mental Health Services Administration[7]	$51,858,000	$62,542,390	$63,779,872	$67,953,616
Office of Juvenile Justice and Delinquency Prevention[8]	$24,809,483	$25,000,000	$20,708,500	$4,862,895
National Highway Traffic Safety Administration	$900,000	$625,000	$600,000	$645,000
TOTAL	$173,977,507	$187,948,385	$151,912,102	$136,542,711

[1] ED received significant reductions in appropriations for its substance abuse prevention programs in FYs 2011 and 2012; therefore the FY 2011 figure of $8,782,000 includes $6,907,000 of continuation costs for the Grants to Reduce Alcohol Abuse (GRAA) program, which was no longer funded in FY 2012, as well as 1,875,000 for the Higher Education Center for Alcohol and Other Drug Abuse and Violence Prevention, which focused in part on underage drinking on college campuses. In FY 2012 ED consolidated the functions of that Center into a new technical assistance center, the National Center on Safe Supportive Learning Environments. However, the exact amount of funding of that Center specific to underage drinking cannot be determined. Similarly, while underage drinking prevention was one activity among many in certain grant projects funded by ED in FYs 2011 and 2012, the exact amount of funding specific to underage drinking cannot be determined.

[2] NIAAA FY 2009 non-ARRA funded expenditures

[3] NIAAA FY 2009 ARRA funded expenditures

[4] NIAAA FY 2010 non-ARRA funding

[5] NIAAA FY 2010 ARRA funding

[6] NIAAA FY 2011 actual levels

[7] FY 2009-2012 figures include SPF/SIG, UAD, Adult Media Campaign, STOP Act grants, and ICCPUD. FY 2009 figure also includes Leadership for UAD. FY 2010 – 2012 also includes PFS, which is a subset of SPF/SIG.

[8] OJJDP's Enforcing the Underage Drinking Laws (EUDL) program received significant budget cuts in FY 2012. Support for EUDL programming was $25,000,000 annually from FY 1998 until FY 2011, when there was a reduction to $5 million, which resulted in the elimination of the EUDL block grant program for all State and territories.

CHAPTER 4
Report on State Programs and Policies Addressing Underage Drinking

CHAPTER 4.1
Introduction

The Sober Truth on Preventing Underage Drinking (STOP) Act recognizes the critical role that states play in the national effort to reduce underage drinking, particularly in their role as regulators of the alcohol market. Its preamble includes this statement of the sense of Congress:

> Alcohol is a unique product and should be regulated differently than other products by the States and Federal Government. States have primary authority to regulate alcohol distribution and sale, and the Federal Government should support and supplement these State efforts. States also have a responsibility to fight youth access to alcohol and reduce underage drinking. Continued State regulation and licensing of the manufacture, importation, sale, distribution, transportation, and storage of alcoholic beverages are ... critical to ... preventing illegal access to alcohol by persons under 21 years of age.

To this end, the Act directs the Secretary of the Department of Health and Human Services (HHS), working with the Interagency Coordinating Committee on the Prevention of Underage Drinking (ICCPUD), to provide an annual report on state activities pertaining to underage drinking prevention programs, policies, related enforcement efforts, and state expenditures.

This year's report provides the following information for the 50 states and the District of Columbia (henceforth referred to as "states"):

1. Information on 25 underage drinking prevention policies focused on reducing youth access to alcohol and youth involvement in drinking and driving. Consistent with the STOP Act requirement to report on "evidence-based best practices to prevent and reduce underage drinking and provide treatment services to those youth who need them," most policies have been identified as best practices by a variety of relevant federal agencies (see below).

2. Data from a survey addressing underage-drinking-enforcement programs; programs targeted to youth, parents, and caregivers; collaborations, planning, and reports; and state expenditures on the prevention of underage drinking.

Underage Drinking Prevention Policies

This section presents summaries of the 25 policies that describe each policy's key components, the status of the policy across states, and trends over time. Summaries are followed by a state-by-state analysis of each policy. The policy variables for each state are linked electronically to both the relevant policy summaries and the definitions of each variable. New for this year's report are analyses of Outlet Siting Near Schools and Retailer Interstate Shipment.

Seventeen of these policies were included in original STOP Act legislation or were recommended by Congress during the 2009–2010 appropriations process. The remaining six policies were added at the request of SAMHSA following input from various stakeholders. The report obtained data for 13 of the policies, including the 6 added by SAMHSA, from the National Institute on Alcohol Abuse and Alcoholism (NIAAA) Alcohol Policy Information System (APIS).

It is important to note that not all of these state policies will apply on Tribal lands. Some will vary by Tribe and land type. Such variations are beyond the scope of this report.

The following policies are included (underlined policies are available on APIS):

Laws Addressing Minors in Possession of Alcohol

1. <u>Underage possession</u>
2. <u>Underage consumption</u>
3. <u>Internal possession by minors</u>
4. <u>Underage purchase and attempted purchase</u>
5. <u>False identification</u>

Laws Targeting Underage Drinking and Driving

6. <u>Youth blood alcohol concentration limits</u>
7. <u>Loss of driving privileges for alcohol violations by minors</u>
8. <u>Graduated driver's licenses</u>

Laws Targeting Alcohol Suppliers

9. <u>Furnishing of alcohol to minors</u>
10. Compliance check protocols
11. Penalty guidelines for sales to minors
12. <u>Responsible beverage service</u>
13. <u>Minimum ages for off-premises sellers</u>
14. <u>Minimum ages for on-premises servers and bartenders</u>
15. Outlet siting near schools
16. <u>Dram shop liability</u>
17. <u>Social host liability</u>
18. <u>Hosting underage drinking parties</u>
19. Retailer interstate shipment
20. <u>Direct sales/shipments</u>
21. <u>Keg registration</u>
22. Home delivery

Laws Affecting Alcohol Pricing

23. <u>Alcohol taxes</u>
24. <u>Drink specials</u>
25. <u>Wholesale pricing</u>

State Survey

This section provides both the complete responses of the states to the survey (included in the state-by-state analysis described above) and a cross-state report. The cross-state report summarizes the findings across states and presents data on variables amenable to quantitative analysis.

The survey content was derived directly from the STOP Act, covering topics and using terminology from the Act. The survey questions were structured to allow states maximum flexibility in deciding which initiatives to describe and how to describe them. Open-ended questions were used whenever possible to allow states to "speak with their own voices." The survey addressed four main areas:

1. Enforcement programs
2. Programs targeted to youth, parents, and caregivers
3. Collaborations, planning, and reports
4. State expenditures on prevention of underage drinking

Best Practices

The majority of the underage drinking prevention policies analyzed in this chapter have been identified as best practices by one or more of the following four sources:

- Community Preventive Services Task Force (*Guide to Community Preventive Services. Preventing excessive alcohol consumption,* http://www.thecommunityguide.org/alcohol/index.html. Last updated: 05/16/2011).

- The Surgeon General (*The Surgeon General's Call to Action To Prevent and Reduce Underage Drinking*, 2007).

- Institute of Medicine (IOM) (*Reducing Underage Drinking: A Collective Responsibility*, 2004).

- National Institute on Alcohol Abuse and Alcoholism (*A Call to Action: Changing the Culture of Drinking at U.S. Colleges,* 2002).

Exhibit 4.1.1 lists the 25 policies analyzed in Chapter 4. An X indicates that a given policy is endorsed as a best practice by one or more of the four federal sources.

As can be seen in Exhibit 4.1.1, 18 of the policies are endorsed as best practices by at least one source document, and more than half of the policies are endorsed as best practices by two or more source documents. Seven policies were not endorsed by any of the sources. Four of these (Direct Sales, Minimum Age for On-Premises Servers, Minimum Age for Off-Premises Servers, and Internal Possession) are included on NIAAA's APIS website. As relatively recent concerns, these policies likely had not been thoroughly studied at the time the federal source documents were prepared. One policy (Outlet Siting Near Schools) not specifically endorsed by any of the sources examined was addressed at a more general level by two sources—the Community Services Prevention Task Force and the NIAAA *Call to Action.* These sources included restrictions on alcohol outlet density as a best practice without specifically endorsing the reduction of alcohol outlet density near schools. Retailer Interstate Shipment, the final policy not endorsed by the four sources, is closely linked to the Home Delivery policy (which is endorsed).

It is important to note that, although all 25 of the policies can be described as evidence based, the data that support each of them are different. Some policies find greater or lesser support in the research literature and in the source documents.

Exhibit 4.1.1: Underage Drinking Prevention Policies – Best Practices

Underage drinking prevention policies	Recommended by the Community Preventive Services Task Force	Addressed in the Surgeon General's Call to Action	IOM Report, Reducing Underage Drinking: A Collective Responsibility	A Call to Action: Changing the Culture of Drinking at U.S. Colleges (NIAAA)
Policies included in original STOP Act legislation or added in 2009–2010 appropriations				
Purchase or attempt to purchase alcohol by minor		x	x	
Consumption by minor		x	x	
Possession by minor		x	x	
False identification/Incentives for retailers to use ID scanners or other technology		x	x	
Penalty guidelines for violations of furnishing laws by retailers				x
Furnishing or sale to a minor		x	x	
Hosting underage drinking parties		x	x	
Dram-shop liability	x		x	
Social-host liability			x	
Compliance checks	x	x	x	
Mandatory-voluntary server-seller training (Responsible Beverage Service programs)		x	x	x
Direct sales (internet/mail order)				
Home delivery			x	
Graduated drivers' licenses		x	x	x
Increasing alcohol tax rates	x		x	x
Restrictions on drink specials		x	x	x
Wholesaler pricing provisions				
Policies added at the request of SAMHSA				
Keg registration		x	x	
Minimum age for on-sale server				
Minimum age for off-sale server				
Internal possession				
Youth BAC limits ("Zero Tolerance Law")		x	x	x
Loss of privileges for alcohol violations				x
Outlet siting near schools				
Retailer interstate shipment				

CHAPTER 4.2
Cross-State Survey Report

Overview

The 2012 Sober Truth on Preventing Underage Drinking (STOP) Act State Survey of the 50 states and the District of Columbia involved the same questions as those asked in the 2011 survey to gather information on the following three topics:

- Enforcement programs to promote compliance with underage drinking laws and regulations
- Programs targeted to youth, parents, and caregivers to deter underage drinking, and the number of individuals served by these programs
- The amount that each state invests, per youth capita, on the prevention of underage drinking

The survey content was derived directly from the STOP Act, covering topics and using terminology from the Act itself. The survey instrument comprised approximately 90 questions divided into 4 sections.

1. Enforcement of underage drinking laws, including:
   - The extent to which states implement random checks of retail outlets, assessing compliance with laws prohibiting the sale of alcohol to minors, and the results of these checks
   - The extent to which the states implement other underage-drinking-enforcement strategies, including Minors in Possession, Cops in Shops, Shoulder Taps, party patrol/party dispersal, and underage alcohol-related fatality investigations (see the definitions on the next page)
   - Sanctions imposed for violations

2. Underage drinking prevention programs targeted to youth, parents, and caregivers, including data on state best-practice standards and collaborations with tribal governments, and the number of people served by these programs

3. State interagency collaborations used to implement the above programs

4. State funds invested in the following categories, along with descriptions of any dedicated fees, taxes, or fines used to raise funds:
   - Compliance checks and provisions for technology to aid in detecting false IDs at retail outlets
   - Checkpoints and saturation patrols
   - Community-based, school-based, and higher-education-based programs
   - Programs that target youth within the juvenile justice and child welfare systems
   - Other state efforts as deemed appropriate

The survey questions were structured to allow states maximum flexibility in deciding which initiatives to describe and how to describe them. Open-ended questions were used, whenever possible, to allow states to "speak with their own voices."

Survey instructions emphasized that states were expected to rely on readily available data, rather than initiate data collection for the sole purpose of answering the survey questions. In all cases, the survey offered the opportunity to respond "Data Not Available."

Definitions for Enforcement Strategies

- *Compliance Checks/Decoy Operations:* Trained underage operatives ("decoys"), working with law enforcement officials, enter retail alcohol outlets and attempt to purchase alcohol.

- *Cops in Shops:* A well-publicized enforcement effort in which undercover law enforcement officers are placed in retail alcohol outlets.

- *Shoulder Tap:* Trained young people (decoys) approach individuals outside of retail alcohol outlets and ask them to make an alcohol purchase.

- *Party Patrol/Party Dispersal:* Operations that identify underage drinking parties, and/or safely make arrests and issue citations at underage drinking parties.

- *Underage Alcohol–Related Fatality Investigations:* Investigations to determine the source of alcohol ingested by fatally injured minors.

Methods

The state governors and the Office of the Mayor of the District of Columbia were sent letters requesting confirmation of a designated representative for each jurisdiction to serve as the contact and be responsible for completing the survey. In most cases, this representative was the same person designated for the 2011 survey. In all cases, designated contacts were typically staff members from state substance abuse program agencies and state alcohol beverage control (ABC) agencies. Two sections of the survey were uploaded to a web-based platform, and the designated contacts were sent a link to this platform. They were also sent a Microsoft Word document containing their 2011 responses for two additional sections and were asked to make changes to this file as needed.

The online survey and Word documents were available for completion by the states beginning in February 2012. The CDM Group, Inc., a Substance Abuse and Mental Health Services Administration (SAMHSA) contractor, provided both telephone and online technical support to state agency staff while the survey was in the field. A representative from the National Liquor Law Enforcement Association provided review and support for any questions pertaining specifically to enforcement.

As with the 2011 State Survey, responses were received from all 50 states and the District of Columbia, which resulted in a 100 percent response rate. (Note: henceforth, the states and the District of Columbia are referred to, together, as "states.") Each state's response was reviewed by senior staff members, who made inquiries when necessary about apparent omissions, ambiguities, or other content issues. The responses were also copyedited, and the edited responses were returned to each state by e-mail. The states either approved the proposed copyedits or provided their own copyedits, and they provided any requested clarifications.

Results

Introduction

The individual state reports provide a full presentation of the survey data submitted by each state. This Results section provides summary information about all variables amenable to quantitative analysis. It is important to keep in mind that the states determined how much information to provide, and that the range of information the respondents provided was highly variable. The breadth and depth of the information should not be assumed to reflect all underage drinking prevention activity in any state.

The results are grouped into five broad headings:
1. Enforcement Programs
2. Programs Targeted to Youth, Parents, and Caregivers
3. Collaborations, Planning, and Reports
4. State Expenditures on the Prevention of Underage Drinking
5. Comparison of Enforcement Data: 2011 to 2012

The final section, Comparison of Enforcement Data: 2011 to 2012, provides a limited comparison between state survey data collected in 2011 and the current 2012 data for selected activities. It should be noted that 2 years of data are insufficient to make any definitive statements regarding trends, and not all states reported data for both years. This section should be viewed with these cautions in mind.

In all cases, where numerical estimates are reported, the reporting period is the most recent year for which complete data were available to the state. Average values are reported as medians. The median is the numerical value separating the higher half of a sample from the lower half and is the best representation of the "average" value when, as is often the case with the state survey responses, the data include outliers (a data point that is widely separated from the main cluster of data points in a dataset).

Enforcement Programs

The STOP Act State Survey requested enforcement data in four areas:
1. Whether the state encourages and conducts comprehensive enforcement efforts—such as random compliance checks and shoulder tap programs—to prevent underage access to alcohol at retail outlets.
2. The number of compliance checks conducted on alcohol retail outlets.
3. The results of these compliance checks.
4. Enforcement of a variety of state laws aimed at deterring underage drinking (see Chapter 4.3: Policy Summaries). In the current survey, arrest data for minor in possession (MIP) offenses have been used to index enforcement of these laws.

Exhibit 4.2.1 shows the percentage of states that collect data on compliance checks, MIP charges, and penalties levied against retail establishments for furnishing alcohol to minors.

Exhibit 4.2.1: Percentage of Jurisdictions that Reported Enforcement Data Collection at the State and Local Levels

	State collects data on compliance checks		State collects data on MIP arrests/ citations	State collects data on MIP, including arrests/ citations by local law enforcement agencies	State collects data on penalties imposed on retail establishments		
	State-conducted	Locally conducted			Fines	License suspensions	License revocations
Percentage	80	37	82	37	73	73	69

The large majority of states collect data on state compliance checks, MIP charges, and penalties imposed on retail establishments. However, the number of states that collect data on local enforcement efforts is limited. Thus, it is likely that the enforcement statistics that follow underestimate the total amount of underage drinking enforcement occurring in the states.

Enforcement Strategies, Statistics, and Results

Compliance Checks

As reported in Exhibit 4.2.1, 80 percent (41 states) reported that they conduct compliance checks and collect associated data. Exhibit 4.2.2 illustrates the results for the states that provided data on state compliance checks and failures. Localities in 19 states also conduct compliance checks and collect data. Fourteen states report conducting and collecting data for both state and local compliance checks, 32 states conduct and collect data on either state or local compliance checks, and 5 states conduct neither state nor local checks. As shown in Exhibit 4.2.2, the number of licensees checked and licensee failures varies widely.

Exhibit 4.2.2: Compliance Checks

	Number of licensees upon which checks were conducted		Percentage of licensees upon which checks were conducted that failed the checks	
State agencies (*n*=38)*	Median for those that collect data	1,347	Median for those that collect data	13%
	Minimum	37	Minimum	5%
	Maximum	11,977	Maximum	84%
Local agencies (*n*=19)	Median for those that collect data	568	Median for those that collect data	15%
	Minimum	7	Minimum	7%
	Maximum	6,108	Maximum	100%
*Three states are omitted from the analysis because, although they reported that they collect compliance check data, they did not provide these data.				

Exhibits 4.2.3 and 4.2.4 provide state-by-state licensee failure rates for compliance checks conducted by state and local agencies based on data reported by the states. Most state-level checks report failure rates of 20 percent or less, with 10 states reporting higher rates. Exhibit 4.2.4 highlights the lack of data on local compliance checks for most states—only 15 states report any data, with 13 of those states reporting rates of 20 percent or less.

The data in Exhibits 4.2.3 and 4.2.4 must be viewed with considerable caution. First, the current data provide no information on cases in which multiple checks are made on the same outlet. Second, the survey did not request data that would allow comparison of the total number of outlets in a jurisdiction with the total number of outlets checked during this period. Future surveys will address these limitations. Finally, compliance check protocols vary by state. For example, states use differing procedures and requirements for choosing underage decoys (see Compliance Check Protocols in Chapter 4.3, Policy Summaries). States may also conduct compliance checks randomly in response to complaints or as a result of a previous compliance check failure. Hence, differences in compliance check protocols may affect the number of outlets checked, the frequency of checks at a particular establishment, and the failure rates.

Exhibit 4.2.3: State Compliance Checks Failure Rate

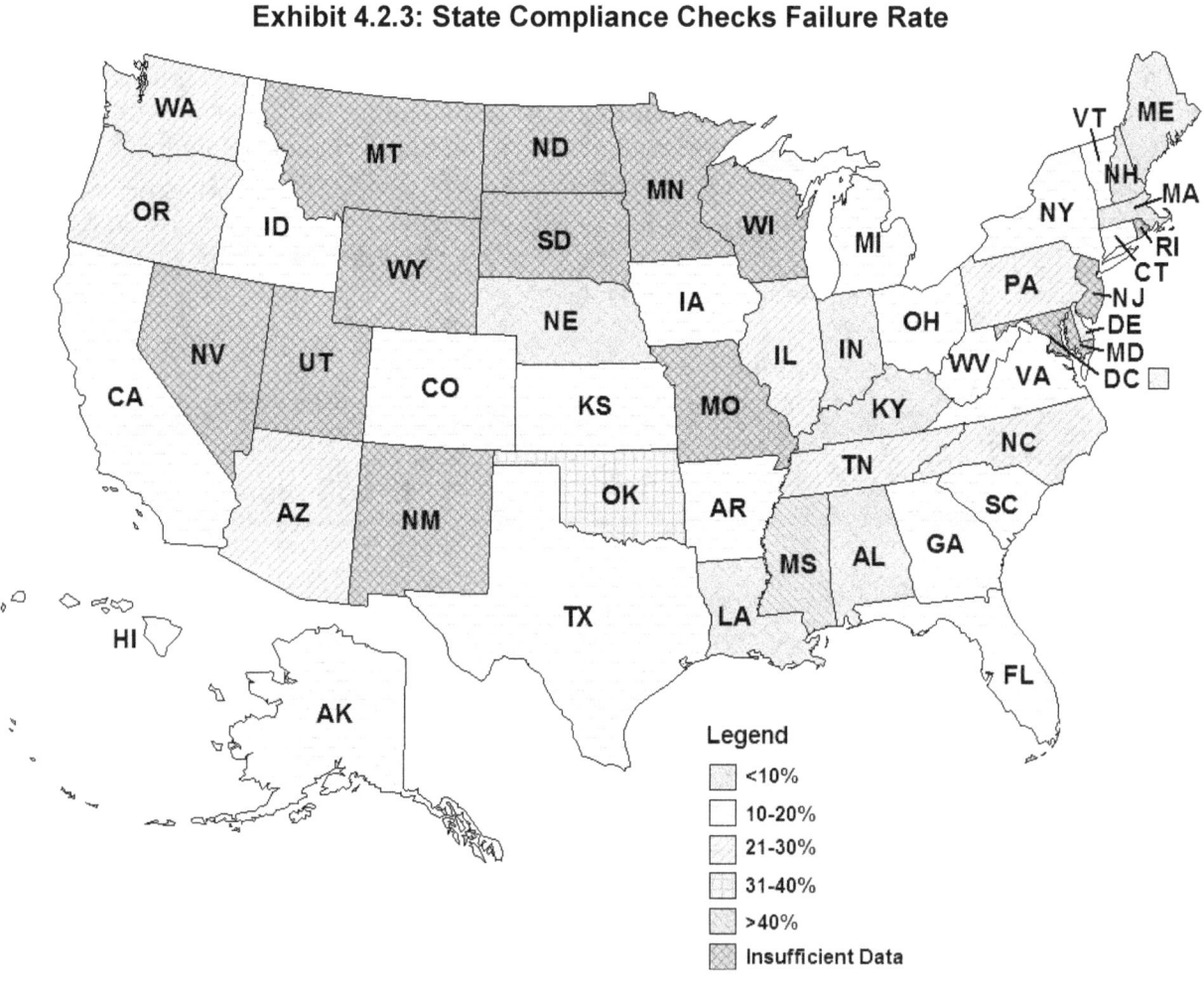

Exhibit 4.2.4: Local Compliance Checks Failure Rate

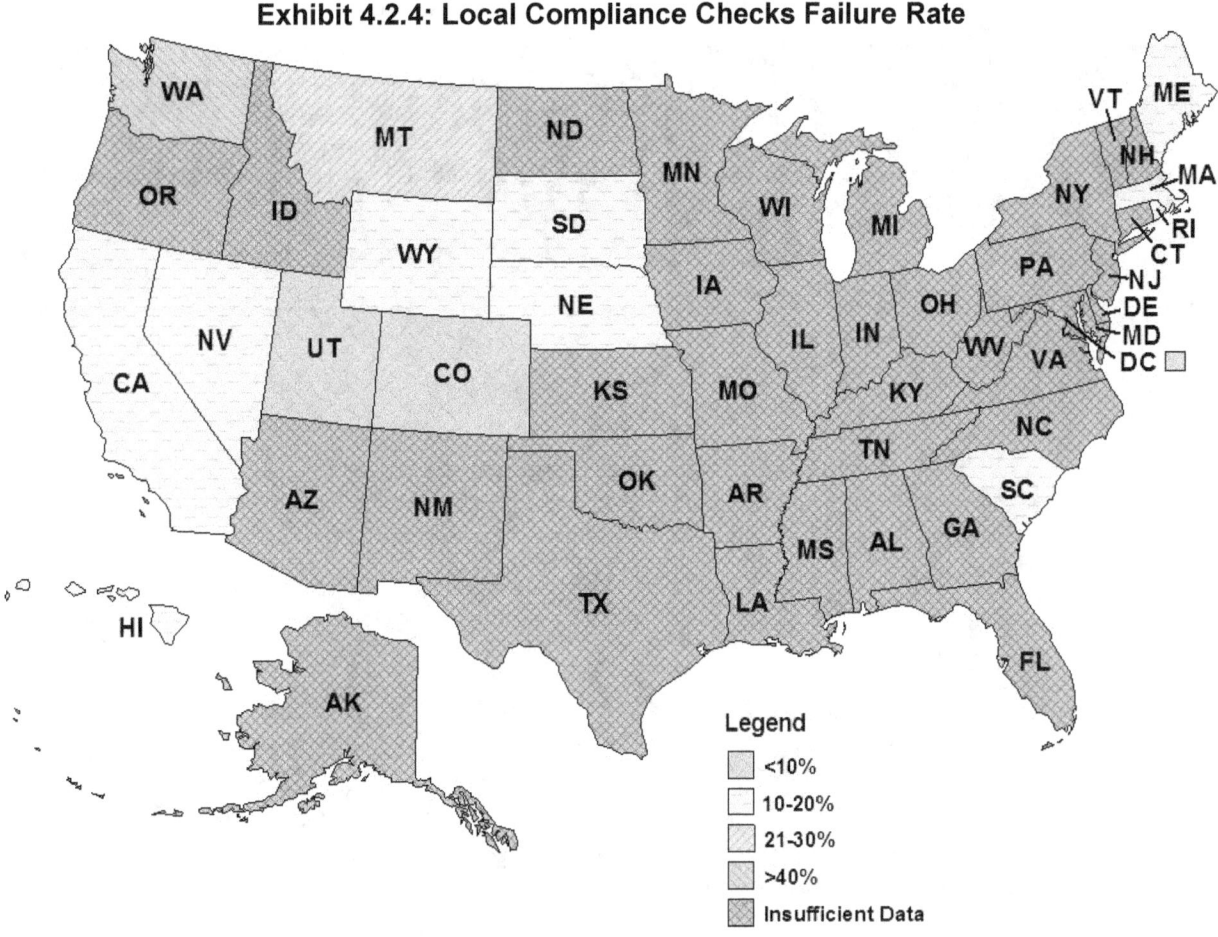

Legend

- <10%
- 10-20%
- 21-30%
- >40%
- Insufficient Data

Other Enforcement Activities

States were asked to report on four other state and local strategies to enforce underage drinking laws: Cops in Shops, Shoulder Tap operations, party patrol operations or programs, and underage alcohol–related fatality investigations.

As shown in Exhibit 4.2.5, the most common enforcement activities at both the state and local levels are party patrol operations or programs and underage alcohol–related fatality investigations. Given that much of the enforcement of laws pertaining to minors in possession occurs at the local level, it is not surprising that more states report implementation of related programs (shoulder tap and party patrol operations) by localities than at the state level. Exhibit 4.2.6 displays states that implement one, two, three, or all four of the strategies listed in Exhibit 4.2.5. Exhibit 4.2.7 displays states in which localities implement one, two, three, or all four of the strategies.

Exhibit 4.2.5: Enforcement Activities

State enforcement: Percentage of states that implement				Local enforcement: Percentage of states in which localities implement			
Cops in Shops	Shoulder Tap operations	Party patrol operations or programs	Underage alcohol-related fatality investigations	Cops in Shops	Shoulder Tap operations	Party patrol operations or programs	Underage alcohol–related fatality investigations
45	27	55	69	39	45	75	67

Exhibit 4.2.6: States that Implement Strategies

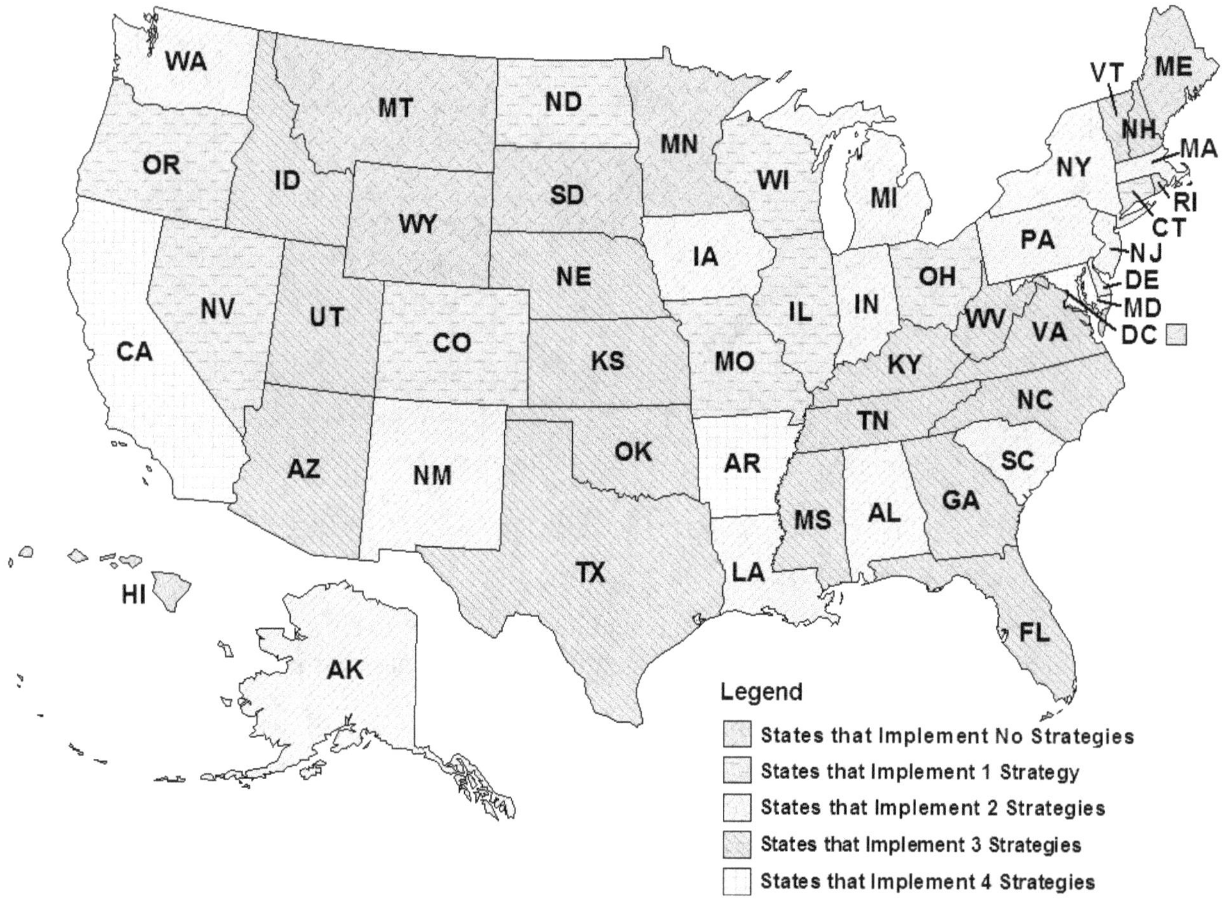

Legend
- States that Implement No Strategies
- States that Implement 1 Strategy
- States that Implement 2 Strategies
- States that Implement 3 Strategies
- States that Implement 4 Strategies

Exhibit 4.2.7: States Where Local Agencies Implement Strategies

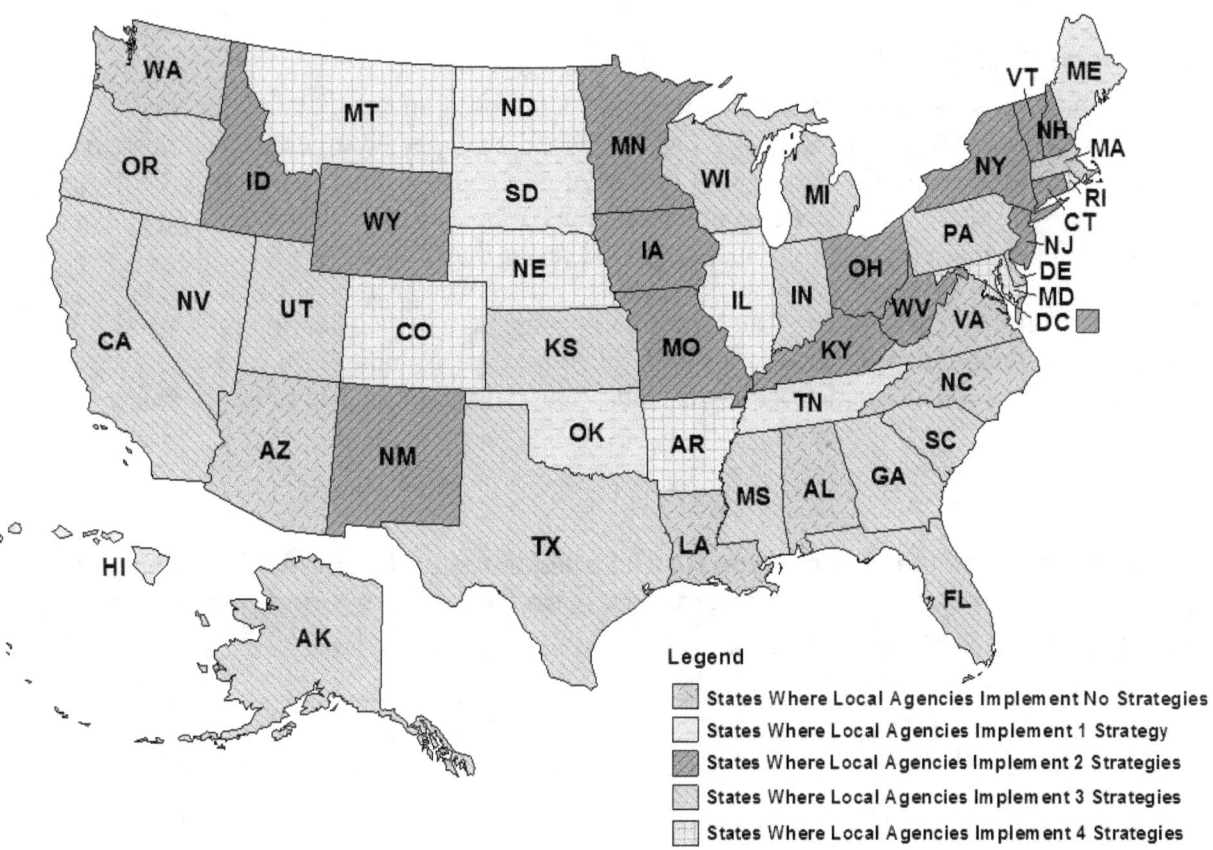

Legend

- States Where Local Agencies Implement No Strategies
- States Where Local Agencies Implement 1 Strategy
- States Where Local Agencies Implement 2 Strategies
- States Where Local Agencies Implement 3 Strategies
- States Where Local Agencies Implement 4 Strategies

In addition, all states regulate or prohibit direct sales and direct shipment of alcohol from producers to consumers, typically through internet orders and delivery by common carriers. (These laws do not address home delivery or internet sales by retailers.) States were asked whether they have a program to investigate and enforce direct-sales or direct-shipment laws and whether these laws are also enforced by local law enforcement agencies. As shown in Exhibit 4.2.8, approximately three fifths of the states have direct-shipment enforcement programs, but only 12 percent report local enforcement.

Exhibit 4.2.8: Enforcement of Direct-Shipment Laws

	State has a program to investigate and enforce direct-sales/shipment laws (%)	Laws are also enforced by local law enforcement agencies (%)
Yes	59	12
No	25	39
Don't know/No answer	16	49

Sanctions Imposed for Violations

Penalties on Retail Establishments

The State Survey requested information on penalties imposed on retail establishments for furnishing to minors (Exhibits 4.2.9–4.2.11). As would be expected, fines are the most common sanction, and they are imposed about six times as often as suspensions. However, revocations are rare. Of the states that collect data on revocations, more than two thirds revoked one or no licenses. Eighty-four percent of the states revoked fewer than six licenses.

Sanctions for furnishing to minors can be put into perspective by considering rates per 1,000 drinking occasions among youth who are 16 to 20 years old. Exhibit 4.2.12 presents these rates for 32 states that collect complete sanctions data (fines, suspensions, and revocations).

Exhibit 4.2.9: Fines Imposed on Retail Establishments for Furnishing to Minors

Number of outlets fined for furnishing		Total amount of fines in dollars across all licensees
Median for those that collect data (*n*=37)	155	$160,738
Minimum	0	$0
Maximum	1,111	$3,429,950

Exhibit 4.2.10: License Suspensions Imposed on Retail Establishments for Furnishing to Minors

Number of outlets suspended for furnishing		Total days of suspension across all licensees
Median for those that collect data (*n*=37)	27	109
Minimum	0	0
Maximum	263	4,349

Exhibit 4.2.11: License Revocations Imposed on Retail Establishments for Furnishing to Minors

Number of outlets revoked for furnishing	
Median for those that collect data (*n*=35)	0*
Minimum	0
Maximum	129
*The median will be zero if more than half the responses are zero.	

Exhibit 4.2.12: Retailer Sanctions for Furnishing to Minors

Sanctions per 100,000 drinking occasions	
Median for those that collect data (*n*=32)	7
Minimum	0.05
Maximum	29

Minor in Possession Offenses

States were also asked to provide statistics on MIP offenses. As noted earlier, arrest data for MIP offenses provide an index of the enforcement of laws designed to deter underage persons from drinking.

Some states reported data that included arrests/citations issued by local law enforcement agencies; others did not.

The first three rows of Exhibit 4.2.13 present the number of arrests/citations reported by all states that collect such data. These data may not provide an accurate picture of MIP enforcement, because much of it is conducted at the local level and, therefore, is not represented in state data. The second three rows present data only from those states that collect both state and local data. When only those states that collect local data are considered, the median number of arrests/citations increases by 93 percent, highlighting the importance of local enforcement efforts and data.

To explore the meaning of these data, two indices were calculated for states with both state and local MIP enforcement. The first index compares the rates of MIP arrests/citations with an estimate of yearly drinking occasions among 16- to 20-year-olds.[29] The second index reflects arrests per 100,000 youth who are 16 to 20 years old. The results appear in Exhibit 4.2.14. Because the data in Exhibit 4.2.14 are from states with both state and local MIP enforcement, the rates for the nation as a whole will be lower.

Exhibit 4.2.13: Number of Minors Found In Possession of (or Having Consumed or Purchased per State Statutes) Alcohol

	Number of arrests/citations
Median for all states that collect data (*n*=42)	1,302
Minimum	65
Maximum	13,355
Median for states that collect both state and local data (*n*=19)	2,515
Minimum	226
Maximum	13,355

---

[29] This estimate is based on the calculations of Wagenaar and Wilson (1994). Using Monitoring the Future data, they estimated a rate of 90 drinking occasions per 100 youth per month.

**Exhibit 4.2.14: State and Local Arrests/Citations for Minors in Possession:
16- to 20-Year-Olds**

	Number of arrests/citations	Arrests/Citations per 1,000 drinking occasions	Arrests/Citations per 100,000 population 16–20
Median for those that collect data (*n*=19)	2,515	1.33	1,437
Minimum	226	0.13	145
Maximum	13,355	9.31	10,049

Sanctions Against Youth vs. Sanctions Against Retailers

Comparing rates of MIP arrests and rates of retailer sanctions (totals of fines, suspensions, and revocations) highlights enforcement priorities. Twenty-two states provided the complete dataset needed for this analysis (Exhibit 4.2.15).

In most states, MIP arrests greatly outnumber retailer sanctions, indicating that priority is given to individual arrests over enforcement at the retail level. The ratio of MIP arrests to retailer sanctions was less than one in only one state.

Programs Targeted to Youths, Parents, and Caregivers

States were asked to describe their underage drinking prevention programs. Information was requested about the following:

1. Programs *specific* to underage drinking (e.g., prevention of underage drinking is the primary objective)
2. Programs *related* to underage drinking (e.g., address other drug use [including tobacco] in addition to alcohol use):

- School-based drug and alcohol education
- Programs that address individual risk and protective factors
- Programs to strengthen families

Exhibit 4.2.15: Ratio of State and Local MIP Arrests to Retailer Sanctions

	MIP arrests per retailer sanctions
Median for those that collect data (*n*=22)	14
Minimum	0.99
Maximum	267

The survey provided space to describe up to 20 specific programs and 2 related programs, and to list 8 additional related programs. For the specific programs, space was also provided to indicate:

- The numbers of youth, parents, and caregivers served by each program.
- Whether the program has been evaluated.
- Whether an evaluation report is available and where the report can be found.

In addition to program descriptions, states were asked whether they had programs to measure and/or reduce youth exposure to alcohol advertising and marketing, and best practice standards for selecting or approving underage-drinking programs.

Exhibit 4.2.16 lists the survey's definitions for youth, parents, and caregivers.

Program Content

States varied widely in the number of programs described, in part because some states provided detailed information on local variations of some program types (e.g., community coalitions), whereas others described the general program.

Many well-known programs were reported, including those focused on life skills, refusal skills, media advocacy, community organizing, and environmental change. Also well represented were indigenous initiatives that appear, at least for the moment, to be unique to their states of origin.

As a method for summarizing the types of programs states are implementing, all programs were coded into one of four categories:

- *Programs focused on individuals*—Programs designed to impart knowledge, change attitudes and beliefs, or teach skills. Although individual youths or adults (usually parents) are the focus of these programs, the programs are almost always conducted with groups (e.g., classrooms, Boys/Girls Clubs, PTAs, members of a congregation). Also in this category are programs for offenders (MIP, driving while intoxicated [DWI]). Certain kinds of education and skills development were considered part of the environment. These include training for alcohol sellers and servers, health care workers, public safety personnel, and others whose activities affect large numbers of people.

- *Programs focused on the environment*—Programs that seek to alter physical, economic, and social environments, which may be focused on entire populations (e.g., everyone in a state or community) or a subpopulation (e.g., underage people, youth who drive). The main mechanisms for environmental change include state laws and local ordinances and their enforcement, institutional policies (e.g., enforcement priorities or prosecutorial

Exhibit 4.2.16: Definitions of Youth, Parents, and Caregivers from Survey

> **Youth:** People younger than 21 years old
>
> **Parents:** People who have primary responsibility for the well-being of a minor (e.g., biological and adoptive parents, grandparents, foster parents, extended family)
>
> **Caregivers:** People who provide services to youth (e.g., teachers, coaches, health and mental health care providers, human services and juvenile justice workers)

practice, how alcohol is to be served at public events, carding everyone who looks younger than 35 years old, alcohol screening of all ER injury admissions), and changing norms. These changes are generally designed to decrease physical availability of alcohol (e.g., home delivery bans, retailer compliance checks), raise economic costs (drink special restrictions, taxation), and/or limit social availability, such as policies that affect the extent to which alcohol and alcohol users are visible in the community (e.g., banning alcohol in public places and at community events, banning outdoor alcohol advertising).

- *Mixed*—Cases where both individual and environmental approaches are a substantive part of the effort. So-called "comprehensive" prevention programs are a relevant example.

- *Media campaigns*

In total, 301 programs (78 percent of all programs) were described in sufficient detail to allow coding.[30] The results are presented in Exhibit 4.2.17. As shown in Exhibit 4.2.17, programs focused on individuals were more than twice as common as programs focused on the environment. States tended to favor either an individual or an environmental approach in the programs they described; 42 percent of the states that reported any programs that could be coded focused exclusively on one or the other.

Numbers Served

For each specific program described, states were asked to estimate the numbers of youths, parents, and caregivers served. These data were spotty, with 75 percent of the states ($n=38$) providing data for at least one program for youths served, 59 percent ($n=30$) for parents served, and 43 percent ($n=22$) for caregivers served. These data may be difficult for certain types of programs to estimate. In particular, the target populations for programs focused on the environment may be entire populations or subpopulations. Estimating the actual numbers reached is therefore problematic. Exhibit 4.2.18 gives the reported number of youths, parents, and caregivers served across all states that reported data.

Exhibit 4.2.17: Types of Programs Implemented by the States

Program category	Percentage of programs implemented
Focused on individuals	58
Focused on the environment	21
Mixed focus	16
Media campaigns	5

Exhibit 4.2.18: Reported Numbers of Youths, Parents, and Caregivers Served

	Youths served	Parents served	Caregivers served
Median	5,526	0	0
Minimum	0	0	0
Maximum	997,257	786,834	664,406

[30] In some cases, the states did not provide enough information about the nature of the program to allow coding. In other cases, space limitations in the survey instrument prevented states from fully describing all their programs.

Evaluation Data

For each specific program, states were asked whether the program has been evaluated and whether an evaluation report is available. Summary data for these questions appear in Exhibit 4.2.19. Clearly, the states vary widely in their emphasis on evaluation.

Programs To Measure and/or Reduce Youth Exposure to Alcohol Advertising and Marketing

States were asked whether they have programs to measure or reduce youth exposure to alcohol advertising and marketing. Twenty-seven percent (*n=14*) of the states reported they had such programs, which tend to implement four approaches:
1. Environmental scans to assess the degree of youth exposure to alcohol advertising
2. Counter-advertising initiatives
3. Eliminating environmental advertising aimed at youth
4. Social marketing

Best Practice Standards

States were asked whether they have adopted or developed best practice standards for underage-drinking-prevention programs. Seventy-six percent (*n=39*) reported they had such standards. States were asked to describe these standards, but the data were of variable quality. Some state responses were ambiguous or too brief to code reliably; however, approximately 46 percent of the 39 states that reported having standards indicated they followed SAMHSA's guidance document on evidence-based practices (*Identifying and Selecting Evidence-Based Interventions for Substance Abuse Prevention,* Revised Guidance Document for the Strategic Prevention Framework State Incentive Grant Program, SAMHSA, January 2009). A few additional states referenced some other federally produced document, and another 26 percent of the states described locally developed guidelines.

Collaborations, Planning, and Reports

The STOP Act Survey included two questions about collaborations. The first asked whether states collaborated on underage drinking issues with federally recognized Tribal governments (if any). Forty-seven percent (*n=24*) said they did collaborate, 25 percent said they did not collaborate, and the remainder reported no federally recognized Tribes in their states.

The second question asked whether the states had a state-level interagency body or committee to coordinate or address underage-drinking-prevention activities. Eighty percent of the states reported that such a committee exists, although the composition of the committee varied somewhat from state to state. Most states' interagency committees included a variety of state

Exhibit 4.2.19: Evaluation of Underage Drinking–Specific Programs

	Percentage of state programs evaluated	Percentage of evaluated programs with reports available
Median	50	0
Minimum	0	0
Maximum	100	100

agencies directly involved in underage-drinking-prevention policy implementation and enforcement, as well as educational- and treatment-program development and oversight. These include the states' departments of health and human services and alcohol beverage control, their substance abuse agency, and their state police/highway patrol. Of interest is the extent to which the committee included representatives of the governor, legislature, and attorney general, given that they are so critical in setting priorities, providing funding, and generating political and public support.

As shown in Exhibit 4.2.20, about one in four states with a committee included the governor and/or attorney general, and one in five included a legislature representative. We also assessed the extent to which the interagency committee included relevant entities and constituencies outside of state government (see Exhibit 4.2.21). Forty-six percent of the states with interagency committees included community coalitions, and 41 percent included college/university administrations, campus life departments, or campus police. About one in four states included youth, and one in five included local law enforcement.

States were asked whether they had prepared a plan for preventing underage drinking and/or issued a report on underage drinking in the past 3 years. About two thirds of the states had prepared a plan, and about three quarters had issued a report. The majority of states provided a source for obtaining the plans or reports (see individual state reports).

State Expenditures on the Prevention of Underage Drinking

States were asked to estimate state expenditures for two categories of enforcement activities and five types of programs targeted to youths, parents, and caregivers. Exhibit 4.2.22 provides the data in $1,000 units reported for the enforcement activities, program activities, and an "other" category. An entry of "zero" in the "Minimum reported" row means that at least one state that maintains data reports no expenditures in that category.

Exhibit 4.2.20: Composition of the Interagency Group—State Government Entities

	Office of the Governor	Legislature	Attorney General
Percentage of states with a committee (*n=41*)	24	20	27

Exhibit 4.2.21: Composition of the Interagency Group—Other Entities

	Local law enforcement	College/university administration, campus life department, campus police	Community coalitions and concerned citizens	Youth
Percentage of states with a committee (*n=41*)	20	41	46	24

Exhibit 4.2.22: 12-Month Expenditures* (in thousands) for Enforcement Activities; Programs Targeted to Youths, Parents, and Caregivers; and Other Programs

	Enforcement activities		Programs targeted to youths, parents, and caregivers					Other programs
	Compliance checks	Checkpoints and saturation patrols	Community-based programs	K–12 programs	College or university programs	Juvenile justice System programs	Child welfare system programs	
Number of states providing data	19	13	37	29	26	21	18	25
Median expenditure**	$112K	$150K	$215K	$18K	$0K	$0*	$0*	$169
Minimum reported	$0	$0	$0	$0	$0	$0	$0	$0
Maximum reported	$868K	$8,248K	$7,316	$33,771K	$511K	$4.220	$702	$5,668
Percentage of states providing data that invest in this category	84	85	78	59	50	38	11	68

* These data must be viewed cautiously. Response rates ranged from about 11 percent to about 85 percent. Thus the extent to which some of these data reflect national trends is unclear.
** The median is zero if more than half the responses are zero.

The largest expenditure category is for community-based programs, followed by K–12 programs. While the median of expenditures for all enforcement activities ($119,500) is considerably higher than that for all programs targeted to youths, parents, and caregivers (approximately $2,178), the total dollar amount expended for these nonenforcement programs (approximately $108.4 million) is more than seven times the total dollar amount spent on enforcement (approximately $14.3 million).[32]

States were also asked whether funds dedicated to underage drinking are derived from taxes, fines, and/or fees. About 90 percent of the states provided data for these questions. The use of these funding sources for underage-drinking-prevention activities is limited (see Exhibit 4.2.23).

Exhibit 4.2.23: Sources of Funds Dedicated to Underage Drinking

Source	Number of states providing data	Percentage reporting yes*
Taxes	47	19
Fines	47	15
Fees	45	16

*Percentages reflect only those states that provided data for these questions.

---

[32] The median of the combined expenditures for programs targeted to youths, parents, and caregivers is affected by the number of states reporting zero expenditures, as is clear from Exhibit 4.2.22.

Comparison of Enforcement Data: 2011 to 2012

The STOP Act State Survey is now in its second year of data collection. The following exhibits offer a snapshot of the results for 2011 and 2012 for several key components of the enforcement data. This section should be viewed with these cautions in mind: (1) a 2-year time span is insufficient to describe any kind of trend and (2) data collection varies from year to year among the states, so it is not possible to compare all states between these 2 years. Fewer than half the states provided information in both years for five of the datasets.[33]

About 70 percent of the states provided minors in possession arrest and state compliance check data for both 2011 and 2012. As shown in Exhibit 4.2.24, of these states, 60 percent reported an increase in the number of MIP arrests, 37 percent reported a decrease, and 3 percent remained the same. State compliance checks followed a different direction, with 44 percent of the states reporting an increase in compliance checks, 53 percent reporting a decrease, and 3 percent staying the same (Exhibit 4.2.25).

Fewer data are available addressing compliance checks conducted by local law enforcement. Exhibit 4.2.26 illustrates this, with only 10 states providing data for both years. Of this small group, 70 percent reported a decrease in the number of local compliance checks. Given that 32 states did not report in either year, these comparisons must be viewed with caution.

Exhibit 4.2.24: Minors in Possession 2011–2012

	Number	Percentage
States reporting in both years (n=35)		
States showing increased arrests	21	60
States showing decreased arrests	13	37
States showing same # of arrests	1	3
States not reporting in both years (n=16)		
States reporting in 2011, but not in 2012	5	—
States reporting in 2012, but not in 2011	4	—
States reporting in neither year	7	—

---

[33]See Appendix E for detailed charts of all state enforcement data reported in 2011 and 2012.

Exhibit 4.2.25: State Compliance Checks 2011–2012

	Number	Percentage
States reporting in both years (n=36)		
States showing increased compliance checks	16	44
States showing decreased compliance checks	19	53
States showing same # of compliance checks	1	3
States not reporting in both years (n=15)		
States reporting in 2011, but not in 2012	2	—
States reporting in 2012, but not in 2011	3	—
States reporting neither year	10	—

Exhibit 4.2.26: Local Compliance Checks 2011–2012

	Number	Percentage
States reporting in both years (n=10)		
States showing increased compliance checks	3	30
States showing decreased compliance checks	7	70
States not reporting in both years (n=41)		
States reporting in 2011, but not in 2012	4	—
States reporting in 2012, but not in 2011	5	—
States reporting in neither year	32	—

A small number of states (11) reported 2011 and 2012 data on total expenditures for compliance checks (Exhibit 4.2.27). Of these states, 55 percent indicated that expenditures increased, with the remaining 45 percent reporting that these expenditures had either decreased or remained the same. These data should be viewed with the caveat that 21 states did not report on compliance check expenditures in either 2011 or 2012.

Exhibit 4.2.28 describes state reporting on penalties for retail establishments between 2011 and 2012. In all penalty categories, larger percentages of the states reported reduced use of these penalties than reported increased use. However, given the great variation in reporting rates for both years (31 percent up to nearly 60 percent), these data should be viewed with caution.

Exhibit 4.2.27: Compliance Check Expenditures 2011–2012

	Number	Percentage
States reporting in both years (n=11)		
States showing increased expenditures	6	55
States showing decreased expenditures	4	36
States showing same amount of expenditures	1	9
States not reporting in both years (n=40)		
States reporting in 2011, but not in 2012	11	—
States reporting in 2012, but not in 2011	8	—
States reporting in neither year	21	—

Exhibit 4.2.28: Penalties on Retail Establishments 2011–2012

Penalty	Percentage of states reporting increase*	Percentage of states reporting decrease*	Percentage of states reporting no change*	Number of states reporting 2011 only	Number of states reporting 2012 only	Number of states reporting neither year
Fines: total number	43 (n=9)	57 (n=12)	0	7	10	13
Fines: total dollar amount	48 (n=11)	52 (n=12)	0	9	8	11
Suspensions: total number	38 (n=10)	62 (n=16)	0	6	6	13
Suspensions: total number of days	38 (n=6)	63 (n=10)	0	11	10	14
Revocations: total number	17 (n=5)	45 (n=13)	38 (n=11)	9	3	10
* Includes only those states that reported in both years.						

Discussion

The extent and richness of state activities related to underage drinking can be fully appreciated only through examination of the state survey responses in this chapter. This report summarizes data on variables amenable to quantitative analysis. Four broad categories of initiatives are discussed:

1. Enforcement Programs
2. Programs Targeted to Youth, Parents, and Caregivers
3. Collaborations, Planning, and Reports
4. State Expenditures on the Prevention of Underage Drinking

A key conclusion to be drawn from the STOP Act State Survey is that the states have demonstrated a commitment to the reduction of underage drinking and its consequences. This commitment is evident in the fact that all states and the District of Columbia completed the survey, reported numerous program activities, and in many cases provided substantial detail about those activities (see individual state summaries).

The results presented above must be viewed with caution. In many cases, substantial missing data decrease the extent to which a meaningful conclusion can be drawn. Caution must also be exercised in interpreting the changes from 2011 to 2012. Single between-year trends are rarely stable and may or may not hold up over time.

Enforcement Programs

The large majority of states collect data on state compliance checks, MIP charges, and penalties imposed on retail establishments. However, only about one third of the states collect data on local enforcement efforts. Thus, the ability to draw conclusions about enforcement activities and effectiveness is limited, because a substantial portion of underage drinking law enforcement happens at the local level. Improvements in state enforcement data systems would increase the accuracy of these analyses in future years.

Overall, enforcement activities appear highly variable across the states. Compliance checks and other enforcement activities related to furnishing (Cops in Shops, Shoulder Tap operations, underage alcohol–related fatality investigations, and enforcement of direct-shipment laws) are fairly widely implemented, although not necessarily at both the state and local levels. However, the total number of checks is modest. The effectiveness of these enforcement activities is difficult to assess from the current data. Sanctions for furnishing are predominantly fines, which are about six times more common than suspensions. Revocations are extremely rare; more than two thirds of the states revoked one or no licenses. Data on MIP actions (an index of the enforcement of a variety of laws aimed at deterring underage drinking) revealed medians of 1.33 arrests per 1,000 underage drinking occasions, and 1,437 arrests per 100,000 in a population of 16- to 20-year-olds.

Programs Targeted to Youth, Parents, and Caregivers

States reported implementing a wide variety of underage-drinking-prevention programs for youth, parents, and caregivers. Many well-known programs were reported, including those focused on life skills, refusal skills, media advocacy, community organizing, and environmental change. The programs are predominantly focused on individuals, and approximately one in five programs focused on environmental change. Data on numbers of program participants were limited, owing perhaps to inherent difficulties in estimating program participation for programs focused on entire populations or subpopulations (e.g., environmental change programs). About one in four states (27 percent) reported implementing programs to measure and/or reduce youth exposure to alcohol advertising and marketing.

Evaluation of underage drinking prevention programs is limited. Only about half of the programs the states described have been evaluated, and reports are available for only about 16 percent of these. As with enforcement, assessments of program effectiveness are limited by a lack of relevant data.

Seventy-six percent of states reported they had best practice standards for underage-drinking-prevention programs. Seventy-nine percent of states with standards reported that they followed a federal standard or had developed their own standard, and the remaining states described a process for selecting programs or listed the programs themselves that were considered best practices.

Collaborations, Planning, and Reports

Eighty percent of states reported the existence of a state-level interagency body or committee to coordinate or address underage-drinking-prevention activities. However, of the states with such a committee, only about one in four included the governor and/or attorney general, and one in five included a representative of the legislature. Forty-six percent of the states included community coalitions, and around 40 percent included college/university administrations, campus life departments, or campus police. One in four states included youth, and one in five included local law enforcement. Thus, key decisionmakers and local stakeholders were underrepresented on the interagency committees.

States were asked whether they had prepared a plan for preventing underage drinking and/or issued a report on underage drinking in the past 3 years. Approximately two thirds of the states had prepared a plan, and nearly three quarters had issued a report.

State Expenditures on the Prevention of Underage Drinking

States were asked to estimate state expenditures for two categories of enforcement activities and five types of programs targeted to youth, parents, and caregivers. The largest expenditure category is for community-based programs, followed by K–12 programs. While the median of expenditures for all enforcement activities ($119,500) is considerably higher than that for all programs targeted to youth, parents, and caregivers (approximately $2,178), the total dollar amount expended for these nonenforcement programs (approximately $108.4 million) is more than seven times the total dollar amount spent on enforcement (approximately $14.3 million). Data reporting was again spotty, with response rates ranging from 11 to 78 percent (median = 50 percent) across the five expenditure categories for programs targeting youth, parents, and caregivers. Thus, these results must be viewed with some caution. On the other hand, these data may be difficult for states to assemble given multiple funding streams and asynchronous fiscal years, among other issues.

Comparison of Enforcement Data: 2011–2012

In the 2 years in which the STOP Act State Survey has been implemented, the states varied greatly in their completion of datasets for both years. Fewer than half of the states provided information in both years for five of the nine enforcement data categories selected for comparison. Around 70 percent of the states reported data in both years for MIP arrests and for state-conducted compliance checks. Sixty percent of the states reporting for both years indicated that MIP arrests had increased, whereas 53 percent of the states reported a decrease in state compliance checks. Only 20 percent of the states reported on local compliance checks and state expenditures for compliance checks in both years. Larger percentages of the states reported reduced use of retailer penalties than reported increased use.

Comment

The data reveal a wide range of activity in the areas studied, although the activities vary in scope and intensity from state to state. Clearly, all states have areas of strength and areas where improvements can be realized. A recurrent theme is the inadequacy of some state data systems to respond to the data requested in the survey, especially for local law enforcement and expenditures. Accurate and complete data are essential both for describing current activities to prevent underage drinking and for monitoring progress in future state surveys.

Citation

Wagenaar, A., & Wolfson, M. (1994). Enforcement of the legal minimum drinking age in the United States. *Journal of Public Health Policy, 15(1)*, 37–53.

CHAPTER 4.3
Policy Summaries

Laws Addressing Minors in Possession of Alcohol

Underage Possession, Consumption, and Internal Possession

Policy Description

As of January 1, 2012, all U.S. states and the District of Columbia prohibit possession of alcoholic beverages (with certain exceptions) by those under age 21. In addition, most but not all jurisdictions have statutes that specifically prohibit consumption of alcoholic beverages by those under age 21.

In recent years, a number of jurisdictions have passed laws prohibiting "internal possession" of alcohol by persons less than 21 years old. These provisions typically require evidence of alcohol in the minor's body, but they do not require any specific evidence of possession or consumption. Internal possession laws are especially useful to law enforcement in making arrests or issuing citations when breaking up underage drinking parties. Internal possession laws allow officers to bring charges against underage individuals who are neither holding nor drinking alcoholic beverages in the presence of law enforcement officers. As with laws prohibiting underage possession and consumption, jurisdictions that prohibit internal possession may apply various statutory exceptions to these provisions.

Although all jurisdictions prohibit possession of alcohol by minors, some jurisdictions do not specifically prohibit underage alcohol consumption. In addition, some jurisdictions that do prohibit underage consumption allow different exceptions for consumption than those that apply to underage possession. Jurisdictions that may prohibit underage possession and/or consumption may or may not address the issue of internal possession.

Some jurisdictions allow exceptions to possession, consumption, or internal possession prohibitions when a family member consents and/or is present. Jurisdictions vary widely in terms of which relatives may consent or must be present for this exception to apply and in what circumstances the exception applies. Sometimes a reference is made simply to "family" or "family member" without further elaboration.

Some jurisdictions allow exceptions to possession, consumption, or internal possession prohibitions on private property. Jurisdictions vary in the extent of the private property exception, which may extend to all private locations, private residences only, or in the home of a parent or guardian only. In some, a location exception is conditional on the presence and/or consent of a parent, legal guardian, or spouse.

With respect specifically to consumption laws, some jurisdictions prohibit underage consumption only on licensed premises.

Status of Underage Possession Policies

As of January 1, 2012, all 50 states and the District of Columbia prohibit possession of alcoholic beverages by those under age 21. Twenty-six jurisdictions have some type of family exception, 21 have some type of location exception, and 19 have neither (see Exhibit 4.3.1). Four of these

Exhibit 4.3.1: Exceptions to Minimum Age of 21 for Possession of Alcohol as of January 1, 2012

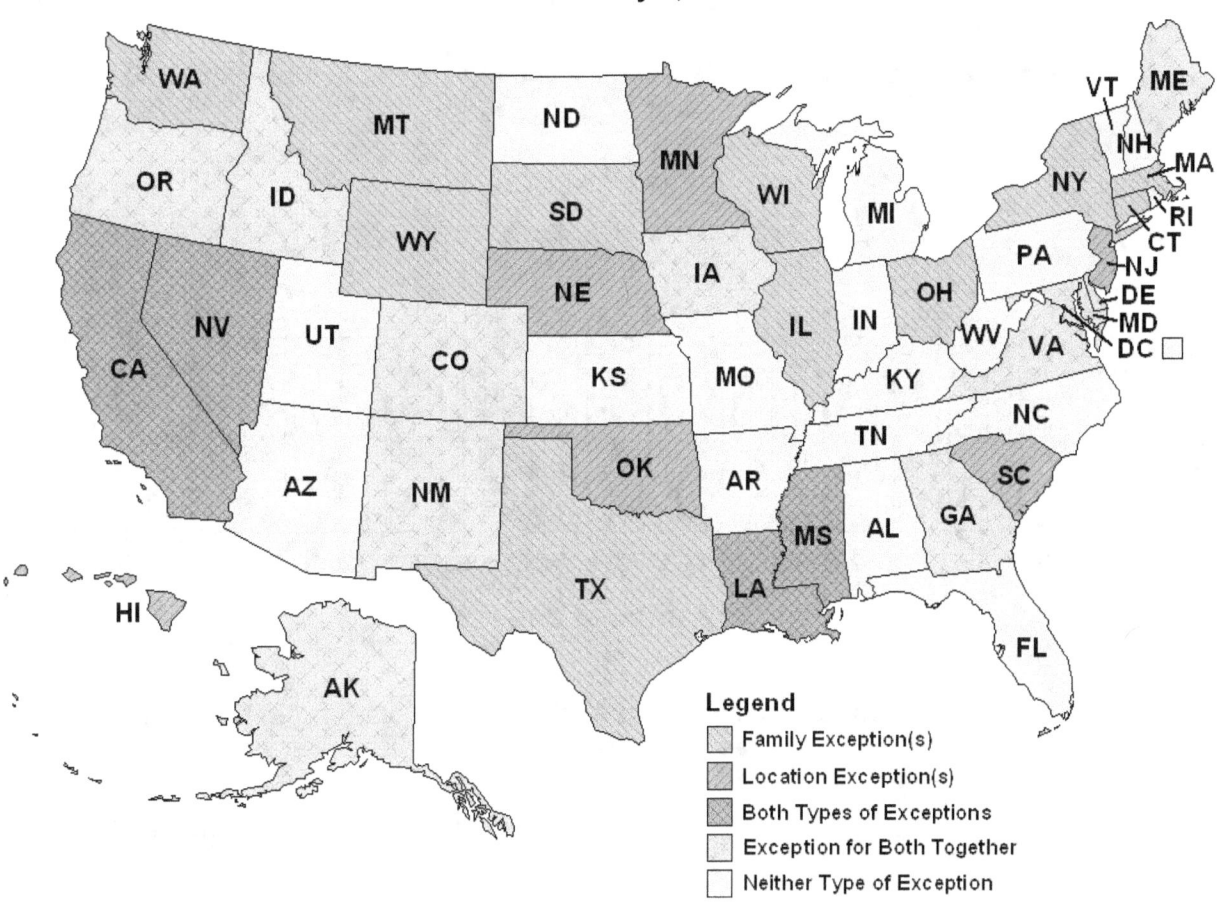

Legend
- Family Exception(s)
- Location Exception(s)
- Both Types of Exceptions
- Exception for Both Together
- Neither Type of Exception

limit the location to the parent/guardian's residence, eight pertain to any private residence, and nine concern any private location.

Trends in Underage Possession Policies

During the period between 1998 and 2012, the number of jurisdictions with family exceptions rose from 23 to 26, the number with location exceptions rose from 20 to 21, and the number of jurisdictions with neither exception decreased from 21 to 19 (see Exhibit 4.3.2).

Status of Underage Consumption Policies

As of January 1, 2012, 35 jurisdictions prohibit consumption of alcoholic beverages by those under age 21. Of those, 17 permit family exceptions to the law, 13 permit location exceptions, and 15 permit neither type of exception (see Exhibit 4.3.3). Seven states (Montana, Ohio, South Dakota, Texas, Washington, Wisconsin, and Wyoming) permit only family exceptions; three states (Hawaii, New Jersey, and Nebraska) permit only location exceptions. Ten states had both types of exceptions, with nine of the states permitting underage consumption only if both family and location criteria are met.

Exhibit 4.3.2: Number of States with Family and Location Exceptions to Minimum Age of 21 for Possession of Alcohol, January 1, 1998, through January 1, 2012

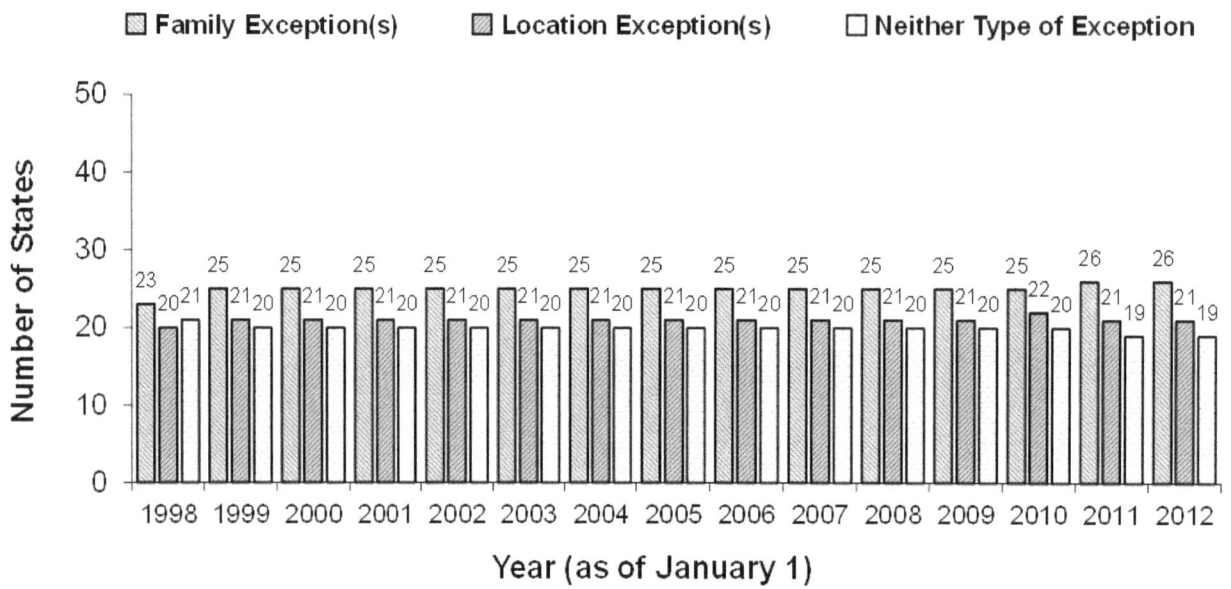

Exhibit 4.3.3: Exceptions to Minimum Age of 21 for Consumption of Alcohol as of January 1, 2012

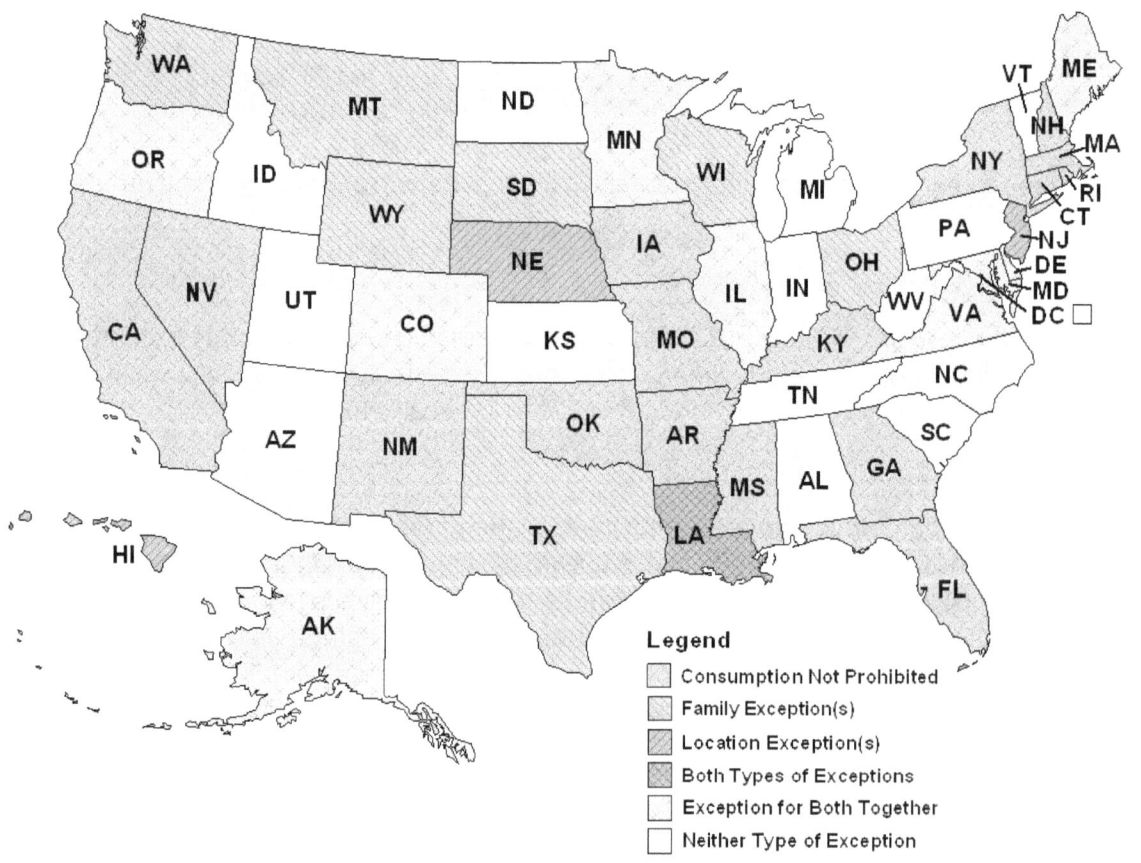

Trends in Underage Consumption Policies

As Exhibit 4.3.4 illustrates, during the period between 1998 and 2012, the number of jurisdictions that did not prohibit underage consumption decreased from 24 to 17. Location exceptions rose from 9 to 13; family exceptions rose from 13 to 17; and the number of jurisdictions with neither type of exception rose from 13 to 14.

Status of Underage Internal Possession Policies

As of January 1, 2012, nine States prohibit internal possession of alcoholic beverages for anyone under age 21 (see Exhibit 4.3.5).. Of the nine States that prohibit internal possession, six do not make any exceptions. In contrast, Colorado has exceptions for situations in which parents or guardians are present and give consent and the possession occurs in any private location. South Carolina's law makes an exception for internal possession in the homes only of parents or guardians. Wyoming makes exceptions for situations in which parents, guardians and spouses are present.

Trends in Underage Internal Possession Policies

As Exhibit 4.3.6 illustrates, during the period between 1998 and 2012, the number of States that prohibit underage internal possession has grown steadily from two to nine. The most recent State to enact a prohibition on internal possession was Wyoming.

Exhibit 4.3.4: Number of States with Family and Location Exceptions to Minimum Age of 21 for Consumption of Alcohol, January 1, 1998, through January 1, 2012

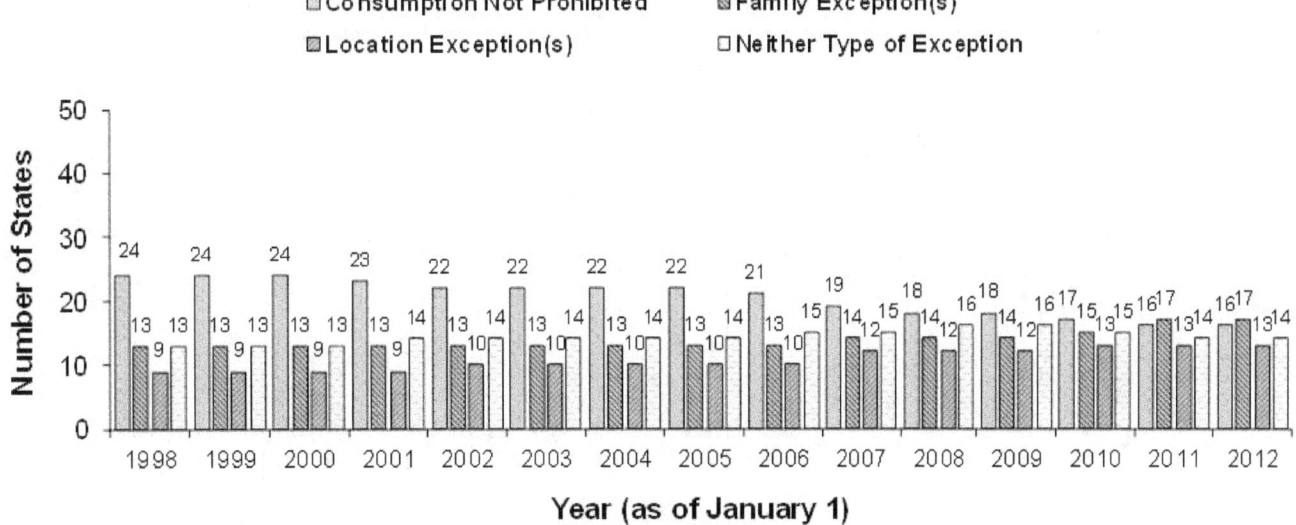

Exhibit 4.3.5: Prohibition of Internal Possession of Alcohol by Persons Under Age 21 as of January 1, 2012

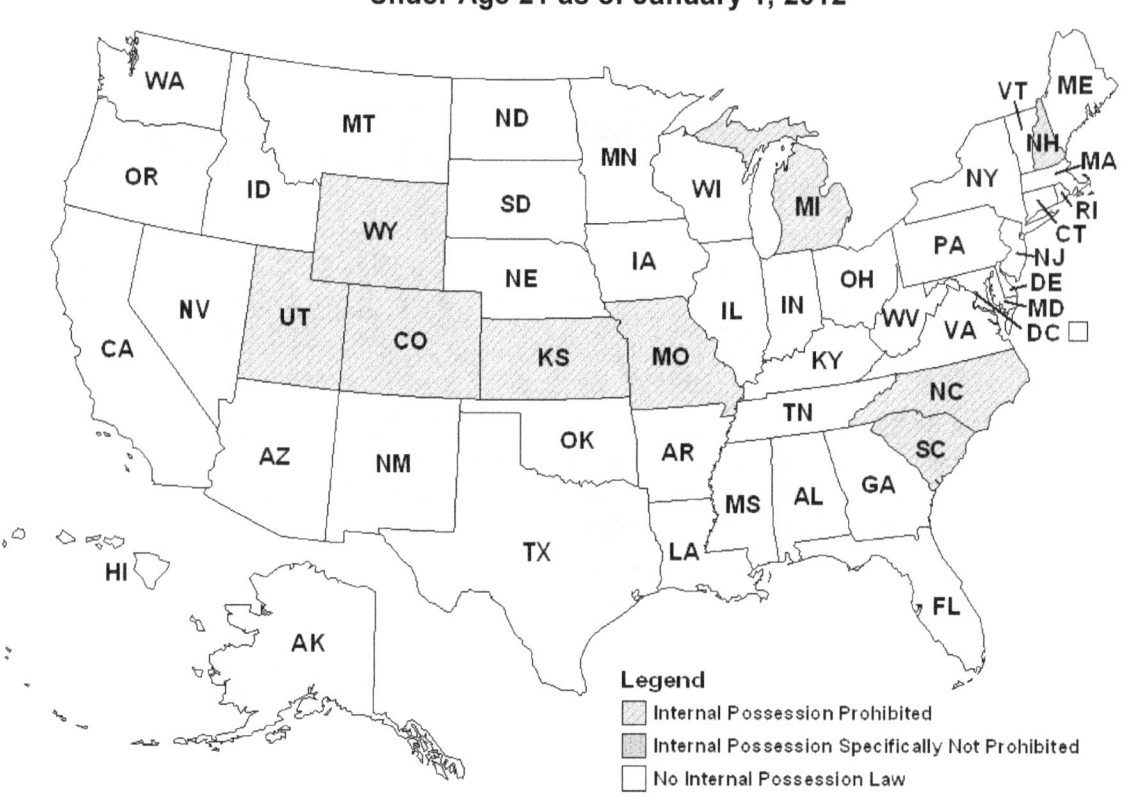

Legend
- Internal Possession Prohibited
- Internal Possession Specifically Not Prohibited
- No Internal Possession Law

Exhibit 4.3.6: Distribution of States with Laws Prohibiting Internal Possession of Alcohol by Persons Under Age 21, January 1, 1998, through January 1, 2012

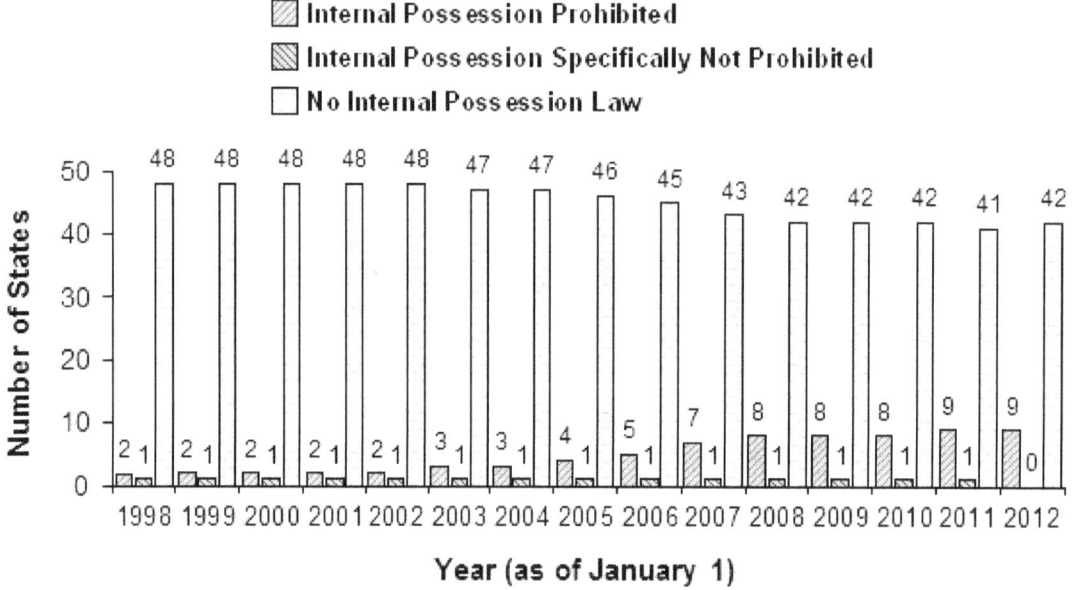

References and Further Information

All data for Underage Possession, Consumption, and Internal Possession policy topics were obtained from the Alcohol Policy Information System (APIS) at http://www.alcoholpolicy.niaaa.nih.gov. Follow links to the policy entitled "Underage Possession/Consumption/Internal Possession of Alcohol." APIS provides further descriptions of this set of policies and its variables, details regarding state policies, and a review of the limitations associated with the reported data. To see definitions of the variables for this policy, go to Appendix B.

Underage Purchase and Attempted Purchase

Policy Description

Most states, but not all, prohibit minors from purchasing or attempting to purchase alcoholic beverages. A minor purchasing alcoholic beverages can be prosecuted for possession because, arguably, a sale cannot be completed until there is possession on the part of the purchaser. Purchase and possession are nevertheless separate offenses. A minor who purchases alcoholic beverages is potentially liable for two offenses in states that have both prohibitions. See the "Underage Possession/Internal Possession/Consumption" section of this report for further discussion.[35] A significant minority of youths purchase or attempt to purchase alcohol for themselves, sometimes using falsified identification (see the "False Identification" section of this report).

Such purchases increase the availability of alcohol to underage persons, which, in turn, increases underage consumption. Prohibitions and associated sanctions on alcohol purchases by underage persons can be expected to depress rates of purchase and attempted purchase by raising the monetary and social costs of this behavior. Such laws provide a primary deterrent (preventing attempted purchases) and a secondary deterrent (reducing the probability that persons sanctioned under these laws will attempt to purchase in the future).

In some states, a person under age 21 is allowed to purchase alcoholic beverages as part of a law enforcement action. Most commonly, these actions are checks on merchant compliance or stings to identify merchants who illegally sell alcoholic beverages to minors. This allowance for purchase in the law enforcement context may exist even though a state does not have a law specifically prohibiting underage purchase.

Status of Underage Purchasing Policies

As of January 1, 2012, 46 states and the District of Columbia prohibit underage purchase or attempted purchase of alcohol; the remaining 4 states (Delaware, Indiana, New York, and Vermont) do not (see Exhibit 4.3.7). Underage persons are allowed to purchase alcohol for law enforcement purposes in 23 states including Indiana, even though Indiana does not have an underage purchase statute. The three other states without underage purchase statutes have no allowances for such purchases made for law enforcement purposes.

Trends in Underage Purchasing Policies

Since 1998, the number of jurisdictions prohibiting underage purchase of alcohol has remained the same (47). During that period, the number of states with allowances for underage purchase for enforcement purposes has steadily increased, from 9 in 1998 to 22 in 2012 (Exhibit 4.3.8).

---

[35] Some states have laws that specifically prohibit both underage purchase and attempted purchase of alcohol. An attempted purchase occurs when a minor takes concrete steps toward committing the offense of purchasing whether or not the purchase is consummated. It is likely that courts in states that only include the purchase prohibition in their statutes would treat attempted purchase as a lesser included offense. It can, therefore, be assumed that all states that prohibit purchase also prohibit attempted purchases. The two offenses are therefore not treated separately in this report.

Exhibit 4.3.7: Underage Purchase of Alcohol for Law Enforcement Purposes as of January 1, 2012

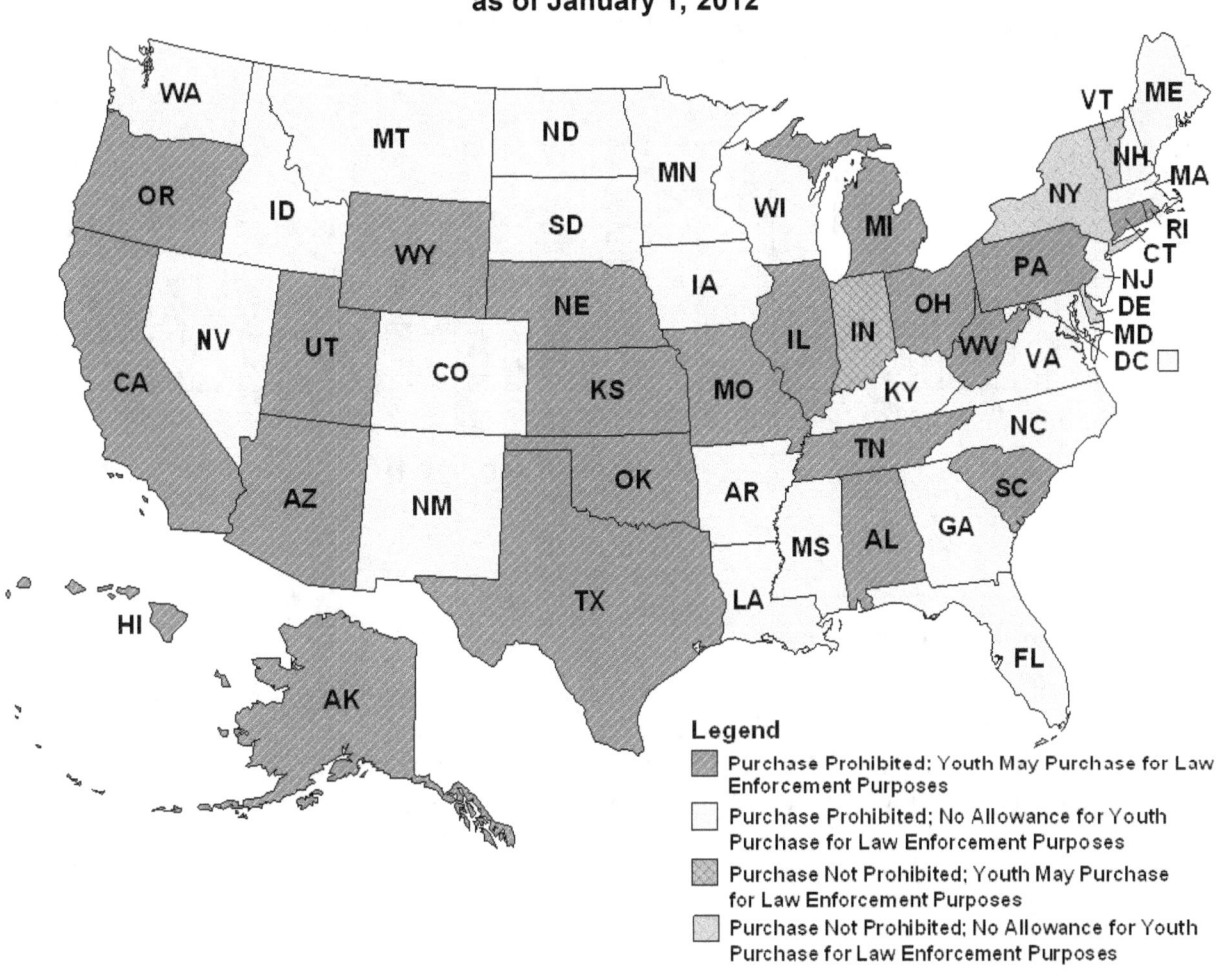

Legend

Purchase Prohibited; Youth May Purchase for Law Enforcement Purposes

Purchase Prohibited; No Allowance for Youth Purchase for Law Enforcement Purposes

Purchase Not Prohibited; Youth May Purchase for Law Enforcement Purposes

Purchase Not Prohibited; No Allowance for Youth Purchase for Law Enforcement Purposes

Exhibit 4.3.8: Underage Purchase of Alcohol for Law Enforcement Purposes, January 1, 1998, through January 1, 2012

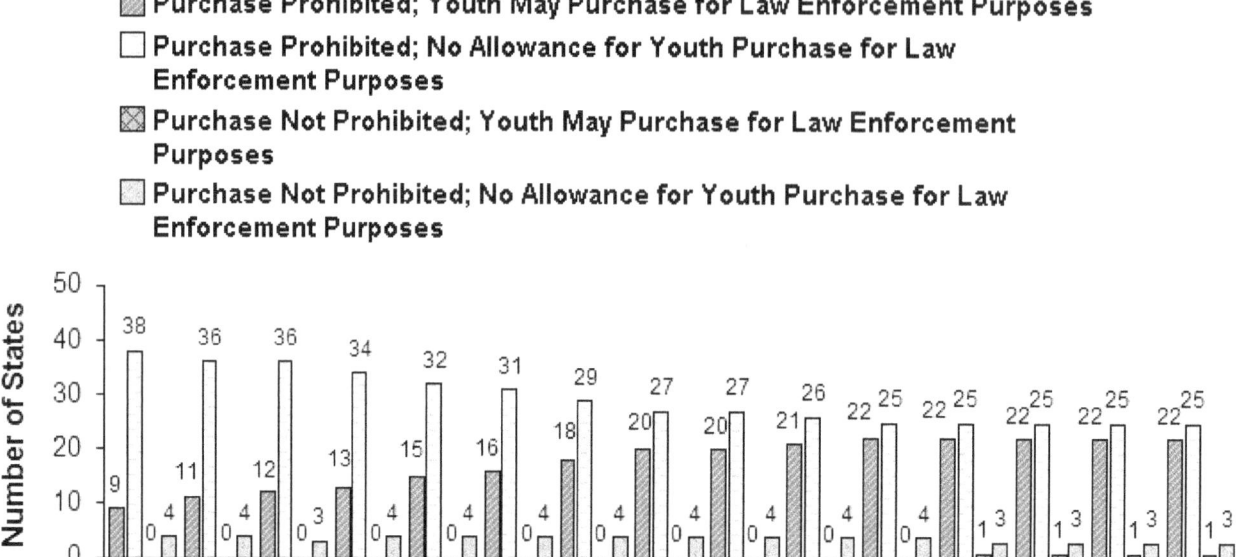

References and Further Information

All data for this policy were obtained from APIS at http://www.alcoholpolicy.niaaa.nih.gov. Follow links to the policy entitled "Underage Purchase of Alcohol." APIS provides further descriptions of this policy and its variables, details regarding state policies, and a review of the limitations associated with the reported data. For definitions for the variables in this policy, go to Appendix B.

False Identification ("false ID")

Policy Description

Alcohol retailers are responsible for ensuring that sales of alcoholic beverages are made only to individuals who are legally permitted to purchase alcohol. Inspecting government-issued identification (driver's license, non-driver identification card, passport, and military identification) is one major mechanism for ensuring that buyers meet minimum age requirements. In attempting to circumvent these safeguards, minors may obtain and use apparently valid ID that falsely states their age as 21 or over. Age may be falsified by altering the birthdate on a valid ID, obtaining an invalid ID card that appears to be valid, or using someone else's ID.

Compliance check studies suggest that underage drinkers may have little need to use false ID because retailers often make sales without any ID inspection. However, concerns about false ID remain high among educators, law enforcement officials, retailers, and government officials. Current technology, including high-quality color copiers and printers, has made false ID easier to fabricate, and the internet provides ready access to a large number of false ID vendors.

All states prohibit use of false identification by minors to obtain alcohol. In addition to the basic prohibitions, states have adopted a variety of legal provisions pertaining to false ID for obtaining alcohol. These provisions can be divided into three basic categories:

- Provisions that target minors who possess and use false identification to obtain alcohol
- Provisions that target those who supply minors with false identification, either through lending of a valid ID or the production of invalid ("fake") IDs
- Provisions that assist retailers in avoiding sales to potential buyers who present false IDs

Government-issued IDs are used for a number of age-related purposes other than the purchase of alcohol: registering to vote, enlisting in the military, entering certain entertainment venues, and so on. APIS confines its analysis to statutes and regulations relating to the use of false identification for the purpose of obtaining alcohol.

For further discussion of policies pertaining to the purchase of alcohol by minors, see the "Underage Purchase and Attempted Purchase" section of this report; policies that mandate training of servers to detect false identification, see the "Responsible Beverage Service" section of this report; and license suspension or revocation, see the "Loss of Driving Privileges for Alcohol Violations by Minors" section of this report.

Status of False ID Policies

Provisions That Target Minors

As of January 1, 2012, all states and the District of Columbia prohibit minors from using false IDs to obtain alcohol (see Exhibit 4.3.9). All but eight states (Delaware, Kansas, Nebraska, Nevada, New Mexico, North Dakota, Vermont, and Wyoming) authorize suspension of minors' driver's licenses for using a false ID in the purchase of alcohol. In all but four states (Alaska, Illinois, Ohio, and West Virginia) the suspension is through judicial proceedings. Two states (Arizona and Iowa) allow for both judicial and administrative proceedings for license sanctions.

**Exhibit 4.3.9: Procedure for Imposing License Sanction for Use of False ID
as of January 1, 2012**

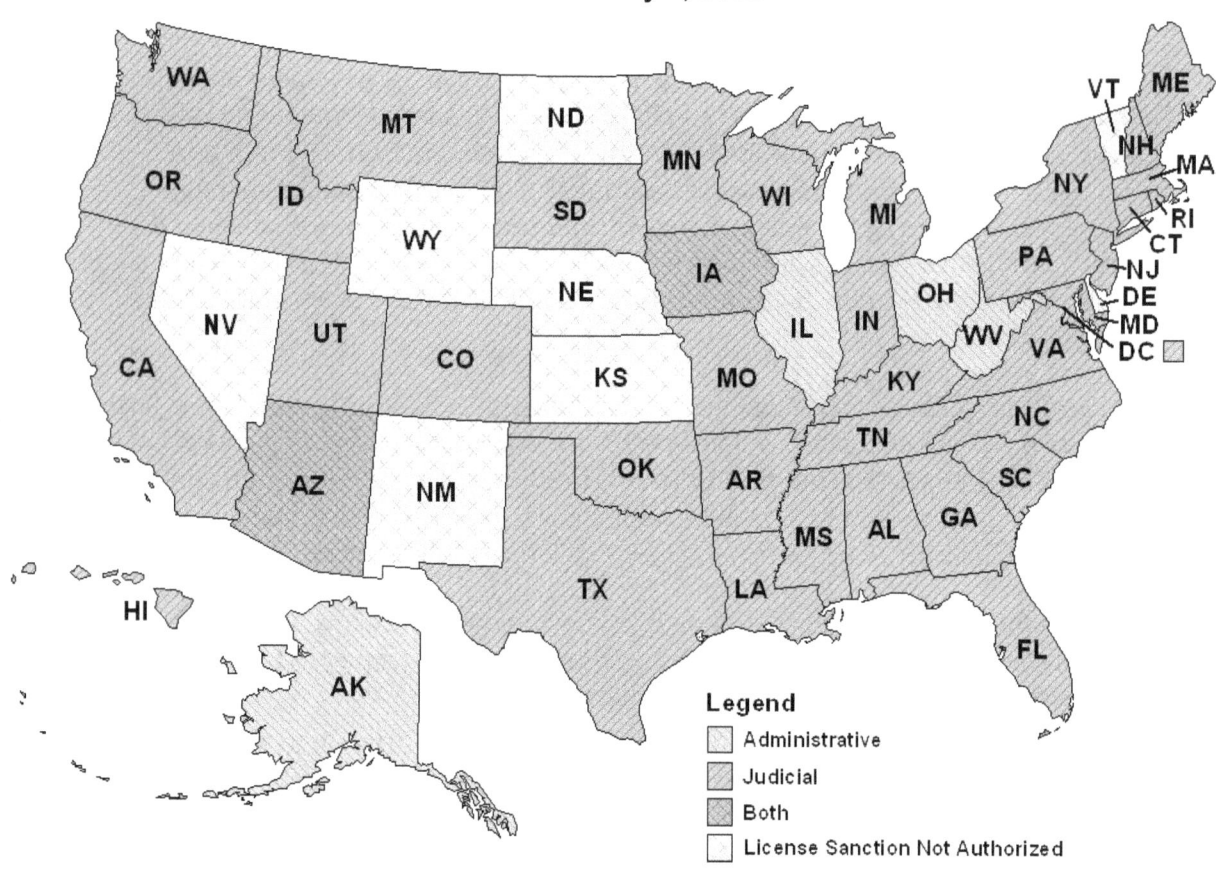

Legend

- Administrative
- Judicial
- Both
- License Sanction Not Authorized

Provisions That Target Suppliers

As of January 1, 2012, 25 states have laws that target suppliers of false IDs; 24 prohibit lending, transferring, or selling false IDs to minors for the purpose of purchasing alcohol; and 13 prohibit manufacturing such licenses.

Retailer Support Provisions

Retailer support provisions vary widely across the states. In prosecution involving an illegal underage alcohol sale, 44 states and the District of Columbia provide for some type of affirmative defense (the retailer shows that he/she reached a good faith or reasonable conclusion that the false ID was valid); 43 states have laws requiring distinctive licenses for persons under age 21; 11 states permit retailers to seize apparently false IDs; 11 states provide incentives for the use of scanners; 4 states (Arkansas, Colorado, South Dakota, and Utah) allow retailers to detain minors; and 4 states (Alaska, Oregon, New Hampshire, and Utah) permit retailers to sue minors for damages.

Trends in False ID State Policies

State false ID policies that target minors and suppliers have been relatively stable for the last 11 years. During this period, Hawaii, Maine, Mississippi, and South Dakota implemented judicial license revocation, and Missouri enacted a law making it illegal to lend, transfer, or sell false IDs to minors. By contrast, states have been actively enacting four of the retailer support provisions. All 11 scanner provisions were enacted over the last 12 years (see Exhibit 4.3.10). Two of the specific affirmative defense laws (Arizona and Vermont), two of the right to detain minors laws (Arkansas and South Dakota), and three of the right to sue minors laws (Alaska, New Hampshire, and Utah) were enacted during this time period. Idaho is an exception to the general trend; in 2007, it rescinded its law permitting retailers to seize apparently false IDs.

References and Further Information

All data for this policy were obtained from APIS at http://www.alcoholpolicy.niaaa.nih.gov. Follow links to the policy entitled "False Identification for Obtaining Alcohol." APIS provides further descriptions of this policy and its variables, details regarding state policies, and a review of the limitations associated with the reported data. Variables are defined in Appendix B.

Exhibit 4.3.10: Number of States with Scanner Provisions in False ID Laws, January 1, 1998, through January 1, 2012

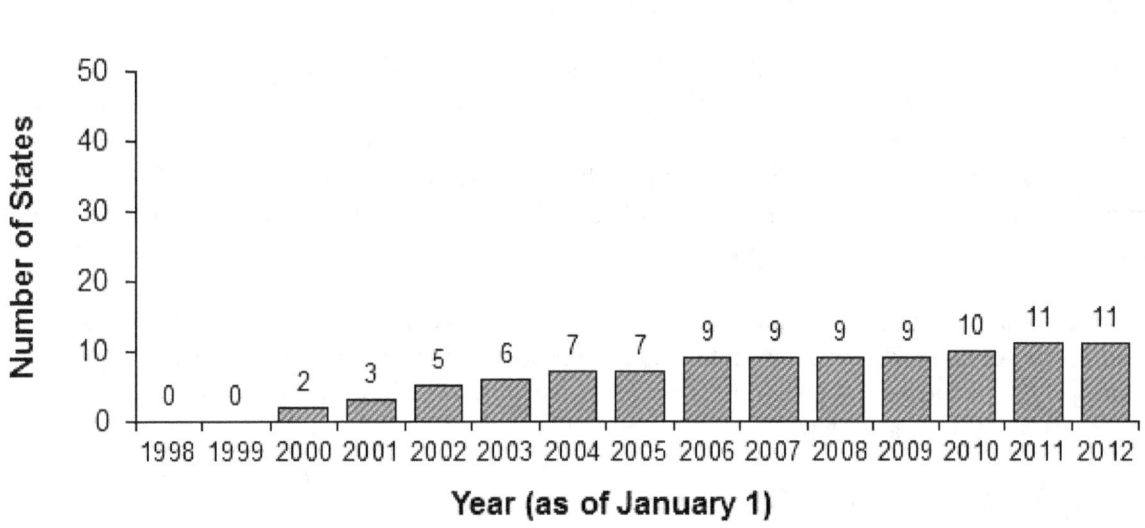

Laws Targeting Underage Drinking and Driving

Youth Blood Alcohol Concentration Limits (underage operators of noncommercial motor vehicles)

Policy Description

Blood alcohol concentration (BAC) limits policies establish the maximum amount of alcohol a minor can have in his/her bloodstream when operating a motor vehicle. BAC is commonly expressed as a percentage. For instance, a BAC of 0.08 percent means that a person has 8 parts alcohol per 10,000 parts blood in the body. State laws generally specify BAC levels in terms of grams of alcohol per 100 milliliters of blood (often abbreviated as grams per deciliter, or g/dL). BAC levels can be detected by breath, blood, or urine tests. The laws of each jurisdiction specify the preferred or required types of tests used for measurement.

There is strong scientific evidence that as BAC increases, the cognitive and motor skills needed to operate a motor vehicle are increasingly impaired. BAC statutes establish criteria for determining when the operator of a vehicle is sufficiently impaired to constitute a threat to public safety and is therefore violating the law. Currently, all states and the District of Columbia mandate a BAC limit of 0.08 g/dL for adult drivers.

Owing to differences between young people and adults (e.g., body mass, physiological development, driving experience), young people's ability to safely operate a motor vehicle is impaired at a lower BAC than for adults. Partly as a result of financial incentives established by the federal government, all jurisdictions in the United States have enacted low BAC limits for underage drivers. Laws establishing very low legal BAC limits of 0.02 g/dL or less for drivers under the legal drinking age of 21 are widely referred to as zero-tolerance laws.

A per se BAC statute stipulates that if the operator has a BAC level at or above the per se limit, a violation has occurred without regard to other evidence of intoxication or sobriety (e.g., how well or poorly the individual is driving). In other words, exceeding the BAC limit established in a per se statute is itself a violation.

Status of Youth BAC Limit Policies

As of January 1, 2012, all states have per se youth BAC statutes (see Exhibit 4.3.11). Thirty-four states set the driving BAC limit for underage persons at 0.02 g/dL. The District of Columbia and 14 states consider any underage alcohol consumption while driving to be a violation of the law and have set the limit to 0.00 g/dL. Two states (California and New Jersey) have set the underage BAC limit to 0.01 g/dL.

Trends in Youth BAC Limit Policies

Since 1998, all states have had zero tolerance (0.02 g/dL or lower) youth BAC limit laws (see Exhibit 4.3.12). In the period between 1999 and 2012, the number of states mandating specific BAC limits for underage drivers remained constant with the exception of one state (Maryland), which lowered its underage BAC limit from 0.02 to 0.00 g/dL. Prior to 1998, three states (South Carolina, South Dakota, and Wyoming) had no youth BAC limits and one (Mississippi) set the limit to 0.08 g/dL.

**Exhibit 4.3.11: Youth Operators Blood Alcohol Concentration Limit Laws
as of January 1, 2012**

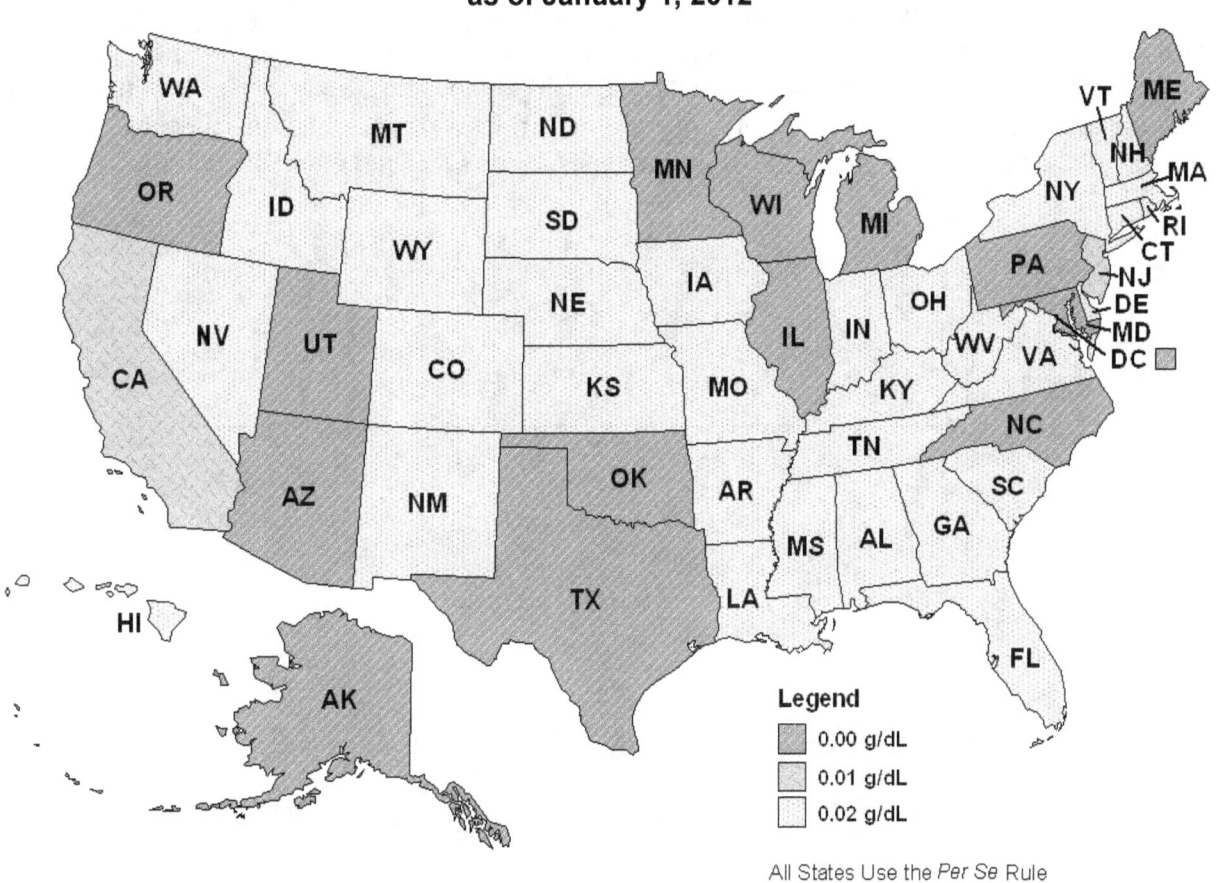

**Exhibit 4.3.12: Distribution of Youth (Underage Operators of Noncommercial
Motor Vehicles) BAC Limit Laws, January 1, 1998, through January 1, 2012**

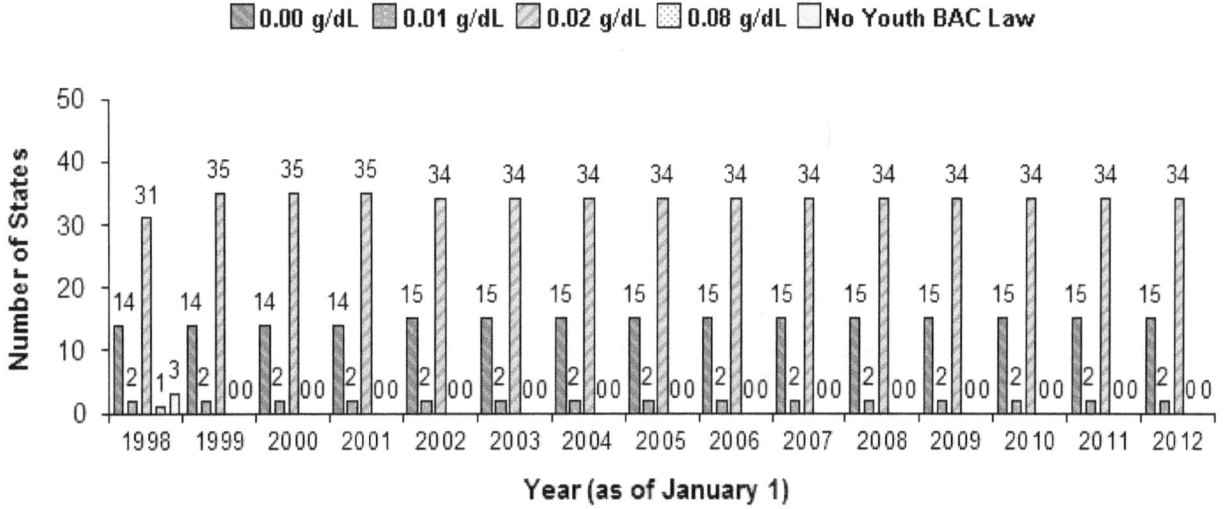

References and Further Information

All data for this policy were obtained from APIS at http://www.alcoholpolicy.niaaa.nih.gov. Follow links to the policy entitled "Blood Alcohol Concentration Limits: Youth (Underage Operators of Noncommercial Motor Vehicles)." APIS provides further descriptions of this policy and its variables, details regarding state policies, and a review of the limitations associated with the reported data. To see definitions of the variables for this policy, go to Appendix B.

Loss of Driving Privileges for Alcohol Violations by Minors ("use/lose" laws)

Policy Description

Use/lose laws authorize suspension or revocation of driving privileges as a penalty for underage purchase, possession, or consumption of alcoholic beverages. States began enacting these statutes in the mid-1980s to deter underage drinking by imposing a punishment that young people would consider significant: the loss of a driver's license. In most states, use/lose laws make it mandatory to impose driver's license sanctions in response to underage alcohol violations. State laws vary as to the type of violation (purchase, possession, or consumption of alcohol) that leads to these sanctions and how long suspensions or revocations stay in effect.

State laws specific to minors (purchase, possession, and consumption of alcoholic beverages) are described in the "Underage Purchase and Attempted Purchase," "Underage Possession," "Underage Consumption," and "Internal Possession by Minors" sections of this report.

Status of Loss of Driving Privileges Policies

Upper Age Limit

Twenty-five states and the District of Columbia set age 21 as the upper limit for which use/lose laws apply. Ten states set the upper limit at age 18, and one state (Wyoming) sets the limit at age 19. In four states (Arkansas, Hawaii, Tennessee, and Virginia), some sanction conditions vary depending on whether the violator is under age 18 or under age 21.

Authority To Impose License Sanction

The vast majority of jurisdictions (36 states and the District of Columbia) have made license suspension or revocation mandatory in cases of underage alcohol violations (see Exhibit 4.3.13). Nine states have made this a discretionary penalty for such violations, and 10 states have no use/lose law. One state (Hawaii) makes this a discretionary penalty for minors below age 18, but mandatory for violators ages 18 through 20. (The total of states is greater than 51 because some have both mandatory and discretionary laws.)

Trends in Loss of Driving Privileges Policies

Between 1998 and 2012, the number of jurisdictions that made license suspension or revocation mandatory in cases of underage alcohol violations increased from 25 to 34 (see Exhibit 4.3.14). During this same time period, the number of jurisdictions with no use/lose laws decreased from 17 to 10, and the number with discretionary authority to impose use/lose sanctions dropped from 10 to 9.

References and Further Information

Data for this policy were obtained from APIS at http://www.alcoholpolicy.niaaa.nih.gov. Follow links to the policy entitled "Loss of Driving Privileges for Alcohol Violations by Minors ("Use/Lose" Laws)." APIS provides further descriptions of this policy and its variables, details regarding state policies, and a review of the limitations associated with the reported data. To see definitions of the variables for this policy, go to Appendix B.

Exhibit 4.3.13: License Suspension/Revocation for Alcohol Violations by Minors as of January 1, 2012

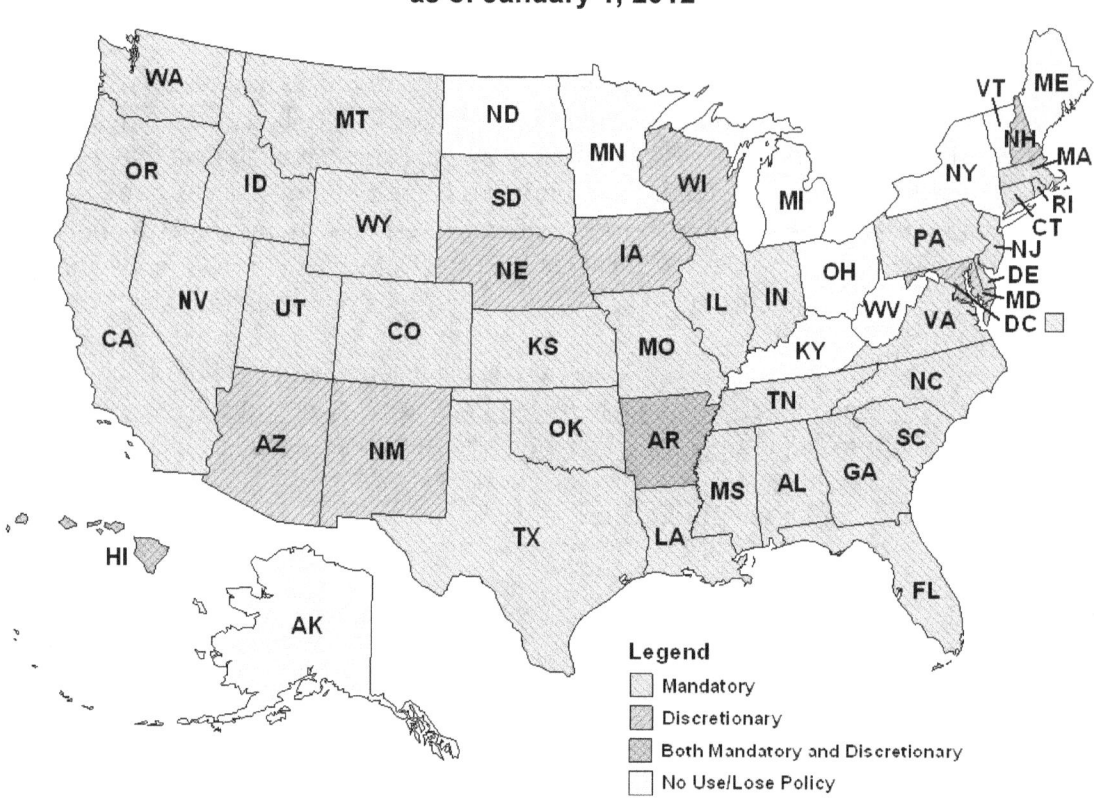

Exhibit 4.3.14: Distribution of License Suspension/Revocation Procedures for Alcohol Violations by Minors, January 1, 1998, through January 1, 2012

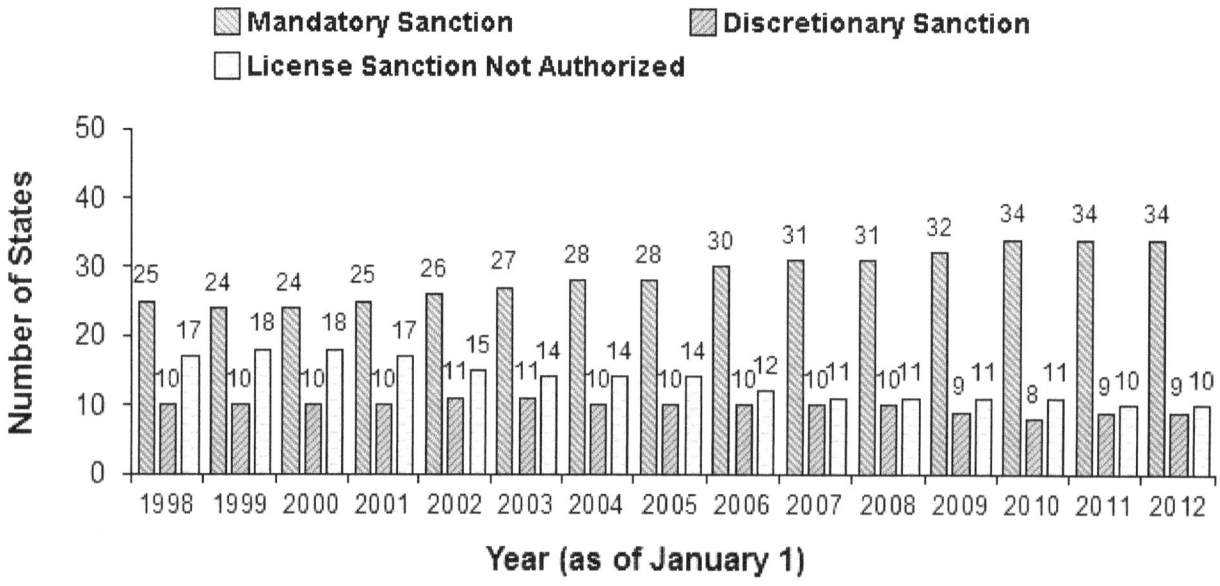

Graduated Driver's Licenses

Policy Description

Graduated driver licensing (GDL) is a system designed to delay full licensure for teenage automobile drivers, thus allowing beginning drivers to gain experience under less risky conditions. Teenagers are targeted because they are at the highest risk for motor vehicle crashes, including alcohol-related crashes. By imposing restrictions on driving privileges, GDL reduces the chances of teenagers driving while intoxicated.

A fully developed GDL system has three stages: a minimum supervised learner's period, an intermediate license (once the driving test is passed) that limits unsupervised driving in high-risk situations, and a full-privilege driver's license available after completion of the first two stages. Beginners must remain in each of the first two stages for set minimum time periods.

The learner's stage has three components:

- Minimum age at which drivers can operate vehicles in the presence of parents, guardians, or other adults
- Minimum holding periods during which learner's permits must be held before drivers advance to the intermediate stage of the licensing process
- Minimum age at which drivers become eligible to drive without adult supervision

The intermediate stage of GDL law has five components:

- Minimum age at which drivers become eligible to drive without adult supervision
- Unsupervised night-driving prohibitions
- Primary enforcement of night-driving provisions
- Passenger restrictions, which set the total number of passengers allowed in vehicles driven by intermediate-stage drivers
- Primary enforcement of passenger restrictions

"Primary enforcement" refers to the authority given to law enforcement officers to stop drivers for the sole purpose of investigating potential violations of night-driving or passenger restrictions. Law enforcement officers in states without primary enforcement can investigate potential violations of these provisions only as part of an investigation of some other offense. Primary enforcement greatly increases the chance that violators will be detected. The single component for the license stage of GDL is the minimum age at which full licensure occurs and both passenger and night-driving restrictions are lifted.

Status of Graduated Driver Licensing Policies

All 51 jurisdictions have some form of GDL policy and all states have full three-stage criteria (see Exhibit 4.3.15). The minimum ages for each stage and the extent to which the other restrictions are imposed vary across jurisdictions. An important GDL provision related to traffic safety is the minimum age for full licensure. Fourteen jurisdictions allow full licensure on the 18th birthday; three jurisdictions permit it at age above 17 but under 18; and 18 permit it on the 17th birthday. The remaining 16 jurisdictions permit full licensure to those who are under 17 but at least 16 years old. All but one jurisdiction has night-driving restrictions; the hours during

Exhibit 4.3.15: Minimum Age of Full Driving Privileges Laws as of January 1, 2012

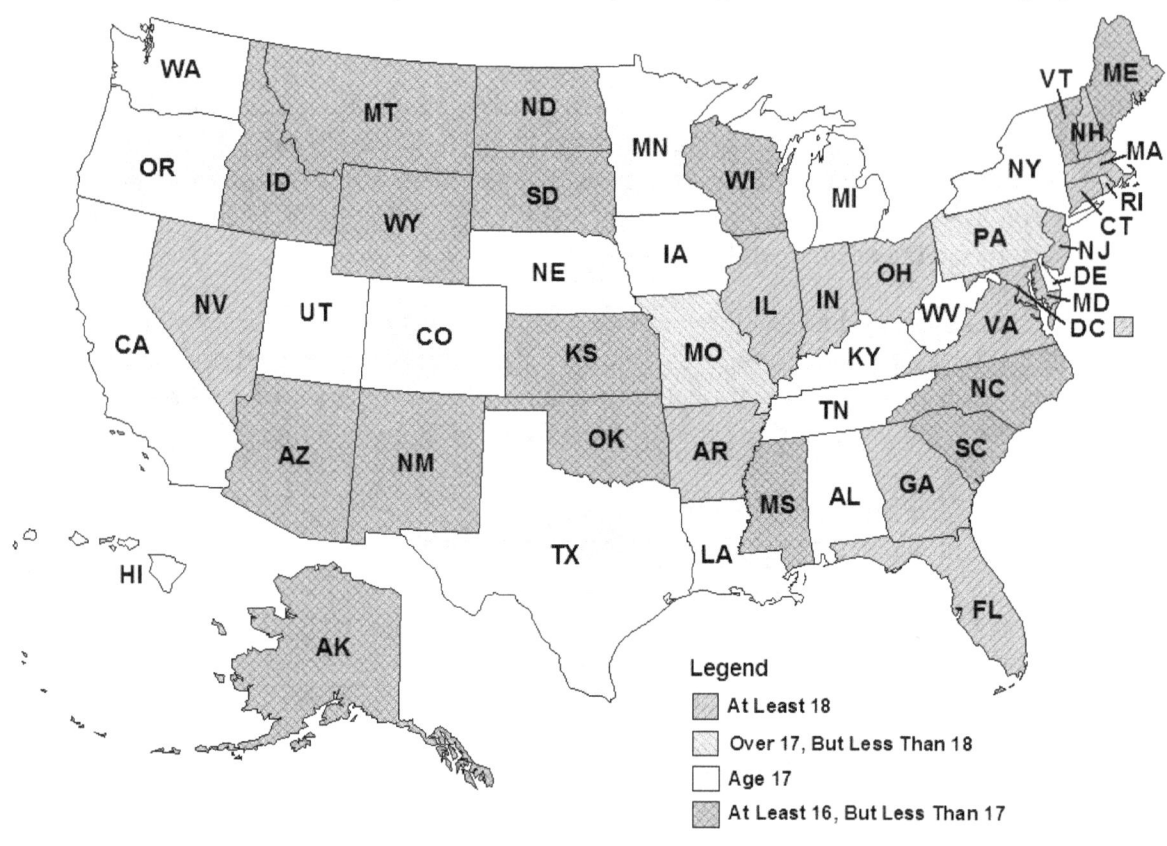

which these restrictions apply vary widely among jurisdictions, but fall largely between 6 p.m. and 1 a.m. Thirty-eight jurisdictions have primary enforcement of night-driving restrictions. Forty-six jurisdictions place passenger restrictions on drivers with less than full licensure, and 31 of those have primary enforcement of these restrictions.

Trends in Graduated Driver Licensing Policies

Since the mid-1990s, states enacting three-stage GDL laws have steadily increased (see Exhibit 4.3.16). On January 1, 1996, only one state (Maryland) had such a law, but by 2000, 23 jurisdictions had enacted three-stage GDL laws and by 2012, that number had risen to 51.

References and Further Information

Legal research for this topic is planned and managed by SAMHSA and conducted under contract by The CDM Group, Inc. Historical data for the years 1996 through 2004 were obtained from "Graduated Driver Licensing Programs and Fatal Crashes of 16 year old Drivers: A National Evaluation" (Baker, S.P., Chen, L.-H., & Li, G. (2006); National Highway Transportation Safety Administration DOT HS 810 614). Data from January 1, 2005, until December 31, 2008, were obtained from the Insurance Institute for Highway Safety (http://www.iihs.org/laws/pdf/us_licensing_systems.pdf). Data through January 1, 2012, were collected by SAMHSA. To see definitions of the variables for this policy, go to Appendix B.

Exhibit 4.3.16: Number of States (and District of Columbia) with Three-Stage Graduated Driver Licensing Policies, July 1, 1996, through January 1, 2012

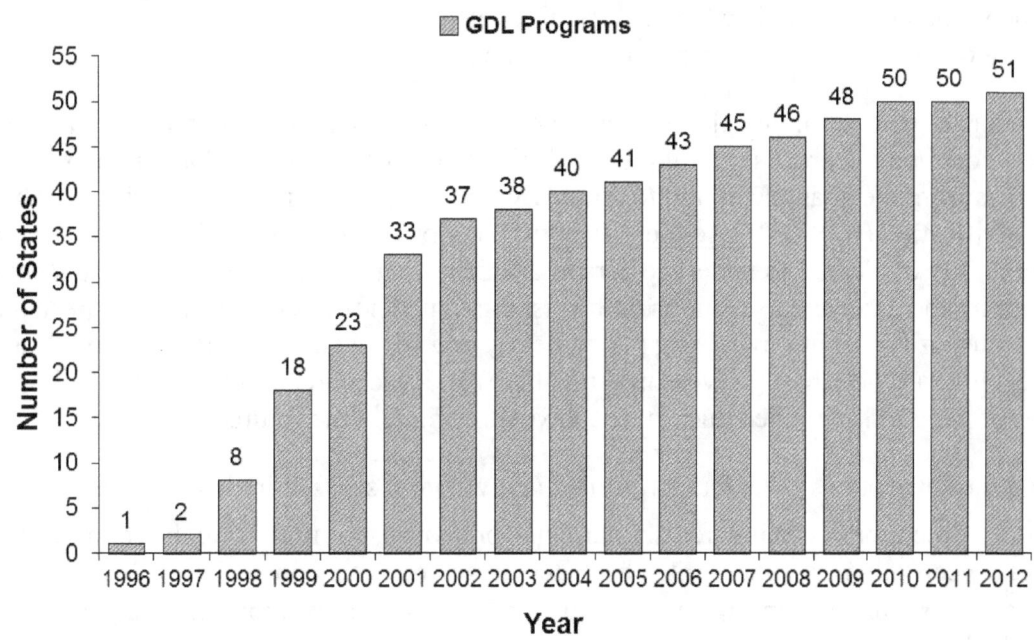

Laws Targeting Alcohol Suppliers

Furnishing Alcohol to Minors

Policy Description

All states prohibit furnishing alcoholic beverages to minors by both commercial servers (bars, restaurants, retail sales outlets) and noncommercial servers. However, examination of case law would be required to determine with certainty that the prohibition applies to both commercial and noncommercial servers in all states. Additionally, most states include some type of exception to their furnishing laws of the types listed below.

Most underage persons obtain alcohol from adults including parents, older siblings and peers, or strangers solicited to purchase alcohol for the minor. Fewer youths purchase alcohol for themselves from merchants who fail to comply with laws prohibiting sale to minors or by using false identification (see the "False Identification" section of this report). These sources increase the availability of alcohol to underage persons, which, in turn, increases underage consumption. Prohibitions and associated sanctions on furnishing to underage persons can be expected to depress rates of furnishing by raising the monetary and social costs of this behavior. Such laws provide a primary deterrent (preventing furnishing) and a secondary deterrent (reducing the chances of persons sanctioned under these laws furnishing in the future).

Two types of exceptions to underage furnishing laws are discussed in this analysis:

- Family exceptions permit parents, guardians, or spouses to furnish alcohol to minors; some states specify that the spouse must be of legal age and others do not.
- Location exceptions permit furnishing alcohol in specified locations and may limit the extent to which family members can furnish to minors. No state has an exception for furnishing on private property by anyone other than a family member.

Some states provide sellers and licensees with one or more defenses against a charge of furnishing alcoholic beverages to a minor. Under these provisions, a retailer who provides alcohol to a minor will not be found in violation of the furnishing law if he or she can establish one of these defenses. This policy topic tracks one such defense: some states require that the minor who initiated a transaction be charged for possessing or purchasing the alcohol before the retailer can be found in violation of the furnishing law. (Defenses associated with minors using false ID can be found in the "False Identification" section of this report.) Many states also have provisions that mitigate or reduce the penalties imposed on retailers if they have participated in responsible beverage service (RBS) programs; see the Responsible Beverage Service" section of this report for further discussion.

In some states, furnishing laws are closely associated with laws that prohibit hosting underage drinking parties. These laws target hosts who allow underage drinking on property they own, lease, or otherwise control. (See the "Hosting Underage Drinking Parties" section of this report for further discussion.) Hosts of underage drinking parties who also supply the alcohol consumed or possessed by minors may be in violation of two distinct laws: furnishing alcohol to minors, and allowing underage drinking to occur on property they control.

Also addressed in this report are social host liability laws, which impose civil liability on hosts for injuries caused by their underage guests. Although related to party hosting laws, social host liability laws are distinct. They do not establish criminal or civil offenses, but instead allow injured parties to recover damages by suing social hosts of events during which minors consumed alcohol and later were responsible for injuries. The commercial analog to social host liability laws is dram shop laws, which prohibit commercial establishments—bars, restaurants, and retail sales outlets—from furnishing alcoholic beverages to minors. See the "Social Host Liability" and "Dram Shop Liability" portions of this report for further discussion.

Status of Underage Furnishing Policies

Exceptions to Furnishing Prohibitions

As of January 1, 2012, all states prohibit the furnishing of alcoholic beverages to minors (see Exhibit 4.3.17). Nineteen states and the District of Columbia have no family or location exceptions to this prohibition. The remaining 31 states permit parents, guardians, and/or spouses to furnish alcohol to their underage children and/or spouses. Of these, 12 states limit the exception to certain locations (3 states, any private location; 7 states, any private residence; 2 states, parents' or guardians' homes only).

Exhibit 4.3.17: Exceptions to Prohibitions on Furnishing Alcohol to Persons Under Age 21 as of January 1, 2012

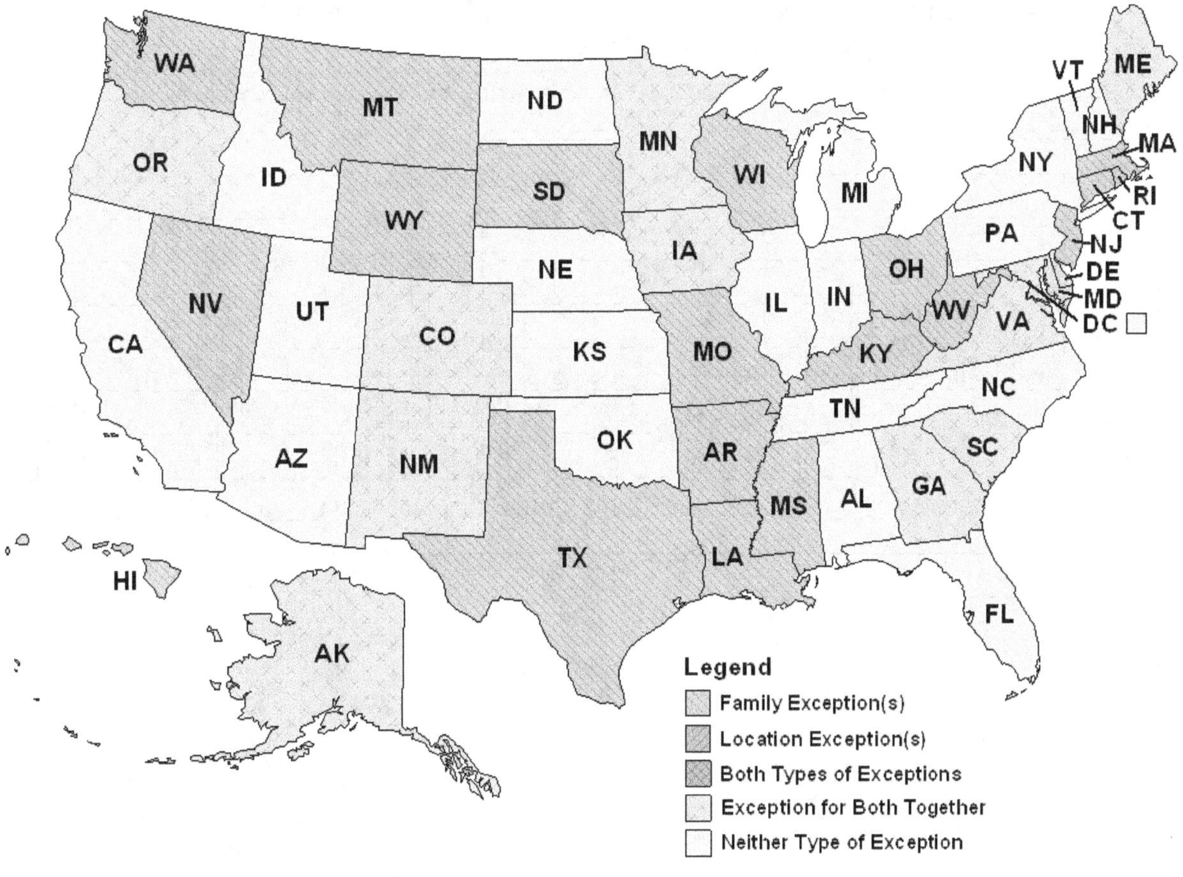

Legend
- Family Exception(s)
- Location Exception(s)
- Both Types of Exceptions
- Exception for Both Together
- Neither Type of Exception

Affirmative Defense for Sellers and Licensees

As of January 1, 2012, the underage furnishing laws of two states (Michigan and South Carolina) include provisions requiring that the seller/licensee be exonerated of charges of furnishing alcohol to a minor unless the minor involved is charged.

Trends in Underage Furnishing Policies

State policies prohibiting the furnishing of alcohol to minors have remained stable over the last decade. As of January 1, 1998, all states prohibited underage furnishing (see Exhibit 4.3.18).

References and Further Information

All data for this policy were obtained from APIS at http://www.alcoholpolicy.niaaa.nih.gov. See the policy entitled "Furnishing Alcohol to Minors." APIS provides further descriptions of this policy and its variables, details regarding state policies, and a review of the limitations associated with the reported data. To see definitions of the variables for this policy, go to Appendix B.

Exhibit 4.3.18: Number of States with Family and Location Exceptions to Prohibition on Furnishing Alcohol to Persons under Age 21, January 1, 1998, through January 1, 2012

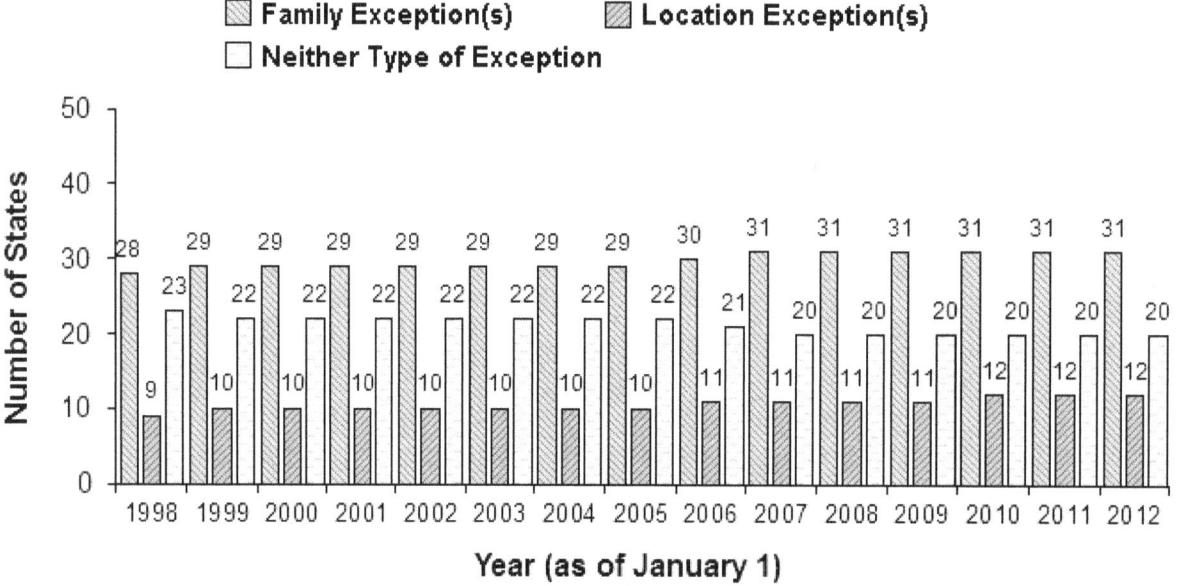

Compliance Check Protocols

Policy Description

Compliance checks involve an underage operative (a "decoy") working with either law enforcement officials or agents from the state alcoholic beverage control (ABC) agency, who enters an alcohol retail establishment and attempts to purchase an alcoholic beverage from a server, bartender, or clerk. The protocols for these checks vary from state to state, but in general follow a similar outline. An underage person (allowable ages vary by state) serves as a decoy in the compliance check. Decoys are generally instructed to act and dress in an age-appropriate manner. The decoy enters an alcohol retail outlet to attempt to purchase a predetermined alcohol product (e.g., a six-pack of beer at an off-sale establishment or a mixed drink at an on-sales establishment). Typically, the decoy is observed by an undercover enforcement officer from a local police department or the state ABC agency. Audio and video recording equipment may also be used or required. State rules vary regarding a decoy's use of legitimate identification cards (driver's licenses, etc.), although a few states allow decoys to verbally exaggerate their age. If a purchase is made successfully, the establishment and/or the clerk or server may be subject to an administrative or criminal penalty.

Most, but not all, states permit law enforcement agencies to conduct compliance checks on a random basis. A few states permit them only when there is a basis for suspecting that a particular licensee has sold alcohol to a minor in the past. To ensure that state and local law enforcement agencies are following uniform procedures, most states have issued formal compliance check protocols or guidelines. If the protocols are not adhered to, then the administrative action against the licensee may be dismissed. The protocols are therefore designed to ensure that law enforcement actions are fair and reasonable and to provide guidelines to licensees for avoiding prosecution.

Compliance checks of off- and on-premise licensed alcohol retailers are an important community tool for reducing illegal alcohol sales to minors and to promote community normative change. The Institute of Medicine (IOM) 2003 report, *Reducing Underage Drinking: A Collective Responsibility*, calls for (1) regular, random compliance checks; (2) administrative penalties, including fines and license suspensions that increase with each offense; (3) enhanced media coverage for the purposes and results of compliance checks; and (4) training for alcohol retailers regarding their legal responsibility to avoid selling alcohol to underage youths.

Compliance checks have both educational and behavior change goals:

- Change or reinforce social norms that underage drinking is not acceptable by publicizing noncompliant retailers.
- Educate the community, including parents, educators, and policymakers, about the ready availability of alcohol to youth, which may not be considered a major issue.
- Increase alcohol retailers' perception that violation of sales to minors laws will be detected and punished, creating a deterrent effect.

Status of Compliance Check Protocols

Data for this policy were coded from formal compliance check protocols or guidelines. A total of 31 states have formal, written protocols; the remaining states either do not have them or do not have them readily available to the public. Compliance check protocols are generally issued by the state police or the state ABC agency. These guidelines vary somewhat in specificity and detail, possibly reflecting differences in the purposes of the checks and the evidentiary standards in each jurisdiction.

The maximum age of the decoy varies from 18 to just under 21, with the majority of states requiring that the maximum age of the decoy be 19 or 20 (see Exhibit 4.3.19). The minimum age of the decoy ranges from 15 to 18, with the majority of the states requiring the minimum age of the decoy to be 17 or 18. Thirty jurisdictions have guidelines for the decoys' appearance (e.g., no facial hair on males, no makeup on females). These requirements vary widely by state. One state uses an age panel to ensure that the decoys appear underage. Four states allow decoys to verbally exaggerate their age. Decoy training is mandatory in 13 states. About one half of the states (16) require decoys to have valid identification in their possession at the time of the check.

References and Further Information

Legal research and data collection for this topic is planned and managed by SAMHSA and conducted under contract by The CDM Group, Inc. To see variables for this policy, go to Appendix B. For further information and background, see:

Pacific Institute for Research and Evaluation. (2007). *Reducing alcohol sales to underage purchasers: A practical guide to compliance investigations.* Washington, DC: U.S. Department of Justice, Office of Justice Programs, Office of Juvenile Justice and Delinquency Prevention.

Exhibit 4.3.19: Maximum Age of Compliance Check Decoys in 2012

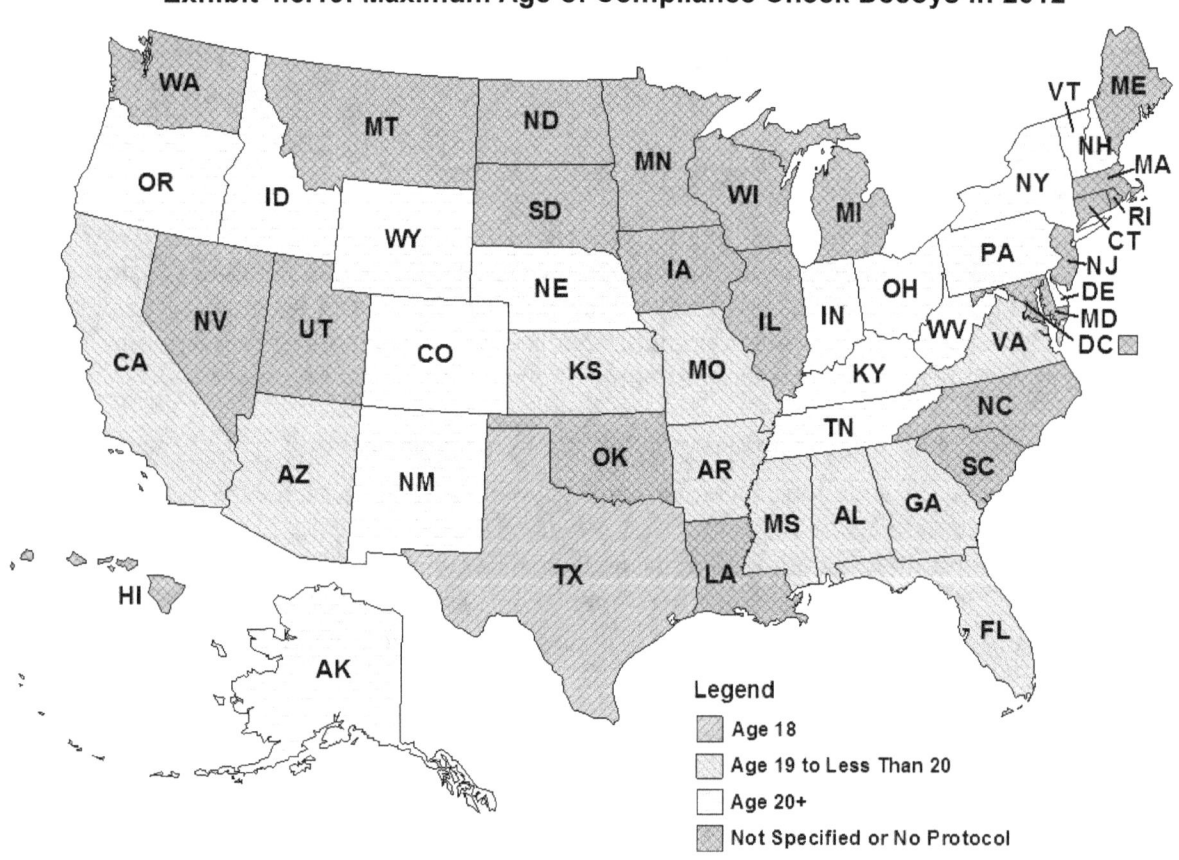

Legend
- Age 18
- Age 19 to Less Than 20
- Age 20+
- Not Specified or No Protocol

Penalty Guidelines for Sales/Service to Minors

Policy Description

In the majority of states, ABC agencies are responsible for adjudicating administrative charges against licensees, including violations for sales or service to those under age 21. Alcohol law enforcement seeks to increase compliance with laws by increasing the level of perceived risk of detection and sanctions. Such deterrence involves three key components: perceived likelihood that a violation will lead to apprehension and sanction, swiftness with which the sanction is imposed, and severity of the sanction (Ross, 1992). As stated in the 2003 IOM report, *Reducing Underage Drinking: A Collective Responsibility*, the effectiveness of alcohol control policies depends heavily on the "intensity of implementation and enforcement and on the degree to which the intended targets are aware of both the policy and its enforcement." The report recommends, "Enforcement agencies should issue citations for violations of underage sales laws, with substantial fines and temporary suspension of license for first offenses and increasingly stronger penalties thereafter, leading to permanent revocation of license after three offenses."

States typically include administrative penalties in their statutory scheme prohibiting sales to minors. The penalty provisions are usually very broad, allowing for severe penalties but delegating responsibility for determining actual penalties in particular cases to the ABC agencies. Penalties may include warning letters, fines, license suspensions, a combination of fines and suspensions, or license revocation. The agencies may consider both mitigating and aggravating circumstances as well the number of violations within a given time period, with repeat offenders usually receiving more severe sanctions.

Many ABC agencies issue penalty guidelines to alert licensees to the sanctions that will be imposed for first, second, and subsequent offenses, providing a time period for determining repeat offenses. The agency may treat the guidelines as establishing a set penalty or range of penalties or may treat them as providing guidance, allowing for deviation at the agency's discretion.

Penalty guidelines that establish firm, relatively severe penalties (particularly for repeat offenders) can increase the deterrent effect of the policy and its enforcement and can increase licensees' awareness of the risks associated with violations.

Status of Penalty Guidelines for Sales/Service to Minors

At least 24 jurisdictions have defined administrative penalty guidelines for licensees who sell alcohol to an underage youth (see Exhibit 4.3.20). The remaining 27 states either do not have penalty guidelines or do not make them readily available to the public. The guidelines may be based on statute, regulations, and/or internal policies developed by the agency.

The guidelines vary widely across states. For example, two states issue warning letters for first offenses if there are no aggravating circumstances. Other states impose fines and/or suspensions. Minimum fines for a first offense range from $250 to $5,000, with most states in the $500 to $1,000 range. Fines are typically in lieu of suspensions for first offenses, with some states allowing licensees to choose between the two sanctions. Florida has the strictest first offense guidelines: it imposes a $1,000 fine and a 7-day suspension. New York imposes a $5,000 penalty if the minor served is under age 19.

Exhibit 4.3.20: States with Penalty Guidelines as of January 1, 2012

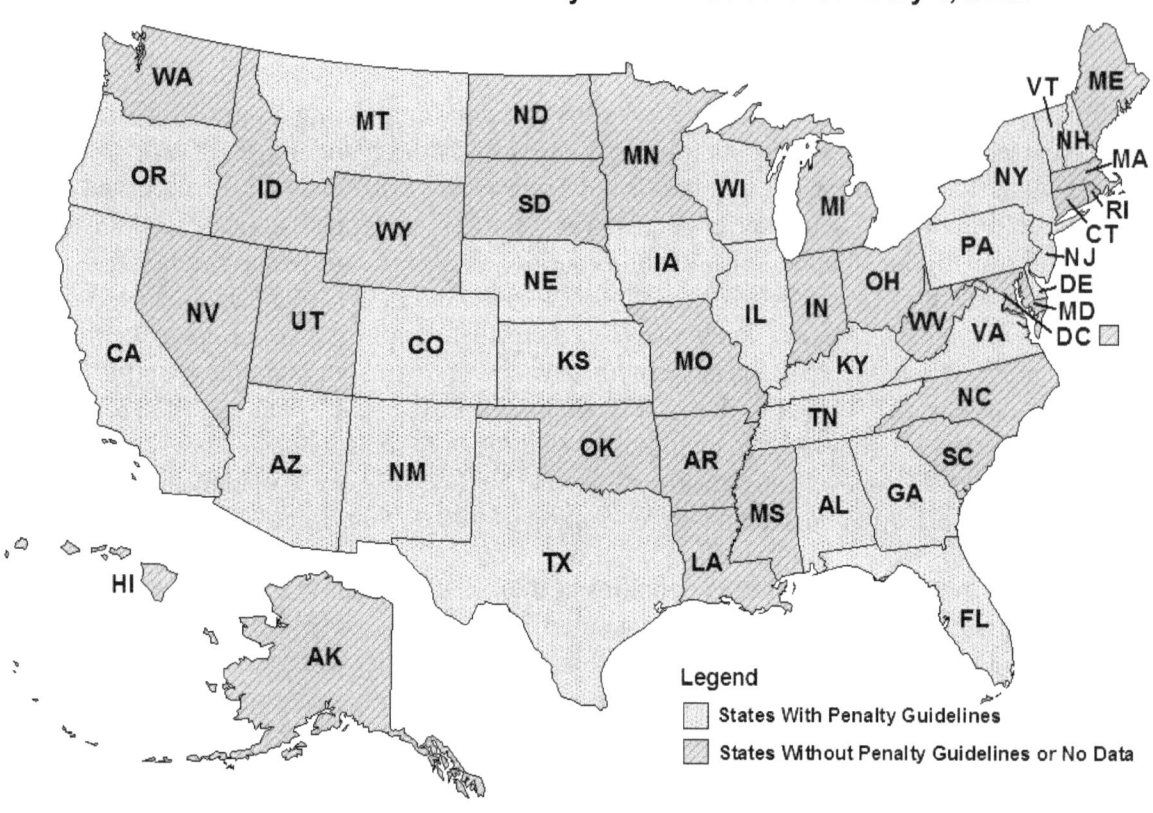

Legend

◻ States With Penalty Guidelines

▨ States Without Penalty Guidelines or No Data

Fines increase to as much as $20,000 for subsequent offenses (in California), with license suspension days increasing to as many as 72 days for subsequent violations (Kentucky). Three states have adopted the IOM recommendation that licenses should be revoked after three offenses (California, Florida, and New Mexico), and an additional six states revoke licenses for a fourth offense. The time periods for defining repeat offenses range from 1 to 5 years.

States also vary in the specificity of their guidelines. Many states list a set penalty or a relatively limited range of penalties. Pennsylvania's guideline, on the other hand, provides for penalties ranging from a $1,000 fine to license revocation for first offenses.

See Chapter 4.4, the Cross-State Survey Report, for a review of penalties actually imposed by states for selling to and serving minors.

References and Further Information

Legal research and data collection for this topic are planned and managed by SAMHSA and conducted under contract by The CDM Group, Inc. To see definitions of the variables for this policy, go to Appendix B. For further information and background see:

National Research Council, Institute of Medicine. (2003). *Reducing underage drinking: A collective responsibility*. Washington, DC: National Academies Press.

Ross, H.L. (1992). *Confronting drunk driving: Social policy for saving lives*. Binghamton, NY: Vail-Ballou Press.

Responsible Beverage Service

Policy Description

Responsible beverage service (RBS) training policies set requirements or incentives for retail alcohol outlet participation in programs that: (1) develop and implement policies and procedures for preventing alcohol sale and service to minors and intoxicated persons, and (2) train licensees, managers, and servers/sellers to implement RBS policies and procedures effectively.

Server/seller training focuses on serving and selling procedures, recognizing signs of intoxication, methods for checking age identification, and techniques for intervening with intoxicated patrons. Manager training includes server/seller training, policy and procedures development, and staff supervision. RBS programs typically have distinct training curricula for on- and off-sale establishments because of the differing characteristics of these retail environments. All RBS programs focus on preventing sale and furnishing to minors.

Responsible beverage service training can be mandatory or voluntary. A program is considered mandatory if state provisions require at least one specified category of individual (e.g., servers/sellers, managers, or licensees) to attend training. States may have either mandatory programs, voluntary programs, or both. For example, a state may make training for new licenses mandatory while also offering voluntary programs for existing licensees. Alternatively, a state may have a basic mandatory program while also offering a more intensive voluntary program that provides additional benefits for licensees choosing to participate in both.

States with voluntary programs usually provide incentives for retailers to participate in RBS training but do not impose penalties for those who decline involvement. Incentives vary by state and include (1) a defense in dram shop liability lawsuits (cases filed by injured persons against retail establishments that provided alcohol to minors or intoxicated persons who later caused injuries to themselves or third parties); (2) discounts for dram shop liability insurance; (3) mitigation of fines or other administrative penalties for sales to minors or sales to intoxicated persons; and (4) protection against license revocation for sales to minors or intoxicated persons.

See the "Dram Shop Liability" section of this report for further discussion of this policy. The "Furnishing of Alcohol to Minors" section has additional information regarding prevention of alcohol sales to minors, and the "False Identification" section includes materials related to age identification policies.

Status of Responsible Beverage Service Training Policies

As of January 1, 2012, 36 states and the District of Columbia have some type of RBS training provision (see Exhibit 4.3.21). Out of these, 18 states and the District of Columbia have some form of mandatory provision, and 24 states provide for voluntary training. Of the 18 mandatory states, 13 states and the District of Columbia apply their RBS training provisions to both on- and off-sale establishments; 4 states (Michigan, Rhode Island, Tennessee, and Washington) apply them to on-premises establishments only; and New Jersey limits its provisions to off-sale establishments. Thirteen of the mandatory states and the District of Columbia apply their provisions to both new and existing establishments, while four states (Michigan, New Hampshire, New Jersey, and Wisconsin) apply them to new establishments only. Six states

Exhibit 4.3.21: Responsible Beverage Service as of January 1, 2012

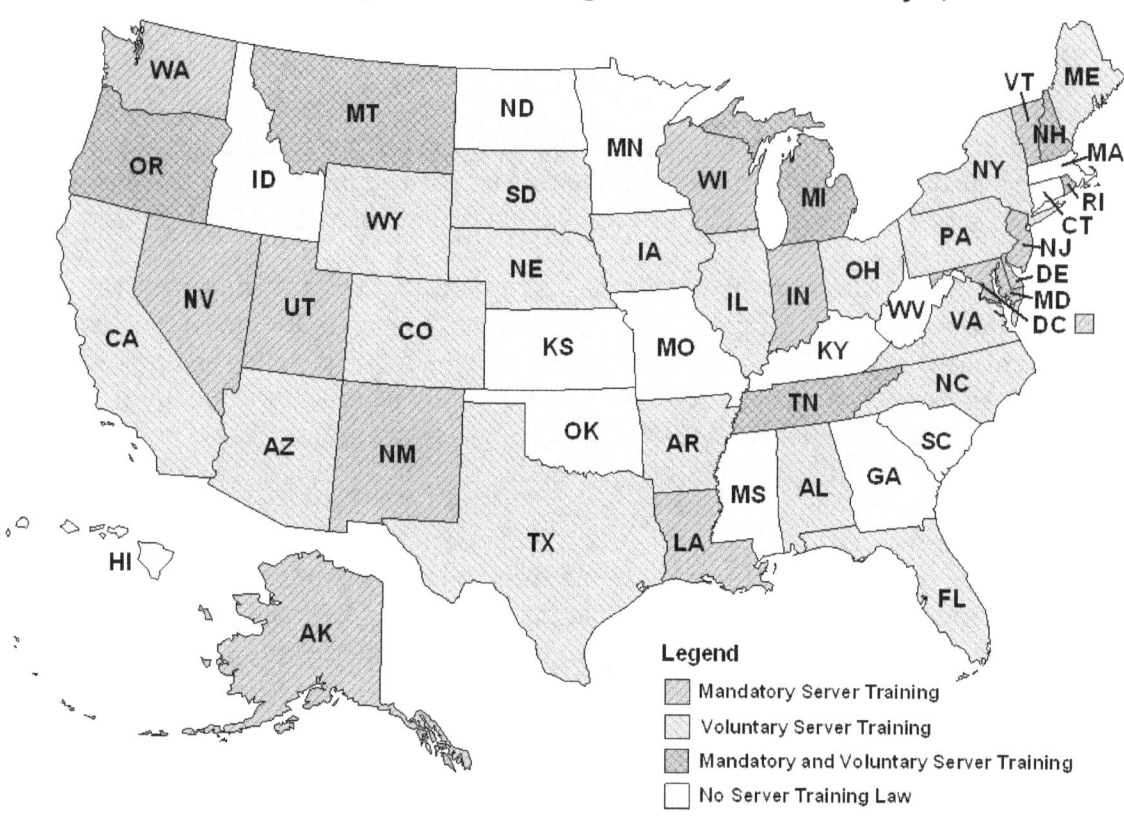

Legend
- Mandatory Server Training
- Voluntary Server Training
- Mandatory and Voluntary Server Training
- No Server Training Law

(Michigan, Montana, New Hampshire, Oregon, Rhode Island, and Tennessee) have both mandatory and voluntary provisions:

- Michigan: The mandatory provisions apply to new on-premises establishments; the voluntary provisions apply to existing on-premises establishments.
- Montana: The mandatory provisions apply to new and existing as well as on- and off-premises establishments; the voluntary incentives also apply to both new and existing and on- and off-premises establishments.
- New Hampshire: The mandatory provisions apply to new on- and off-premises establishments; the voluntary provisions provide incentives available to both types of establishments.
- Oregon: Both the voluntary and mandatory provisions apply to both types of establishments, with the voluntary provisions offering incentives for participation in both.
- Rhode Island: The mandatory provisions apply to existing on-premises establishments. The voluntary provisions offer dram shop liability defense incentives and do not specify which type of establishment may participate.
- Tennessee: The mandatory provisions apply to new and existing on-premises establishments. The voluntary provisions offer incentives available to off-premises establishments, but do not specify whether the incentives are available to new and/or existing establishments.

Trends in Responsible Beverage Service Policies

Between 2003 and 2012, the number of states with mandatory policies increased from 15 to 19, and the number of states with voluntary policies rose from 17 to 24 (see Exhibit 4.3.22). The number of states with no RBS training policy decreased from 22 to 14.

References and Further Information

All data for this policy were obtained from APIS at http://www.alcoholpolicy.niaaa.nih.gov. Follow links to the policy entitled "Beverage Service Training and Related Practices." APIS provides further descriptions of this policy and its variables, details regarding state policies, and a review of the limitations associated with the reported data. To see definitions of the variables for this policy, go to Appendix B.

Exhibit 4.3.22: Number of States with Responsible Beverage Service, January 1, 2003, through January 1, 2012

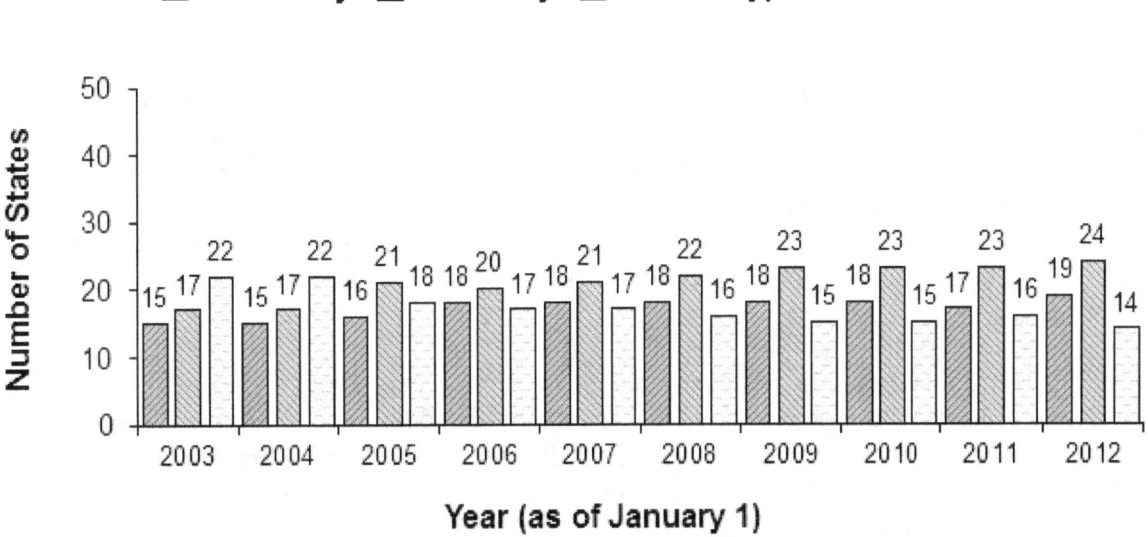

Note: some jurisdictions have both types of laws

Minimum Ages for Off-Premises Sellers

Policy Description

Most states have laws that specify a minimum age for employees who sell alcoholic beverages in off-premises establishments such as liquor stores. A small number require sellers to be at least 21 years old, but most states permit sellers to be younger. Some states allow any person to sell alcohol regardless of age. Other variations across states include minimum age requirements for conducting sales transactions with customers and allowing younger employees to stock coolers with alcohol or bag purchased alcohol. Age restrictions may also vary based on the type of off-premises establishment or type of alcohol being sold. For example, younger persons may be allowed to sell beer but not wine or distilled spirits. Younger persons may also be allowed to sell alcohol in grocery or convenience stores rather than liquor stores. Some states permit younger minimum selling ages only if a manager or supervisor is present.

State laws specifying minimum ages for employees who sell alcoholic beverages for on-premises consumption are described in the "Minimum Ages for On-Premises Servers and Bartenders" section of this report.

Status of Age of Seller Policies

Minimum Age of Sellers and Types of Beverages

Most jurisdictions specify the same minimum age for sellers of all types of alcoholic beverages (see Exhibit 4.3.25). As of January 1, 2012, 10 states specify that off-premises sellers must be 21 years or older. Three states (Idaho, Indiana, and Nebraska) require off-premise sellers to be 19 years or older; 15 states and the District of Columbia have set the minimum age at 18. Four states (Arizona, Maine, Nevada, and New Hampshire) set the minimum age between 16 and 17 years. Four states (California, Georgia, Louisiana, and Virginia) do not specify any minimum age for sellers.

Minimum age requirements in the remaining 14 states vary by type of alcohol, with age requirements generally higher for the sale of distilled spirits and lower for beer. Florida, New York, and North Carolina set a minimum age of 18 for the sale of spirits and have no age minimum for beer or wine. Alabama and South Carolina have a minimum age of 21 for the sale of spirits but no minimum for beer and wine. Vermont sets a minimum age for selling beer and wine (16), but does not specify a minimum age for selling spirits.

Manager or Supervisor Presence

Thirteen states require that a supervisor or manager be present when an underage seller conducts an alcoholic beverage transaction.

Trends in Age of Seller Policies

There were no changes in age of seller policies across states between 2003 and 2012 (see Exhibit 4.3.26).

Exhibit 4.3.25: Minimum Age To Sell Beer for Off-Premises Consumption as of January 1, 2012

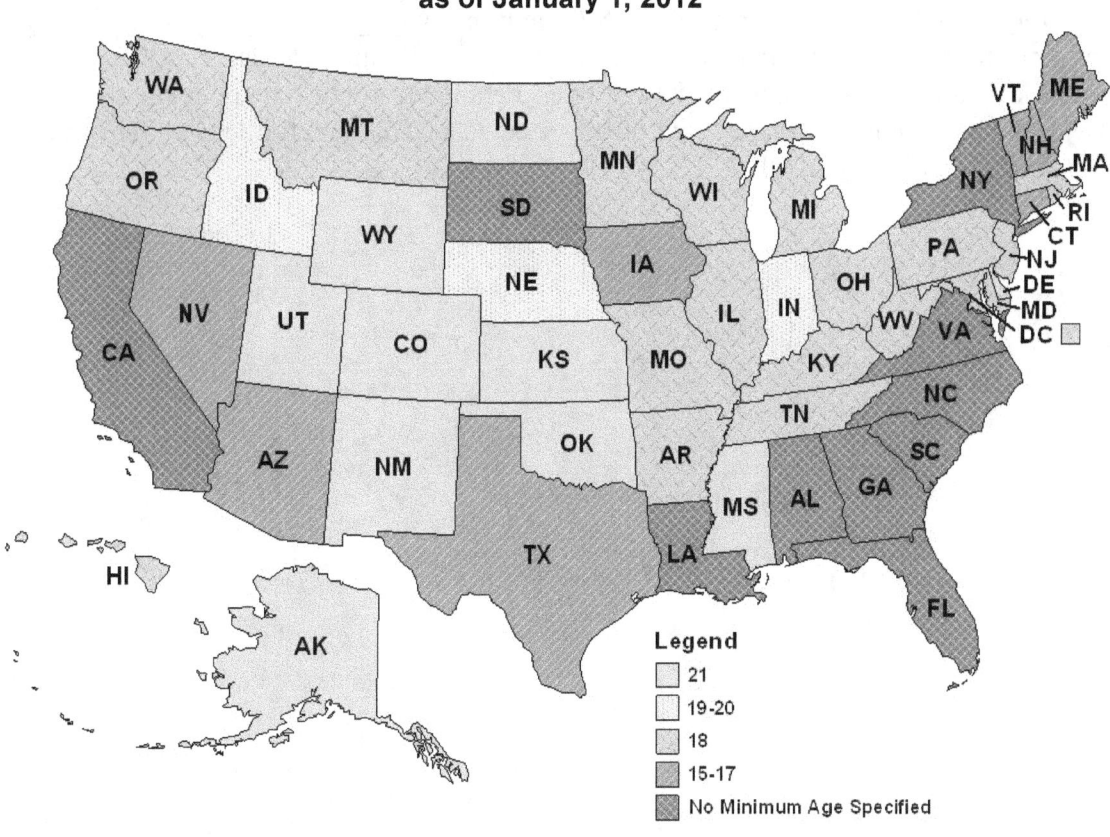

Legend
- 21
- 19-20
- 18
- 15-17
- No Minimum Age Specified

Exhibit 4.3.26: Distribution of Minimum Ages for Off-Premises Sellers of Beer, January 1, 2003, through January 1, 2012

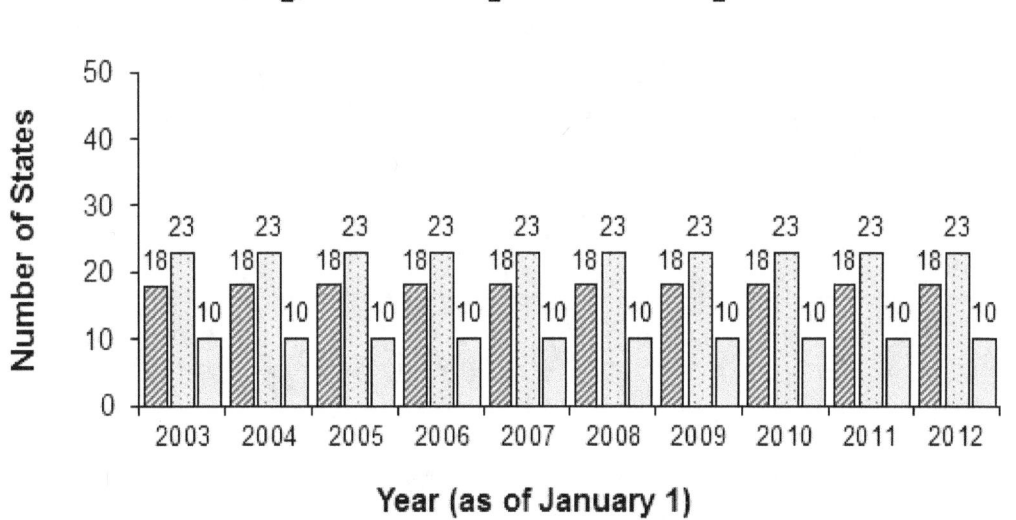

Age < 18   Age 18-20   Age 21

References and Further Information

All data for this policy were obtained from APIS at http://www.alcoholpolicy.niaaa.nih.gov. Follow links to the policy entitled "Minimum Ages for Off-Premises Sellers." APIS provides further descriptions of this policy and its variables, details regarding state policies, and a review of the limitations associated with the reported data. To see definitions of the variables for this policy, go to Appendix B.

Minimum Ages for On-Premises Servers and Bartenders

Policy Description

All states specify a minimum age for employees who serve or dispense alcoholic beverages. Generally, the term "servers" refers to waitpersons, and "bartenders" refers to individuals who dispense alcoholic beverages. These restrictions recognize that underage employees, particularly those who are unsupervised, may lack the maturity and experience to conduct adequate checks of age identification and resist pressure from underage peers to complete illegal sales.

States vary widely in terms of minimum age requirements for servers and bartenders. In some states, the minimum age for both types of employee is 21, but others set lower minimum ages, particularly for servers. No state permits underage bartenders while prohibiting underage servers. Some states permit servers or bartenders younger than 21 to work only in certain types of on-premises establishments, such as restaurants, or to serve only certain beverage types, such as beer or wine. Underage servers and bartenders may be allowed only if legal-age managers or supervisors are present when underage persons are serving alcoholic beverages or tending bar. State laws setting a minimum age for employees who sell alcohol at off-premises establishments are described in the "Minimum Ages for Off-Premises Sellers" section of this report.

Status of Age of Server Policies

Age of Servers

As of January 1, 2012, Alaska, Nevada, and Utah specify that on-premises alcohol servers of beer, wine, or distilled spirits must be age 21 or older (see Exhibit 4.3.23). Only one state (Maine) allows 17-year-olds to be servers. Ten states specify that servers be at least 19 or 20 years old, and the remaining 36 states and the District of Columbia allow 18-year-old servers.

Age of Bartenders

Minimum ages for bartenders are generally higher than for servers across the states. Nineteen states and the District of Columbia limit bartending to persons age 21 or older. Five states (Arizona, Idaho, Kentucky, Nebraska, and Ohio) specify that bartenders be at least 19 or at least 20. Twenty-five states allow 18-year-olds to bartend, while only one state (Maine) allows 17-year-olds to be bartenders. Minimum ages for serving beer, wine, and distilled spirits are identical in all but three states: Maryland, North Carolina, and Ohio. Maryland and North Carolina require bartenders to be 21 to serve spirits, but permit 18-year-olds to dispense beer and wine; Ohio requires bartenders to be 21 to serve wine and distilled spirits, but those ages 19 and older are allowed to dispense beer.

Trends in Age of Server Policies

Manager or Supervisor Presence

Ten states require that a supervisor or manager be present when an underage seller conducts an alcoholic beverage transaction. State policies for ages of servers and bartenders in on-premises establishments have been generally stable over the last decade (see Exhibit 4.3.24). Between 2003 and 2012, Arkansas lowered its minimum age for servers from 21 to 19, and North Dakota lowered its age for servers from 19 to 18.

Exhibit 4.3.23: Minimum Ages for On-Premises Servers (Beer) as of January 1, 2012

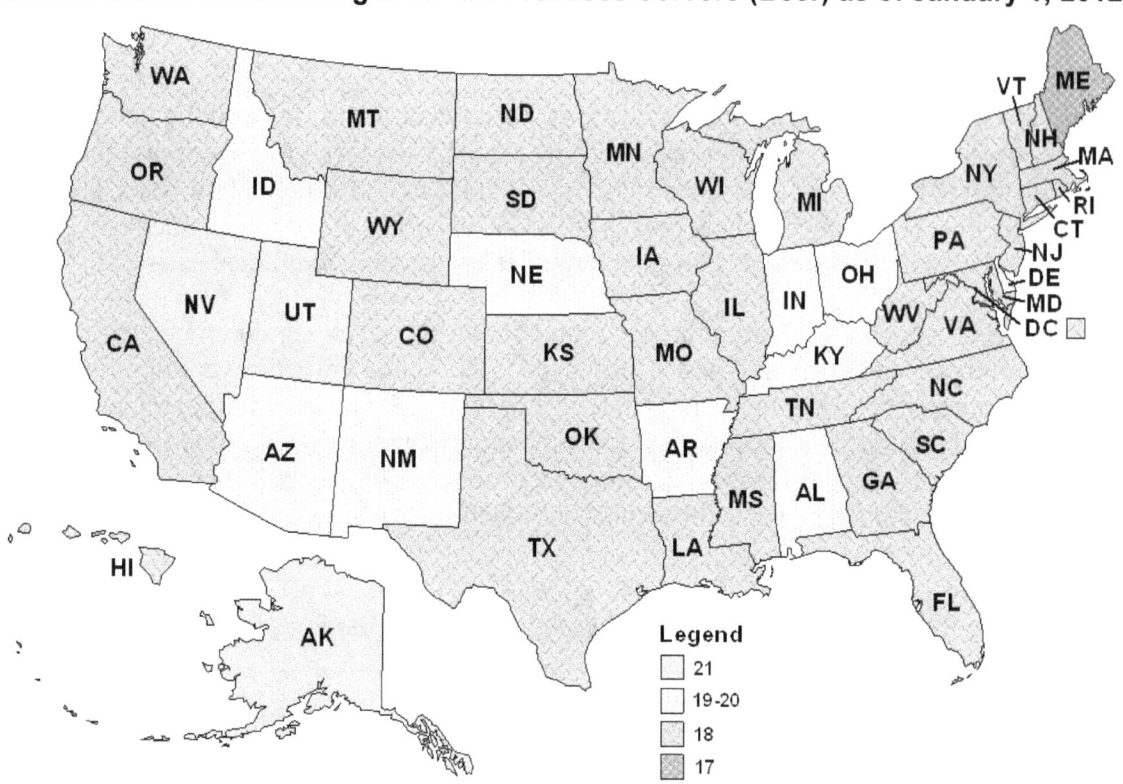

Exhibit 4.3.24: Distribution of Minimum Ages for On-Premises Servers of Beer, January 1, 2003, through January 1, 2012

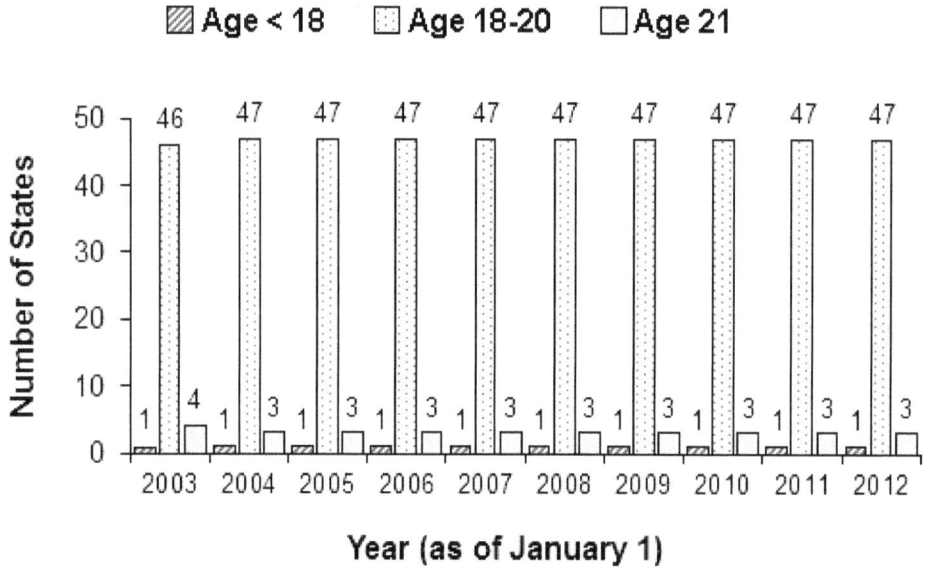

Distance Limitations Applied to New Alcohol Outlets Near Universities, Colleges, and Primary and Secondary Schools

Policy Description

Policies that limit the placement of retail alcohol outlets near colleges and schools are designed to make alcohol less accessible to children and youths by keeping alcohol sales physically distant from locations where underage people congregate. In addition, such policies aim to reduce the social availability of alcohol by limiting youth exposure to alcohol consumption.

Outlets Near Colleges and Universities

Alcohol outlet density in general is linked to excessive alcohol consumption and related harms, according to research collected and evaluated by the Community Preventive Services Task Force and presented in the *Community Guide* (Task Force on Community Preventive Services, 2009; Campbell, 2009). The *Community Guide* recommends the use of regulatory authority, for example through zoning and licensing, to reduce alcohol outlet density.

Limiting the location of retail outlets near colleges and universities, with their high concentrations of underage drinkers, is one way to implement this recommendation in a high-risk setting. The National Institute on Alcohol Abuse and Alcoholism (NIAAA) publication, *A Call to Action: Changing the Culture of Drinking at U.S. Colleges*, includes limiting alcohol outlet density as an evidence-based, recommended strategy for reducing college drinking (NIAAA, 2002).

Research shows a correlation between underage drinking and retail outlet density near college and university campuses. Outlet density was correlated with heavy and frequent drinking among college students, including underage students, in a study of eight universities (Weitzman, 2003). Another study found that both on- and off-premises alcohol outlet densities were associated with campus rape offense rates; the effect of on-campus densities was reduced when student drinking levels were considered (Scribner, 2010). A third study examined "second-hand" effects of drinking on residential neighborhoods near college campuses, and concluded that limiting the number of outlets near colleges, particularly those colleges with high rates of binge drinking, could mitigate the second-hand effects (Wechsler, 2002). A 1996 study found higher rates of drinking and binge drinking among college students when there were higher numbers of alcohol outlets within 1 mile of campus (Chaloupka & Wechsler, 1996).

Outlets Near Primary and Secondary Schools

Limiting outlets near primary and secondary schools is another way to reduce alcohol outlet density in a high-risk setting of underage drinking, although there is no research comparable to that for universities that focuses specifically on the relationship between drinking by K–12 students and the proximity of alcohol outlets to their schools.

Types of Outlet Density Restrictions

Outlet density restrictions typically require that alcohol outlets be located a certain distance from a school. Such restrictions may regulate the location of retail outlets near colleges and universities, near primary and secondary schools, or near both categories of schools.

Some restrictions limit the sale of alcohol directly on university campuses. Outlet density restrictions may apply to off-premises retailers, on-premises retailers, or both types of retailers. Restrictions may also apply to the sale of beer, wine, spirits, or some combination of the three.

Distance requirements vary widely, from 100 feet (the distance a primary or secondary school in Illinois must be from an off-premises outlet) to 1.5 miles (the distance a university in California must be from an outlet selling wine or spirits). Restrictions that mandate greater distances are more likely to promote the goals of keeping alcohol away from underage drinkers and reducing their exposure to alcohol marketing.

Distance restrictions apply to the issuance of new licenses, and retail alcohol outlets that were in business prior to the enactment of the restriction may still be allowed to operate within the restricted zone. In these cases, the distance restriction would prevent increased alcohol outlet density without necessarily reducing density or eliminating the presence of retail establishments in the restricted zone.

Status of Outlet Density Restrictions

Colleges and Universities

Thirteen states have some type of restriction on outlet density near colleges and universities, while 38 have no restrictions. Of the 13 states with restrictions, 11 have restrictions that apply to both on-premises and off-premises outlets. Kansas's restriction applies only to off-premises outlets and West Virginia's applies only to on-premises outlets.

Nearly all of the restrictions apply to beer, wine, and spirits. California and Mississippi restrictions apply only to wine and spirits, North Carolina restriction applies to beer and wine, and West Virginia's applies only to beer. Exhibit 4.3.27 shows the states with restrictions on colleges and universities and shows whether the restrictions apply to off-premises or on-premises outlets.

Primary and Secondary Schools

Many more states have laws restricting outlet location near primary and secondary schools: 34 states have some restriction, while 17 states have none. Out of the 34 states restricting outlet location, 26 apply restrictions to both off-premises locations and on-premises locations. The restrictions apply only to on-premises locations in six states: California, Florida, Hawaii, Maine, Montana, and West Virginia. Arkansas and Kansas restrict only off-premises locations.

Most of the restrictions apply to beer, wine, and spirits. New York, Wisconsin, and Mississippi restrictions apply to wine and spirits; Ohio and North Carolina restrictions apply only to beer and wine, and West Virginia restrictions apply only to beer. Exhibit 4.3.28 shows the states with restrictions on primary and secondary schools and shows whether the restrictions apply to off-premises or on-premises outlets.

Exhibit 4.3.27: States with Restrictions on Placement of Retail Outlets Near Colleges and Universities

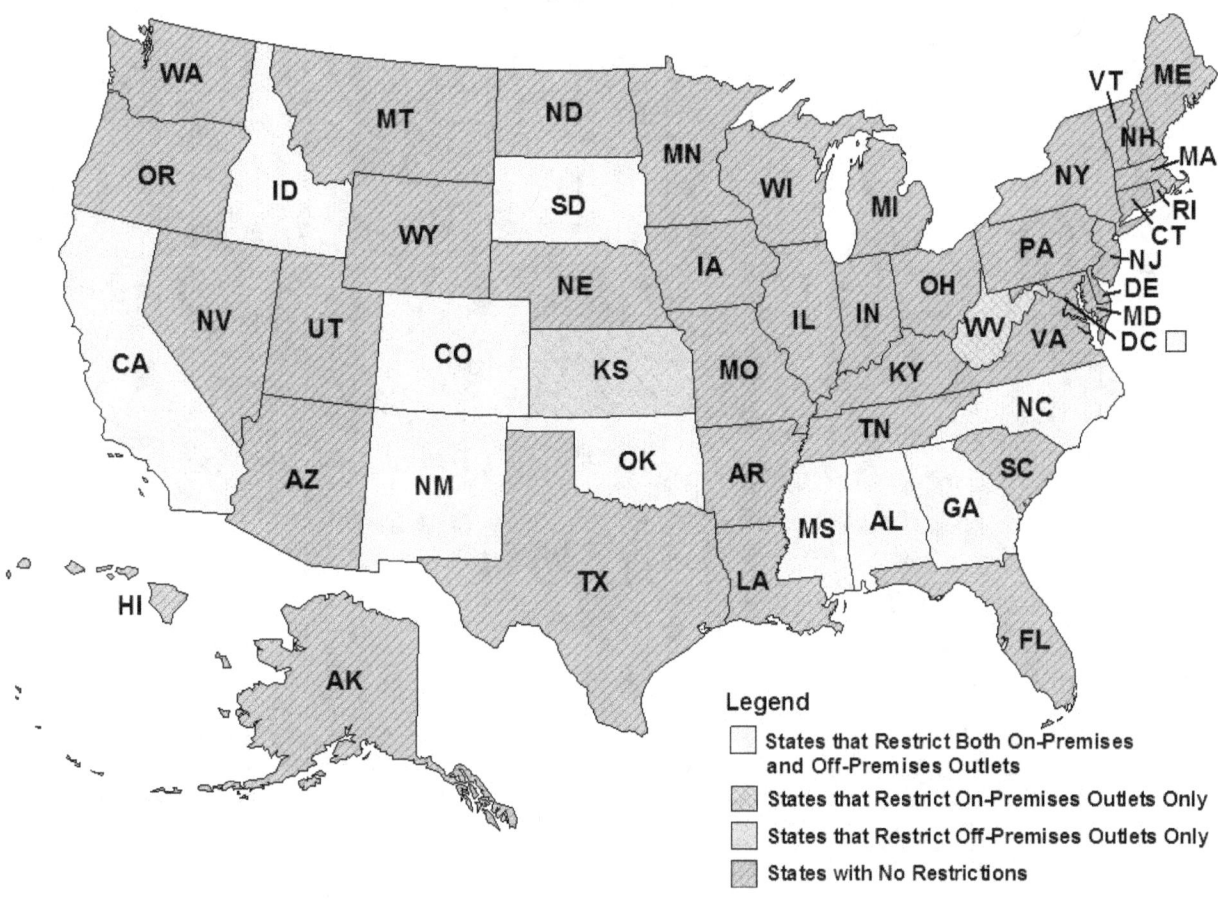

Legend

- ☐ States that Restrict Both On-Premises and Off-Premises Outlets
- States that Restrict On-Premises Outlets Only
- States that Restrict Off-Premises Outlets Only
- States with No Restrictions

References and Further Information

Legal research and data collection for this topic are planned and managed by SAMHSA and conducted under contract by The CDM Group, Inc. To see definitions of the variables for this policy, go to Appendix B. For further information and background see:

Campbell, C., Hahn, R., Elder, R., et al. (2009). The effectiveness of limiting alcohol outlet density as a means of reducing excessive alcohol consumption and alcohol-related harms. *American Journal of Preventive Medicine, 37,* 556–569.

Centers for Disease Control and Prevention, Guide to Community Preventive Services. (2009). Preventing Excessive Alcohol Consumption: Regulation of Alcohol Outlet Density. http://www.thecommunityguide.org/alcohol/outletdensity.html

Chaloupka, F.J., & Wechsler, H. (1996). Binge drinking in college: The impact of price, availability, and alcohol control policies. *Contemporary Economic Policy, 14(4),* 112–124.

National Institute on Alcohol Abuse and Alcoholism. (2002). A Call to Action: Changing the Culture of Drinking at U.S. Colleges, available at http://www.collegedrinkingprevention.gov/media/TaskForceReport.pdf

Exhibit 4.3.28: States with Restrictions on Placement of Retail Outlets Near Primary and Secondary Schools

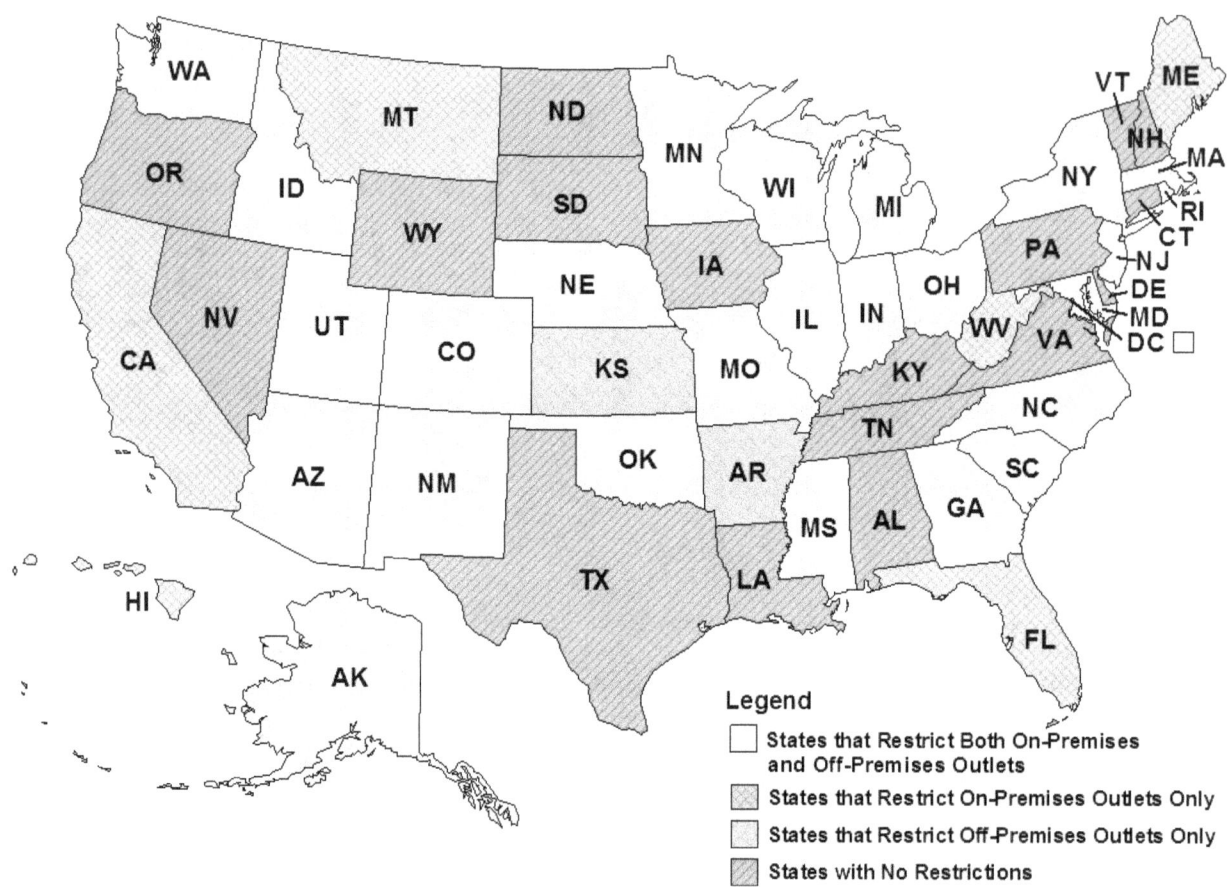

Legend

☐ States that Restrict Both On-Premises and Off-Premises Outlets

▨ States that Restrict On-Premises Outlets Only

☐ States that Restrict Off-Premises Outlets Only

▨ States with No Restrictions

Scribner, R., Mason, K., Simonsen, N., Theall, K., Chotalia, J., Johnson, S., Schneider, S.K., & Dejong, W. (2010). An ecological analysis of alcohol-outlet density and campus-reported violence at 32 U.S. colleges. *Journal of Studies on Alcohol and Drugs, 71*, 184–191.

Task Force on Community Preventive Services. (2009). Recommendations for reducing excessive alcohol consumption and alcohol-related harms by limiting alcohol outlet density. *American Journal of Preventive Medicine, 6*, 570–571.

Wechsler, H., Lee, J.E., Hall, A., Wagenaar, A., & Lee, H. (2002). Secondhand effects of student alcohol use reported by neighbors of colleges: The role of alcohol outlets. *Social Science & Medicine, 55*, 425–435.

Weitzman, E., Folkman, A., Folkman, K.L., & Wechsler, H. (2003). The relationship of alcohol outlet density to heavy and frequent drinking and drinking-related problems among college students at eight universities. *Health & Place, 9*, 1–6.

Dram Shop Liability

Policy Description

Dram shop liability refers to the civil liability faced by commercial alcohol providers for injuries or damages caused by their intoxicated or underage drinking patrons. The analysis in this report is limited to alcohol service to minors.[36] The typical factual scenario in legal cases arising from dram shop liability is a licensed retail alcohol outlet that furnishes alcohol to a minor who, in turn, causes an alcohol-related motor vehicle crash that injures a third party. In states with dram shop liability, the injured third party ("plaintiff") may be able to sue the retailer (as well as the minor who caused the crash) for monetary damages. Liability comes into play only if an injured private citizen files a lawsuit. The state's role is to provide a forum for such a lawsuit; the state does not impose a dram-shop-related penalty directly. (This distinguishes dram shop liability from the underage furnishing policy, which results in criminal liability imposed by the state.)

Dram shop liability is closely related to the policy on furnishing alcohol to minors, but the two topics are distinct. Retailers who furnish alcohol to minors may face fines or other punishment imposed by the state as well as dram shop liability lawsuits filed by parties injured as a result of the same incident. Dram shop liability and social host liability (presented elsewhere in this report) are identical, except that the former involves lawsuits filed against commercial alcohol retailers and the latter involves lawsuits filed against noncommercial alcohol providers.

Dram shop liability serves two purposes: (1) it creates a disincentive for retailers to furnish to minors because of the risk of litigation leading to substantial monetary losses, and (2) it allows parties injured as a result of an illegal sale to a minor to gain compensation from those responsible for the injury. The minor causing the injury is the primary and most likely party to be sued. Typically, the retailer is sued through a dram shop claim when the minor does not have the resources to fully compensate the injured party.

Dram shop liability is established by statute or by a state court through "common law." Common law is the authority of state courts to establish rules by which an injured party can seek redress against the person or entity that negligently or intentionally caused injury. Courts can establish these rules only when the state legislature has not enacted its own statutes, in which case the courts must follow the legislative dictates (unless found to be unconstitutional). Thus, dram shop statutes normally take precedence over dram shop common law court decisions. This analysis includes both statutory and common law dram shop liability for each state.

A common law liability designation signifies that the state allows lawsuits by injured third parties against alcohol retailers for the negligent service or provision of alcohol to a minor. Common law liability assumes the following procedural and substantive rules:

- A negligence standard applies (i.e., the defendant did not act as a reasonable person would be expected to act in like circumstances). Plaintiffs need not show that the defendant acted intentionally, willfully, or with actual knowledge of the minor's underage status.

---

[36] "Dram shop liability" is a legal term that originated in the 19th century. Dram shops were retail establishments that sold distilled spirits by the "dram," a liquid measure that equals 1 ounce. This form of liability is also known as "commercial host liability."

- Damages are not arbitrarily limited. If negligence is established, the plaintiff receives actual damages and can seek punitive damages.

- Plaintiffs can pursue claims against defendants without regard for the age of the person who furnished the alcohol and the age of the underage person furnished with alcohol.

- Plaintiffs must establish only that minors were furnished alcohol and that the furnishing contributed to the injury without regard to the minor's intoxicated state at the time of sale.

- Plaintiffs must establish key elements of the lawsuit via "preponderance of the evidence" rather than a more rigorous standard (e.g., "beyond a reasonable doubt").

A statutory liability designation indicates that the state has a dram shop statute. Statutory provisions can alter the common law rules listed above, restricting an injured party's ability to make successful claims. This report includes three of the most important statutory limitations:

1. Limitations on damages: Statutes may impose statutory caps on the total dollar amount that plaintiffs may recover through dram shop lawsuits.

2. Limitations on who may be sued: Potential defendants may be limited to only certain types of retail establishments (e.g., on-premises but not off-premises licensees), or certain types of servers (e.g., servers above a certain age).

3. Limitations on elements or standards of proof: Statutes may require plaintiffs to prove additional facts or meet a more rigorous standard of proof than would normally apply in common law. The statutory provisions may require plaintiff to:
   - Establish that the retailer knew the minor was underage or that the retailer intentionally or willfully served the minor.
   - Establish that the minor was intoxicated at the time of sale or service.
   - Provide clear and convincing evidence or evidence beyond a reasonable doubt that the allegations are true.

These limitations can restrict the circumstances that can give rise to liability or greatly diminish a plaintiff's chances of prevailing in a dram shop liability lawsuit, thus reducing the likelihood of a lawsuit being filed. Other restrictions may also apply. For example, many states do not allow "first-party claims"—cases brought by the person who was furnished alcohol for his or her own injuries. This report does not track these additional limitations.

Some states have enacted responsible beverage service affirmative defenses. In these states, a defendant can avoid liability if it can establish that its retail establishment had implemented an RBS program and was adhering to RBS practices at the time of the service to a minor. Texas has enacted a more sweeping RBS defense. A defendant licensee can avoid liability if it establishes that (1) it did not encourage the illegal sale and (2) it required its staff, including the server in question, to attend RBS training. Proof that RBS practices were being adhered to at the time of service is not required. See the RBS Training policy topic in this report for more information.

Status of Dram Shop Liability

As of January 1, 2012, 45 jurisdictions imposed dram shop liability as a result of statutory or common law or both (see Exhibit 4.3.29). The District of Columbia and 28 states have either common law liability or statutory liability or both with no identified limitation. The remaining 16 states impose one or more limits on statutory dram shop liability: 7 states limit the damages that may be recovered, 4 states limit who may be sued, and 12 states require stricter standards for proof of wrongdoing than for usual negligence. Seven states provide an RBS defense for alcohol outlets (see Exhibit 4.3.30). Six states provide an affirmative RBS defense and one state provides a complete RBS defense.

Trends in Dram Shop Liability for Furnishing Alcohol to a Minor

Between 2009 and 2012, the number of jurisdictions that permit dram shop liability remained constant and three states (Colorado, Illinois, and Maine) increased the dollar limits on damages.

Exhibit 4.3.29: Common Law/Statutory Dram Shop Liability and Limitations as of January 1, 2012

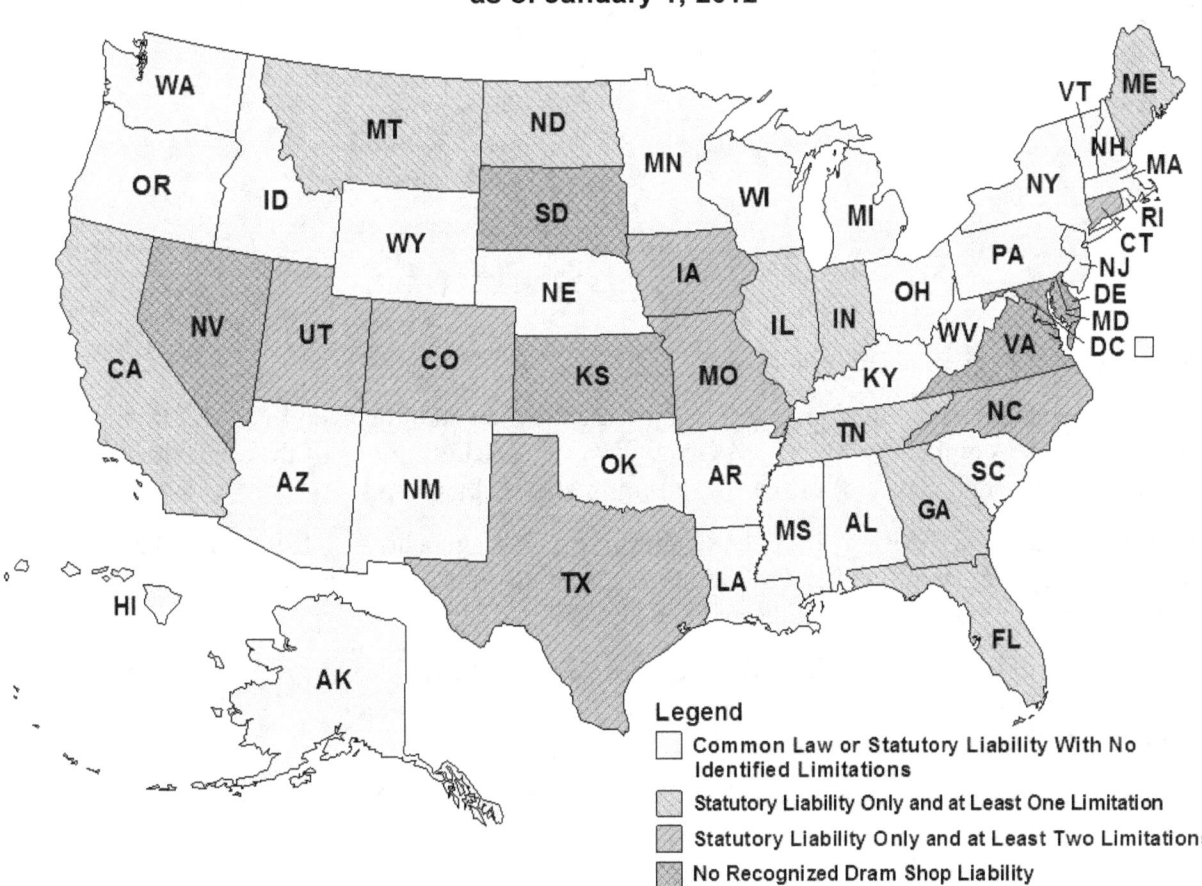

Legend
- Common Law or Statutory Liability With No Identified Limitations
- Statutory Liability Only and at Least One Limitation
- Statutory Liability Only and at Least Two Limitations
- No Recognized Dram Shop Liability

Exhibit 4.3.30: Responsible Beverage Service Program Defenses Against Dram Shop Liability Across the United States as of January 1, 2012

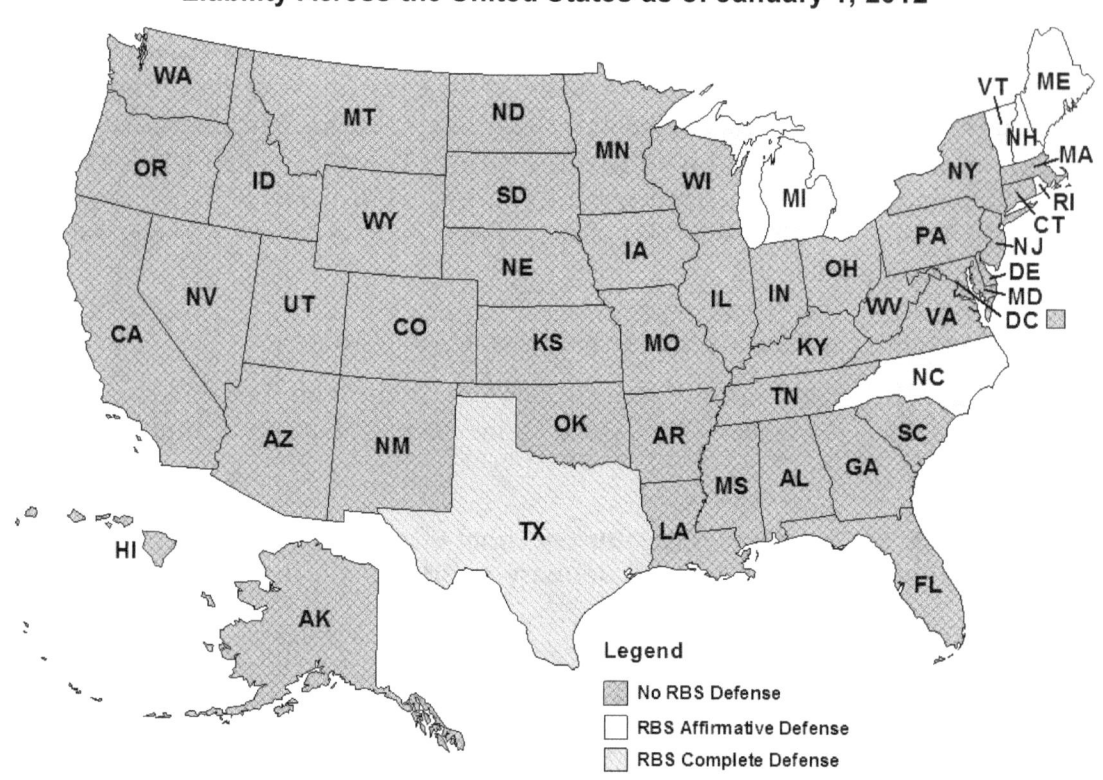

Legend
- No RBS Defense
- RBS Affirmative Defense
- RBS Complete Defense

References and Further Information

Legal research and data collection for this topic are planned and managed by SAMHSA and conducted under contract by The CDM Group, Inc. To see definitions of the variables for this policy, go to Appendix B. For further information and background see:

Holder, H., Janes, K., Mosher, J., Saltz, R., Spurr, S., & Wagenaar, A. (1992). Final report: Evaluation of dram shop liability and the reduction of alcohol-related traffic problems. National Highway Traffic Safety Administration, DTNH22-87-R-07254.

Holder, H., Janes, K., Mosher, J., Saltz, R., Spurr, S., & Wagenaar, A. (1993). Alcoholic beverage server liability and the reduction of alcohol-involved problems. *Journal of Studies on Alcohol, 54,* 23–36.

Mosher, J., et al. (2011). *Liquor liability law.* Newark, NJ: LexisNexis.

Social Host Liability

Policy Description

Social host liability refers to the civil liability faced by noncommercial alcohol providers for injuries or damages caused by their intoxicated or underage drinking guests. The analysis in this report does not address social host liability for serving adult guests. The typical factual scenario in legal cases arising from social host liability involves an underage drinking party at which the party host furnishes alcohol to a minor who in turn injures a third party in an alcohol-related incident (often a motor vehicle crash). In states with social host liability, injured third parties ("plaintiffs") may be able to sue social hosts (as well as the minor who caused the crash) for monetary damages. Liability comes into play only if injured private citizens file lawsuits. The state's role is to provide a forum for such lawsuits; the state does not impose social host–related penalties directly. (As discussed below, this distinguishes social host liability from underage furnishing and host party policies, which can result in criminal liability imposed by the state.)

Social host liability is closely related to the furnishing alcohol to a minor and host party policy topics, but the three topics are distinct. Social hosts who furnish alcohol to minors or allow underage drinking parties on their property may face fines or other punishment imposed by the state as well as social host liability lawsuits filed by injured parties stemming from the same incident. Social host liability and dram shop liability (presented elsewhere in this report) are identical policies except that the former involves lawsuits brought against noncommercial alcohol retailers, and the latter involves lawsuits filed against commercial alcohol providers.

Social host liability serves two purposes: (1) it creates disincentives for social hosts to furnish to minors due to the risk of litigation and potentially substantial monetary losses and (2) it allows those injured as a result of illegal furnishing of alcohol to minors to gain compensation from the person(s) responsible for their injuries. Minors causing injuries are the primary and most likely parties to be sued. Typically, social hosts are sued through social host liability claims when minors do not have the resources to fully compensate the injured parties.

Social host liability is established by statute or by a state court through "common law." Common law refers to the authority of state courts to establish rules by which injured parties can seek redress against persons or entities that negligently or intentionally caused injuries. Courts have the authority to establish these rules only when state legislatures have not enacted their own statutes, in which case the courts must follow legislative dictates (unless found to be unconstitutional). Thus, social host statutes normally take precedence over social host common law court decisions.

Many states require evidence that social hosts furnished alcohol to the underage guest, although others permit liability if social hosts allowed underage guests to drink on the hosts' property even if the hosts did not furnish the alcohol. This analysis does not report the states that have adopted this more permissive standard. The analysis includes both statutory and common law social host liability for each state.

A common law liability designation signifies that the state allows lawsuits by injured third parties against social hosts for the negligent service or provision of alcohol to minors in noncommercial settings. Common law liability assumes the following procedural and substantive rules:

- A negligence standard applies (i.e., defendants did not act as reasonable persons would be expected to act in similar circumstances). Plaintiffs need not show that defendants acted intentionally, willfully, or with actual knowledge of minors' underage status.

- Damages are not arbitrarily limited. If successful in establishing negligence, plaintiffs receive actual damages and have the possibility of seeking punitive damages.

- Plaintiffs can pursue claims against defendants without regard for the age of the person who furnished the alcohol and the age of the underage person furnished with alcohol.

- Plaintiffs must establish only that minors were furnished with alcohol and that the furnishing contributed to injuries without regard to the minors' intoxicated state at the time of the party.

- Plaintiffs must establish the key elements of lawsuits by "preponderance of the evidence" rather than a more rigorous standard (such as "beyond a reasonable doubt").

A statutory liability designation indicates that a state has a social host liability statute. Statutory provisions can alter the common law rules listed above, restricting an injured party's ability to make successful claims. This report includes three of the most important statutory limitations:

1. Limitations on damages: Statutes may impose statutory caps on the total dollar amount that plaintiffs may recover through social host lawsuits.

2. Limitations on who may be sued: Potential defendants may be limited to persons above a certain age.

3. Limitations on elements or standards of proof: Statutes may require plaintiffs to prove additional facts or meet a more rigorous standard of proof than would normally apply in common law. The statutory provisions may require the plaintiff to:
   - Establish that hosts had knowledge that minors were underage or proof that social hosts intentionally or willfully served minors.
   - Establish that the minors were intoxicated at the time of service.
   - Provide clear and convincing evidence or evidence beyond a reasonable doubt that the allegations are true.

These limitations can limit the circumstances that can give rise to liability or greatly diminish plaintiffs' chances of prevailing in a social host liability lawsuit, thus reducing the likelihood of a lawsuit being filed. Other restrictions in addition to the three listed above may also apply. For example, many states do not allow "first-party claims," cases brought by the person who was furnished alcohol for his or her own injuries. This report does not track these additional limitations.

Status of Social Host Liability

As of January 1, 2012, 33 states impose social host liability through statute or common law; 15 states and the District of Columbia do not impose social host liability. In two states, there is no statutory liability and common law liability is unclear (see Exhibit 4.3.31). Eighteen states have either common law liability or statutory social host liability with no identified limitations. Eleven states impose one limit on statutory social host liability and four states impose two limitations. The count for limitations is as follows: 4 states limit the damages that may be

Exhibit 4.3.31: Common Law/Statutory Social Host Liability as of January 1, 2012

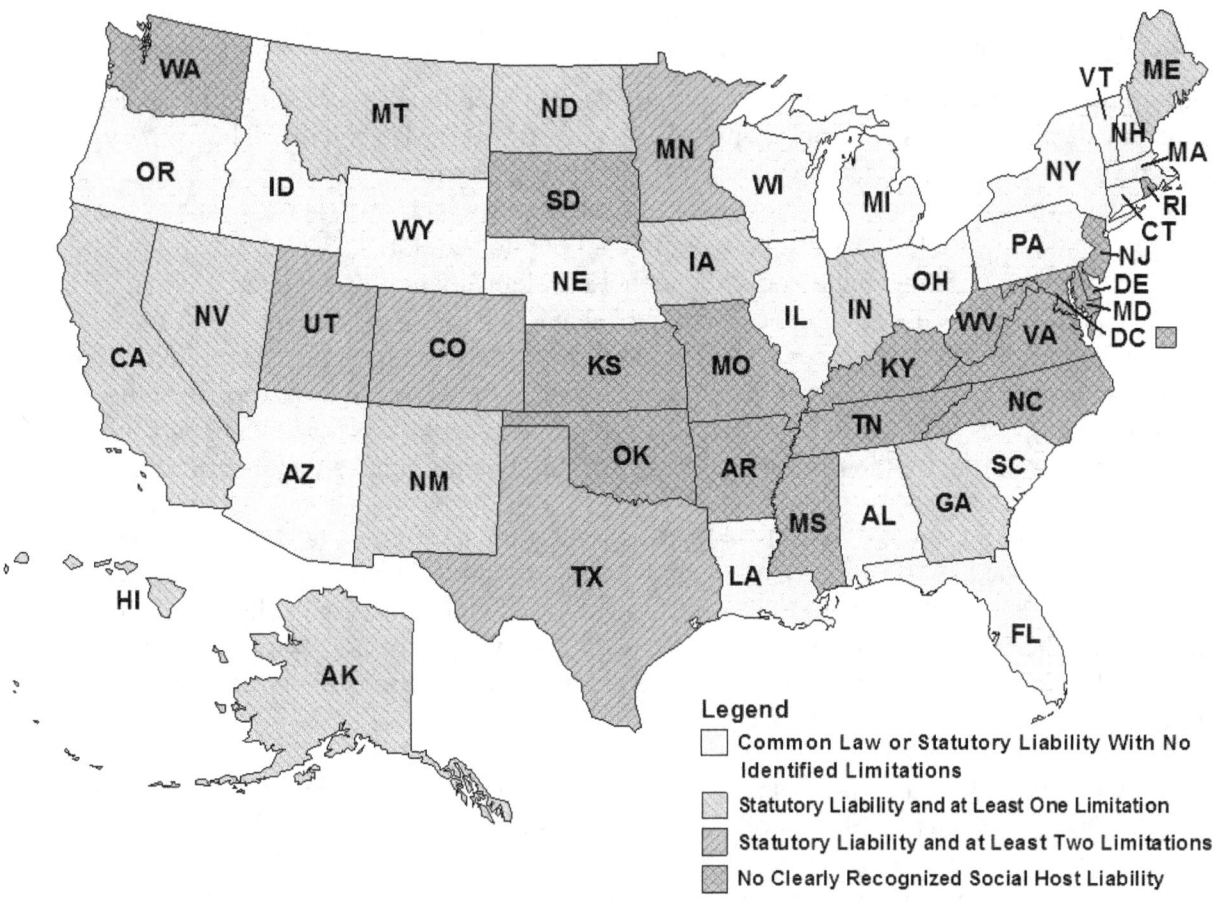

recovered, 4 states limit who may be sued, and 11 states require standards of proof of wrongdoing that are stricter than usual negligence standards.

Trends in Social Host Liability for Furnishing Alcohol to a Minor

In the years between 2009 and 2012, the number of states that permit social host liability increased by one. California requires standards of proof of wrongdoing that are stricter than usual negligence standards. One state (Utah) increased the dollar limits on damages.

References and Further Information

Legal research and data collection for this topic are planned and managed by SAMHSA and conducted under contract with The CDM Group, Inc. To see definitions of the variables for this policy, go to Appendix B. For additional information and background, see:

Mosher, J., et al. (2011). *Liquor liability law.* Newark, NJ: LexisNexis.

Stout, E., Sloan, A., Liang, L., & Davies, H. (2000). Reducing harmful alcohol-related behaviors: Effective regulatory methods. *Journal of Studies on Alcohol, 61,* 402–412.

Hosting Underage Drinking Parties

Policy Description

Host party laws establish state-imposed liability against individuals (social hosts) responsible for underage drinking events on property they own, lease, or otherwise control. The primary purpose of these laws is to deter underage drinking parties by raising the legal risk for individuals who allow underage drinking events on property they own, lease, or otherwise control. Underage drinking parties pose significant public health risks. They are high-risk settings for binge drinking and associated alcohol problems including impaired driving. Young drinkers are often introduced to heavy drinking behaviors at these events. Law enforcement officials report that, in many cases, underage drinking parties occur on private property, but the adult responsible for the property is not present or cannot be shown to have furnished the alcohol. Host party laws address this issue by providing a legal basis for holding persons responsible for parties on their property whether or not they provided alcohol to minors.

Host party laws often are closely linked to laws prohibiting the furnishing of alcohol to minors (analyzed elsewhere in this report), although laws that prohibit the hosting of underage drinking parties may apply without regard to who furnishes the alcohol. Hosts who allow underage drinking on their property and also supply the alcohol consumed or possessed by the minors may be in violation of two distinct laws: furnishing alcohol to a minor and allowing underage drinking to occur on property they control.

Two general types of liability may apply to those who host underage drinking parties. The first, analyzed here, concerns state-imposed liability. State-imposed liability involves a statutory prohibition that is enforced by the state, generally through criminal proceedings that can lead to sanctions such as fines or imprisonment. The second, social host liability (analyzed elsewhere in this report), involves an action by a private party seeking monetary damages for injuries that result from permitting underage drinking on the host's premises.

Although related, these two forms of liability are distinct. For example, an individual may allow a minor to drink alcohol, after which the minor causes a motor vehicle crash that injures an innocent third party. In this situation, the social host may be prosecuted by the state under a criminal statute and face a fine or imprisonment for the criminal violation. In a state that provides for social host civil liability, the injured third party could also sue the host for monetary damages associated with the motor vehicle crash.

State host party laws differ across multiple dimensions, including the following:

- They may limit their application specifically to underage drinking parties (e.g., by requiring a certain number of minors to be present for the law to take effect) or may prohibit hosts from allowing underage drinking on their property generally, without reference to hosting a party.

- Underage drinking on any of the host's properties may be included, or the laws may restrict their application to residences, out-buildings, and/or outdoor areas.

- The laws may apply only when hosts make overt acts to encourage the party, or they may require only that hosts knew about the party or were negligent in not realizing that parties were occurring (i.e., should have known based on the facts available).

- A defense may be available for hosts who take specific preventive steps to end parties (e.g., contacting police) once they become aware that parties are occurring.

- The laws may require differing types of behavior on the part of the minors at the party (possession, consumption, intent to possess or consume) before a violation occurs.

- Jurisdictions have varying exceptions in their statutes for family members or others, or for other uses or settings involving the handling of alcoholic beverages.

Status of Host Party Laws

As of January 1, 2012, 19 jurisdictions have general host party laws, 9 have specific host party laws, and 24 have no laws of either sort (see Exhibit 4.3.32). Of the jurisdictions with host party laws, 23 apply to both residential and outdoor property and 4 apply to residential property but not outdoor property. Twenty-six jurisdictions apply their law to other types of property (e.g., motels, hotels, campgrounds, out-buildings). Seven jurisdictions permit negation of violations when the host takes preventive action; 22 require knowledge standards to trigger liability; 3 rely on a negligence standard; 4 require an overt act on the part of the host to trigger liability; and 1 requires recklessness. Finally, 20 jurisdictions have family exceptions and 4 have resident exceptions.

Trends in Host Party Law Policies

Between 1998 and 2011, the number of jurisdictions that enacted specific host party laws rose from 5 to 9, and the number that enacted general host party laws rose from 11 to 19. In 1998, there were 16 host party laws of both types; in 2012 there are 28 (see Exhibit 4.3.33).

Exhibit 4.3.32: Prohibitions against Hosting Underage Drinking Parties as of January 1, 2012

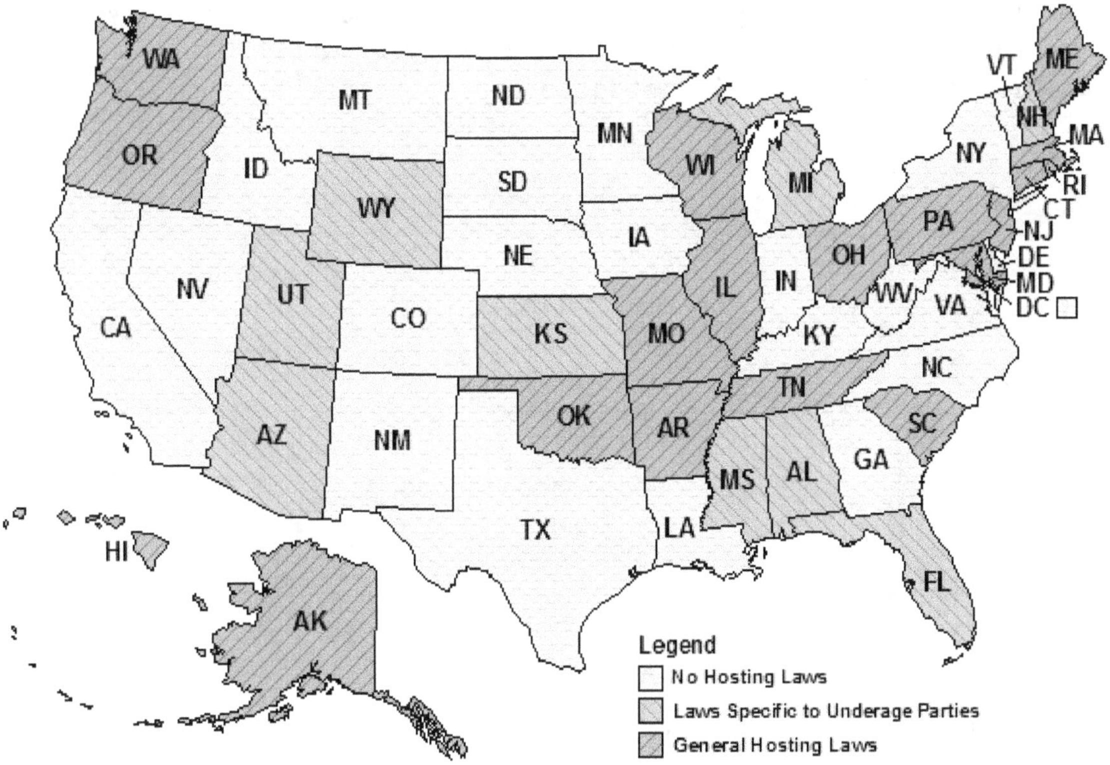

Legend
- No Hosting Laws
- Laws Specific to Underage Parties
- General Hosting Laws

Exhibit 4.3.33: Number of States with Prohibitions Against Hosting Underage Drinking Parties, January 1, 1998, through January 1, 2012

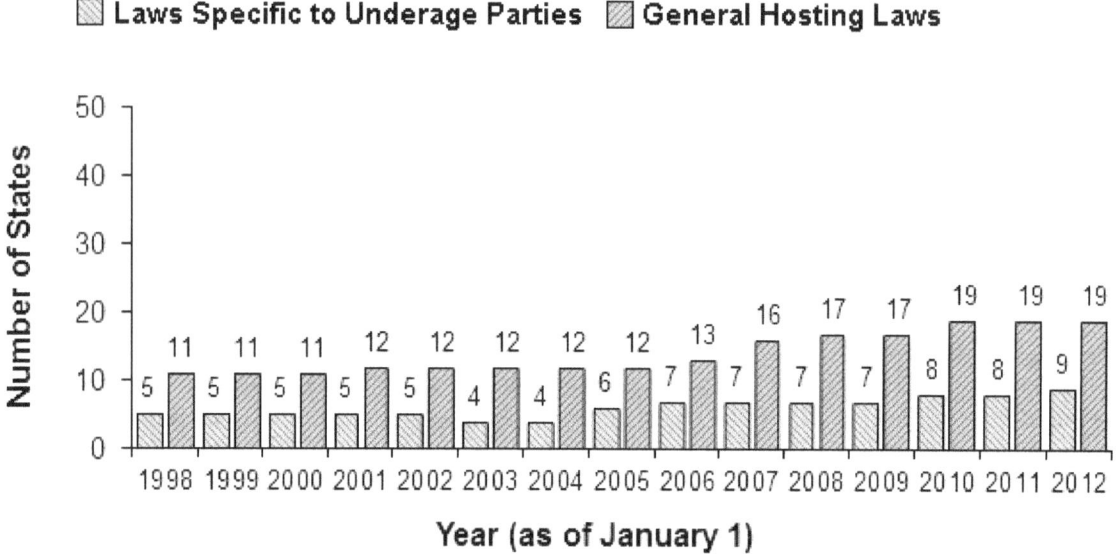

References and Further Information

All data for this policy were obtained from APIS at http://www.alcoholpolicy.niaaa.nih.gov. Follow links to the policy entitled "Prohibitions against Hosting Underage Drinking Parties." APIS provides further descriptions of this policy and its variables, details regarding state policies, and a review of the limitations associated with the reported data. To see definitions of the variables for this policy, go to Appendix B.

Retailer Interstate Shipments of Alcohol

Policy Description

This policy addresses state laws that prohibit or permit retailers to ship alcohol directly to consumers located across state lines, usually by ordering alcohol over the internet. It is related to, but distinct from, both the Direct Shipment policy, which addresses alcohol shipments to consumers by alcohol producers, and the Home Delivery policy, which involves retailer deliveries to consumers within the same state.

Retailer interstate shipments may be an important source of alcohol for underage drinkers. In a recent study (Williams & Ribisl, 2012), a group of 8 18- to 20-year-old research assistants in North Carolina placed 100 orders for alcoholic beverages using internet sites hosted by out-of-state retailers. Forty-five percent of the orders were successfully completed and 39 percent were rejected as a result of age verification. The remaining 16 percent of orders failed for reasons believed to be unrelated to age verification (e.g., technical and communications problems with vendors).

Most vendors (59 percent) used weak, if any, age verification at the point of order, and, of the 45 successful orders, 23 (51 percent) had no age verification at all. Age verification at delivery was also inconsistently applied.

The North Carolina study reported that there are more than 5,000 internet alcohol retailers, and that the retailers make conflicting claims regarding the legality of shipping alcohol across state lines to consumers. For example, one internet alcohol retailer says on its website that only four states (Massachusetts, Nevada, Texas and West Virginia) do not allow internet alcohol retailers to ship directly to individual consumers. Other internet alcohol retailers provide differing lists of states or imply that all shipments are legal.

There were also conflicting claims regarding the role of common carriers. The North Carolina study reported that all deliveries were made by such companies, and many internet alcohol retailers list well-known common carriers on their websites. Yet carriers contacted by the North Carolina researchers stated that they do not deliver packages of alcohol except with direct shipping permits. This suggests confusion regarding state laws addressing interstate retail shipments. North Carolina, where the study took place, prohibits such shipments, which means that at least 43 percent of the retailers in the study appeared to have violated the state law.

The National Research Council/Institute of Medicine report on reducing underage drinking recognized the potential for young people to obtain alcohol over the internet. It recommended that states either ban such sales or require alcohol labeling on packages and signature verification at the point of delivery (National Research Council and Institute of Medicine, 2004).

There are several potential barriers to implementing and enforcing bans on retailer interstate alcohol sales, including:

1. States will have difficulty securing jurisdiction over out-of-state alcohol retailers.

2. States may have little incentive to use limited enforcement resources to crack down on in-state alcohol retailers that are shipping out of state because they are not violating state law, taxes are being collected, and any problems occur out of state.

3. Enforcing bans on retailer interstate shipments may prompt online retailers to locate outside the country (many already are foreign based), creating additional jurisdictional and enforcement problems.

Types of Restrictions on Interstate Internet Sales

The restrictions addressed in this policy vary by beverage type (beer, wine, distilled spirits). Interstate shipments may be prohibited for one beverage type, more than one beverage type, or all three beverage types. Some states place restrictions on interstate internet sales including requiring a direct shipping permit and/or limiting the amount of beverage that may be shipped.

Current Status of Interstate Internet Sales

As shown in Exhibit 4.3.34, 32 states prohibit retailer interstate sales of all 3 beverage types, 8 prohibit sales of 2 beverage types, and 3 prohibit sales of 1 beverage type. Spirits are the most commonly prohibited beverage (43 states), followed by beer (39 states) and wine (33 states). In nine states, retailer interstate sales laws were deemed uncodable for at least one beverage type (beer, wine, liquor). For the purposes of this summary, these states are treated as *not* expressly prohibiting interstate internet sales for the uncodable beverage types.

Exhibit 4.3.34: Number of Beverage Types for which Interstate Internet Sales Are Expressly Prohibited

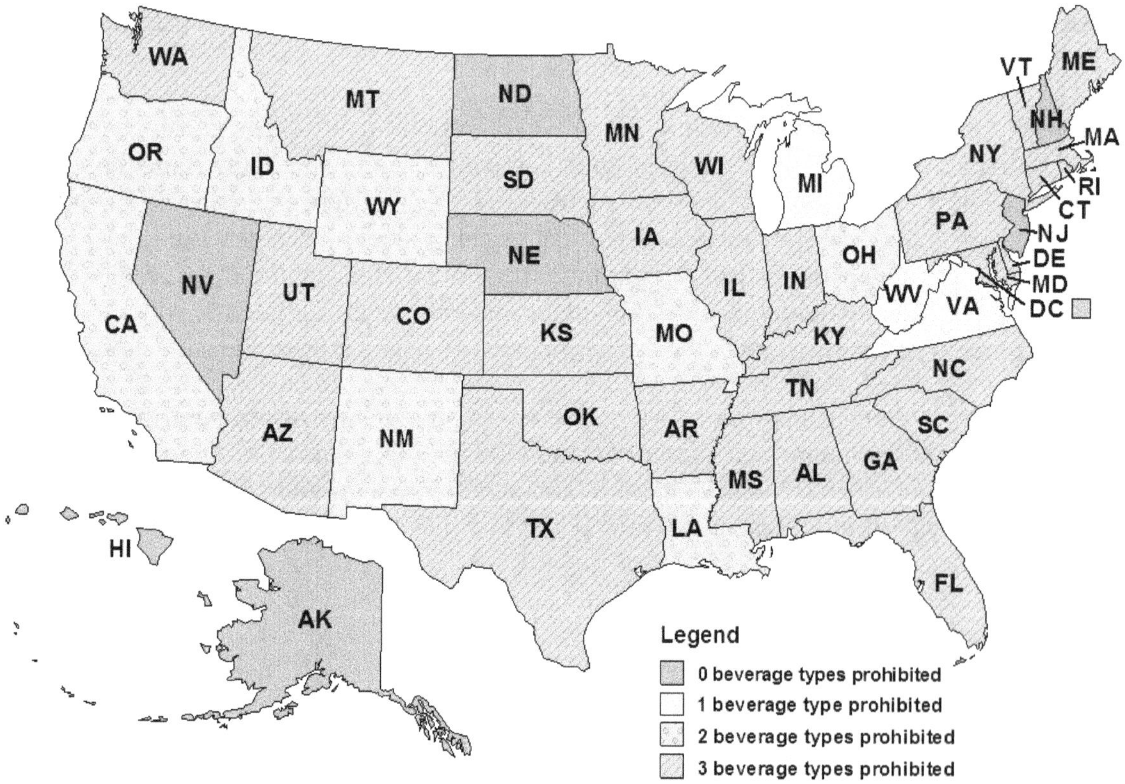

Legend
- 0 beverage types prohibited
- 1 beverage type prohibited
- 2 beverage types prohibited
- 3 beverage types prohibited

References and Further Information

Legal research and data collection for this topic are planned and managed by SAMHSA and conducted under contract by The CDM Group, Inc. To see definitions of the variables for this policy, go to Appendix B. For further information and background see:

"Drink Up New York: The web's best source for fine wine, spirits, sake & more!" (No date). http://www.drinkupny.com

National Research Council and Institute of Medicine. (2004). *Reducing underage drinking: A collective responsibility*. Committee on Developing a Strategy to Reduce and Prevent Underage Drinking, Richard J. Bonnie and Mary Ellen O'Connell, Editors. Board on Children, Youth, and Families, Division of Behavioral and Social Sciences and Education. Washington, DC: National Academies Press.

N.C.Gen. Stat. § 18B-102.1; N.C.Gen. Stat. § 18B-109.

Williams, R S., & Ribisl, K.M. Internet alcohol sales to minors. (2012). *Archives of Pediatrics and Adolescent Medicine 166(9),* 808–813.

Direct Sales/Shipments from Producers to Consumers

Policy Description

State proscriptions against direct sales and shipments of alcohol from producers to consumers date back to the repeal of Prohibition. The initial reason for the proscription was to ensure that the pre-Prohibition-era "tied house system" (under which producers owned and/or controlled retail outlets directly) did not continue after repeal. Opponents of the tied house system argued that producers who controlled retail outlets permitted unsafe retail practices and failed to respond to community concerns. The alternative that emerged was a three-tier production and distribution system with separate production, wholesaling, and retail elements. Consequently, producers must distribute products through wholesalers rather than sell directly to retailers or consumers; wholesalers must purchase from producers; and consumers must purchase from retailers.

Modern marketing practices, particularly internet sales that link producers directly to consumers, have led many states to create laws with exceptions to general mandates that alcohol producers distribute their products only through wholesalers. Some states permit producers to ship alcohol to consumers using a delivery service (usually a common carrier). In some cases, these exceptions are responses to legal challenges by producers or retailers arguing that state law unfairly discriminates between in-state and out-of-state producers. The U.S. Supreme Court has held that state laws permitting in-state producers to ship directly to consumers while barring out-of-state producers from doing so violate the U.S. Constitution's Interstate Commerce Clause, and that this discrimination is neither authorized nor permitted by the 21st Amendment.[37]

One central concern emerging from this controversy is the possibility that direct sales/shipments (either through internet sales or sales made by telephone or other remote communication) will increase alcohol availability to underage persons. Young people may attempt to purchase alcohol through direct sales instead of face-to-face sales at retail outlets, because they perceive that detection of their underage status is less likely. These concerns were validated by a recent study that found that internet alcohol vendors use weak, if any, age verification, thereby allowing minors to successfully purchase alcohol online. In response to these concerns, several jurisdictions that permit direct sales/shipments have included provisions to deter youth access. These may include requirements that:

- Consumers have face-to-face transactions at producers' places of business (and show valid age identification) before any future shipments to consumers can be made.[38]

- Producers/shippers and deliverers verify recipient age, usually by checking recipients' identification.

- Producers/shippers and deliverers obtain permits or licenses or be approved by the state.

- Producers/shippers and deliverers maintain records that must either be reported to state officials or be open for inspection to verify recipients of shipments.

- Direct shipment package labels include statements that the package contains alcohol and/or that the recipient must be at least 21 years old.

---

[37] See, e.g., *Granholm v. Heald*, 544 U.S. 460, 125 S.Ct. 1885 (2005).

[38] Laws that require face-to-face transactions for all sales prior to delivery are treated as prohibitions on direct sales/shipments.

State laws also vary on the types of alcoholic beverages (beer, wine, distilled spirits) that producers may sell directly and ship to consumers. These and other restrictions may apply to all direct shipments. This report includes only those requirements related to preventing underage sales.[39]

Status of Direct Sales/Shipment Policies

As of January 1, 2012, 40 states permit direct sales/shipments from producers to consumers, and 11 prohibit such transactions (see Exhibit 4.3.35). One state (Indiana) requires face-to-face transactions at producers' places of business (and verification of valid age identification) before shipments to the consumer can be made. Thirty-seven states require producers to obtain a shipper's permit or state approval prior to shipping. Of the 40 states permitting direct sales or shipments, 8 require shippers to verify purchaser age, 20 require deliverers to verify recipient age, 5 require age verification by both shippers and deliverers, and 1 requires verification at

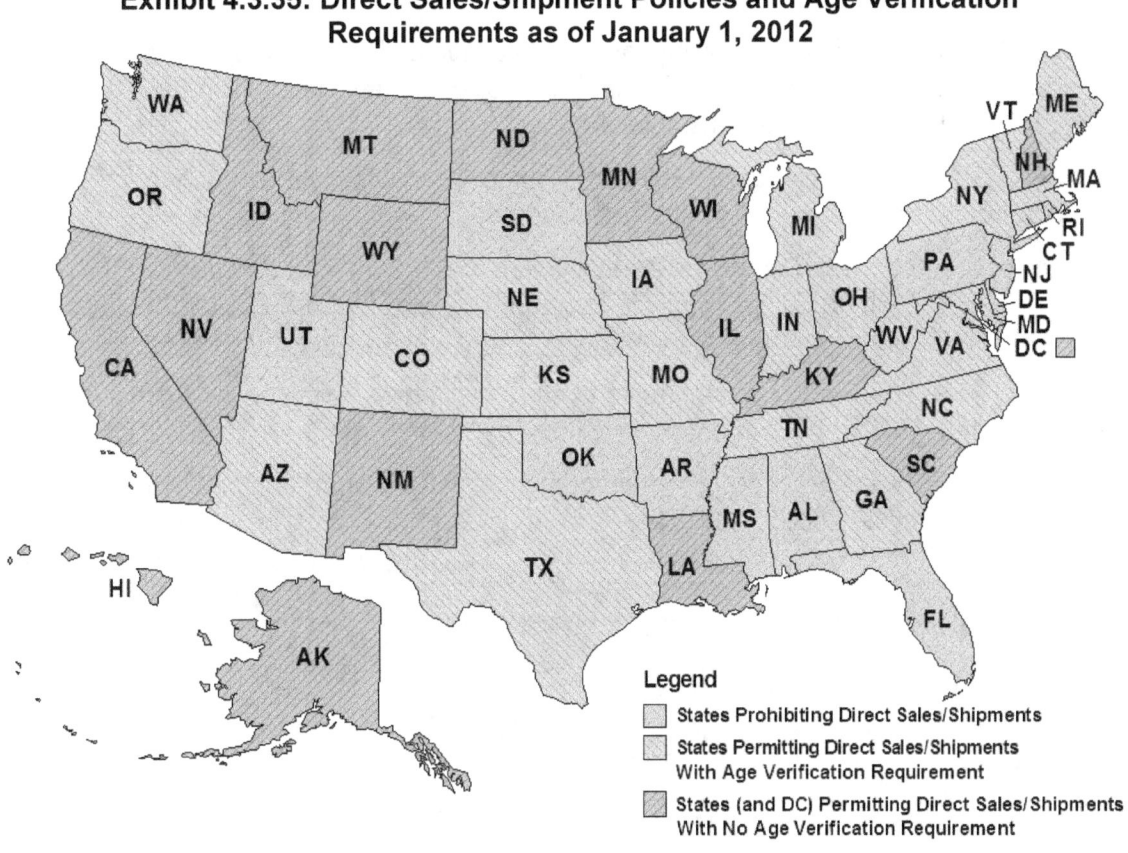

Exhibit 4.3.35: Direct Sales/Shipment Policies and Age Verification Requirements as of January 1, 2012

Legend
- States Prohibiting Direct Sales/Shipments
- States Permitting Direct Sales/Shipments With Age Verification Requirement
- States (and DC) Permitting Direct Sales/Shipments With No Age Verification Requirement

---

[39] These include caps on amount that can be shipped; laws that permit only small producers to sell directly to consumers; reporting and taxation provisions unrelated to identifying potential underage recipients; and brand registration requirements. In some cases, exceptions are so limited that a state is coded as not permitting direct sales (e.g., shipments are allowed only by boutique historical distilled spirits producers).

some point before delivery. Sixteen states and the District of Columbia do not require any age verification. Thirty-three states require a label stating that the package can only be received by a person over age 21, 32 states require a label stating that the package contains alcohol, and 4 states have no labeling requirements related to underage drinking.

Trends in Direct Sales/Shipments Policies

Between January 1, 2009, and January 1, 2012, four states added more regulation to their policies. Five other states (Kansas, Maine, Maryland, New Mexico, and Tennessee) adopted permit systems for allowing the direct shipment of wine from producers to purchasers. Previously, New Mexico had allowed direct shipping by wineries only in those states that offered it reciprocal privileges. Alaska adopted label requirements stating that the recipients of wine shipments must be over 21 and that the package contains alcohol. Iowa adopted age verification requirements at the point of delivery. New Hampshire adopted a provision regarding collecting purchasers' names. In 2011, Ohio expanded direct shipping privileges to include beer.

References and Further Information

Legal research and data collection for this topic are planned and managed by SAMHSA and conducted under contract by The CDM Group, Inc. To see variables for this policy, go to Appendix B. For further information and background, see:

Jurkiewicz, C., & Painter, M. (Eds.). (2008). *Social and economic control of alcohol: The 21st Amendment in the 21st century.* New York: CRC Press.

Moramarto, M. (2008). *The Twenty-First Amendment, Granholm, and the future of the three-tier system.* Working Paper, Social Science Research Network, December 13, 2008. Retrieved February 10, 2009, from papers.ssrn.com/sol3/papers.cfm?abstract_id=1340198

Norton, E. (2006). The Twenty-First Amendment in the twenty-first century: Reconsidering state liquor controls in light of Granholm v. Heald. *Ohio State Law Journal, 67,* 1465–1494.

Williams, R.S., & Ribisl, K.M. (2012). Internet alcohol sales to minors. *Archives of Pediatrics and Adolescent Medicine, 166(9),* 808–813.

Keg Registration

Policy Description

Keg registration laws (also called keg tagging laws) require wholesalers or retailers to attach tags, stickers, or engravings with an identification number to kegs exceeding a specified capacity. These laws discourage purchasers from serving underage persons from the keg by allowing law enforcement officers to trace the keg to the purchaser even if he or she is not present at the location where the keg is consumed.

At purchase, retailers are required to record identifying information about the purchaser (e.g., name, address, telephone number, driver's license). In some states, keg laws specifically prohibit destroying or altering the ID tags and provide penalties for doing so. Other states make it a crime to possess unregistered or unlabeled kegs.

Refundable deposits may also be collected for the kegs themselves, the tapper mechanisms used to serve the beer, or both. Deposits are refunded when the kegs and/or tappers are returned with identification numbers intact. These deposits create an incentive for the purchaser to keep track of the whereabouts of the keg, as a financial penalty is imposed if the keg is not returned.

Some jurisdictions collect information (e.g., location where the keg is to be consumed, tag number of the vehicle transporting the keg) to aid law enforcement efforts, further raising the chances that illegal furnishing to minors will be detected. Some jurisdictions also require retailers to provide warning information at the time of purchase about laws prohibiting service to minors and/or other laws related to the purchase or possession of the keg.

Disposable kegs complicate keg registration laws. Some of these containers meet the capacity definition for a keg but cannot be easily tagged or traced, as they are meant to be disposed of when empty. Most states do not differentiate disposable from nondisposable kegs, although some have modified keg registration provisions to accommodate this container type.

Status of Keg Registration Policies

Keg Registration Laws

The District of Columbia and 30 states require keg registration; 19 states do not require that kegs be registered. Minimum keg sizes subject to keg registration requirements range from 2 to 7.75 gallons with the exception of South Dakota, where the requirements are 8 or 16 gallons. Utah alone prohibits keg sales altogether, making a keg registration law irrelevant.

Prohibited Acts

Ten states prohibit both the possession of unregistered kegs and the destruction of keg labels. Six states prohibit only the possession of unregistered kegs, 8 prohibit only the destruction of keg labels, and 25 states and the District of Columbia prohibit neither act.

Purchaser Information Collected

All 31 jurisdictions with keg registration laws require retailers to collect some form of purchaser information. Of these, 27 require purchasers to provide a driver's license or other government-issued identification. Six jurisdictions (District of Columbia, Georgia, North Carolina, Oregon,

Virginia, and Washington) require purchasers to provide the address at which the keg will be consumed.

Warning Information to Purchaser

Of the 31 jurisdictions with keg registration laws, 23 states and the District of Columbia require that some kind of warning information be presented to purchasers about the violation of any laws related to keg registration (see Exhibit 4.3.36). Fourteen states and the District of Columbia specify "active" warnings (requiring an action on the part of the purchaser, such as signing a document), and nine states specify "passive" warnings (requiring no action on the part of the purchaser). Seven states do not require that any warning information be given to purchasers.

Trends in Keg Registration Policies

The number of states enacting keg registration laws rose steadily between 2003 and 2008, with an increase from 20 to 31 jurisdictions (see Exhibit 4.3.37).

References and Further Information

All data for this policy were obtained from APIS at http://www.alcoholpolicy.niaaa.nih.gov. Follow links to the policy entitled "Keg Registration." APIS provides further descriptions of this policy and its variables, details regarding state policies, and a review of the limitations associated with the reported data. To see definitions of the variables for this policy, go to Appendix B.

Exhibit 4.3.36: Keg Registration Laws as of January 1, 2012

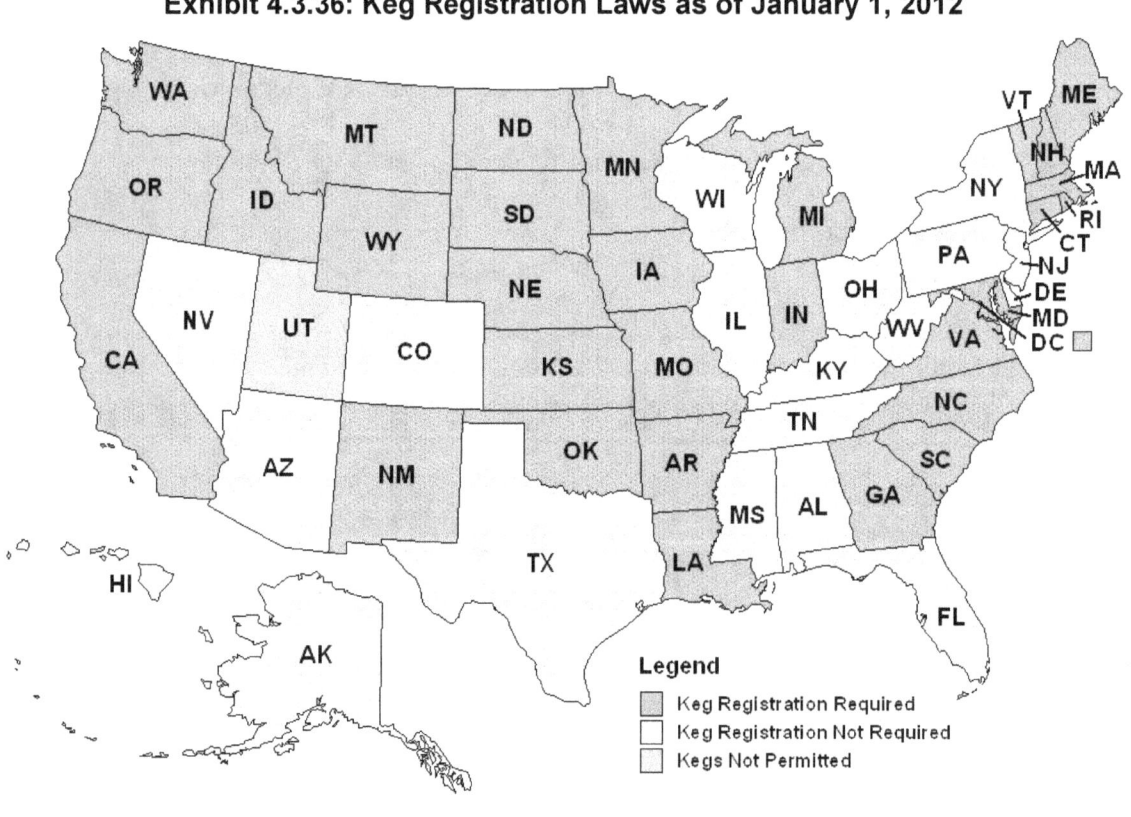

Exhibit 4.3.37: Number of States with Keg Registration Laws, January 1, 2003, through January 1, 2012

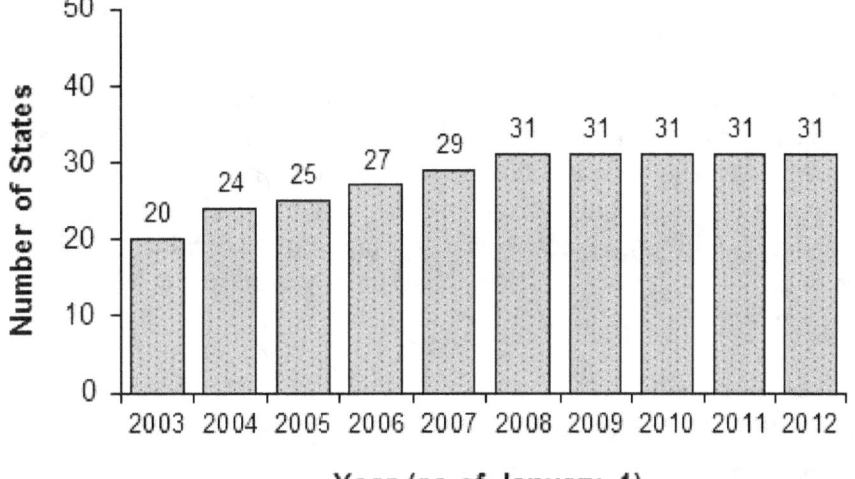

Home Delivery

Policy Description

Home delivery restrictions prohibit or limit the ability of alcohol retailers to deliver alcoholic beverages to customers who are not present at their retail outlet. The University of Minnesota Alcohol Epidemiology Program notes that home delivery of alcohol may increase alcohol availability to youth by increasing opportunities for underage persons to subvert minimum age purchase requirements. Ordering by phone, fax, or e-mail may facilitate deception. Delivery persons may have less incentive to check purchasers' age identification when they are away from the licensed establishment and cannot be watched by a surveillance camera, the liquor store's management, or other customers.

Research on home delivery of alcohol is limited. One study examined the use of home delivery by adult men. The authors report that regular drinkers without a history of alcohol problems were significantly less likely to have had alcohol delivered than problem drinkers. Another study found similar results for underage drinkers. Ten percent of 12th graders and 7 percent of 18- to 20-year-olds in 15 Midwestern communities reported they obtained alcohol through delivery services in the last year. Use of delivery services was more prevalent among young men and among more frequent, heavier drinkers.

A state home delivery law may:

- Specifically prohibit or permit the delivery of beer, wine, and/or spirits to residential addresses, hotel rooms, conference centers, etc.

- Permit home delivery, but with restrictions, including:
  - Limits on the quantity that may be delivered.
  - Limits on the time of day or days of the week when deliveries may occur.
  - A requirement that the retail merchant obtain a special license or permit.

In some states that allow home delivery, local ordinances may restrict or ban home delivery in specific sub-state jurisdictions.

Status of Home Delivery Policies

Exhibit 4.3.38 shows the number of states that permit, prohibit, or have no law regarding home delivery of beer, wine, and spirits. As the exhibit shows, 18 states permit home delivery of all three beverages, 9 prohibit delivery of all three, and 15 have no law for any beverage. Nine states have different laws for different beverages: Five states (New Hampshire, North Carolina, Oregon, Virginia, and Washington) permit delivery of beer and wine but have no law regarding spirits. Michigan permits beer and wine delivery but prohibits spirits, and Kentucky prohibits delivery of wine and spirits but has no law regarding beer. Louisiana and West Virginia permit home delivery of wine but have no law regarding beer and spirits.

Of the 24 states that permit home delivery of *beer and wine*, 11 place at least one restriction on retailers. Of the 18 states that permit home delivery of *spirits*, eight place at least one restriction on retailers. Of the two states that permit delivery of wine only, both impose retailer restrictions. Exhibit 4.3.39 shows the distribution of those restrictions imposed by two or more states on home delivery laws: (1) a state permit is required (Colorado, Texas, Virginia, and West

Exhibit 4.3.38: Home Delivery of Beer, Wine, and Spirits

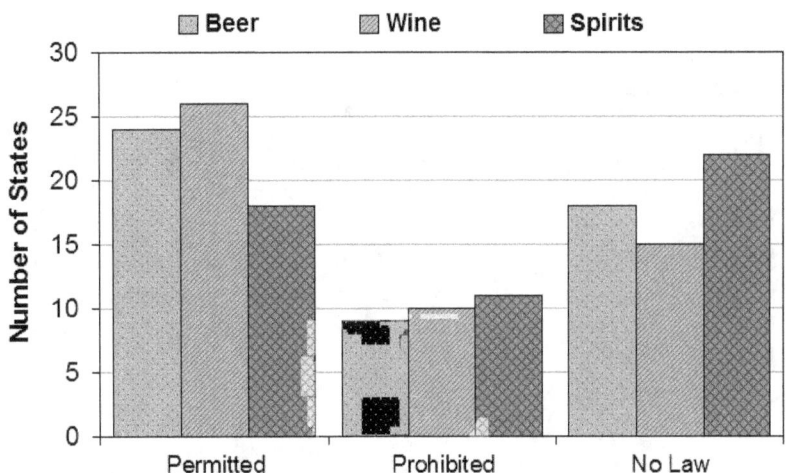

Exhibit 4.3.39: Restrictions Imposed by Two or More States on Delivery of Beer, Wine, and Spirits

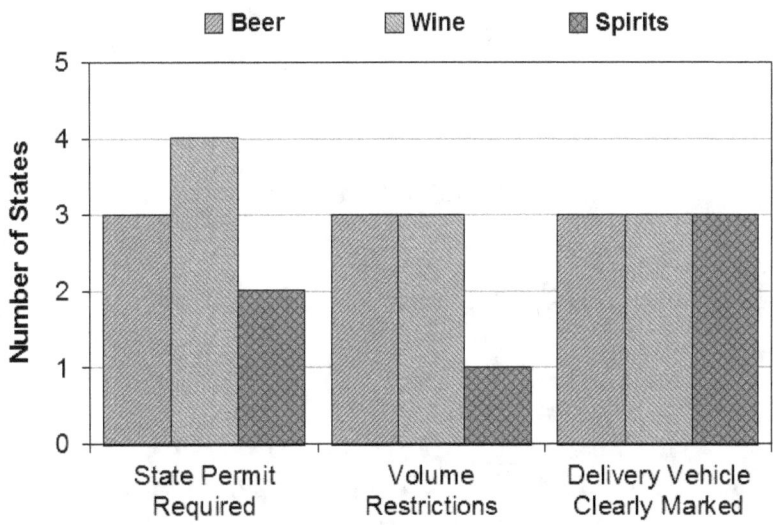

Virginia); (2) volumes that can be delivered are restricted (Indiana, Louisiana, New York, Virginia and West Virginia); and (3) the delivery vehicle must be clearly marked (New Jersey, New York, and Texas). Three additional states that permit delivery of beer, wine, and spirits place a single, unique restriction on retailers: (1) orders must be in writing (Alaska); (2) written information on fetal alcohol syndrome must accompany the delivered product (Alaska); and (3) a local permit is required to deliver to the retailer's county or city (Maryland). One state (Washington) that permits delivery of beer and wine requires a special license only for internet orders. Massachusetts requires that each vehicle used for transportation and delivery have a state-issued permit. Oregon requires "for hire" carriers to be approved by the state.

Exhibits 4.3.40 through 4.3.42 summarize the status of home delivery for beer, wine, and spirits as of January 1, 2012.

Exhibit 4.3.40: Beer

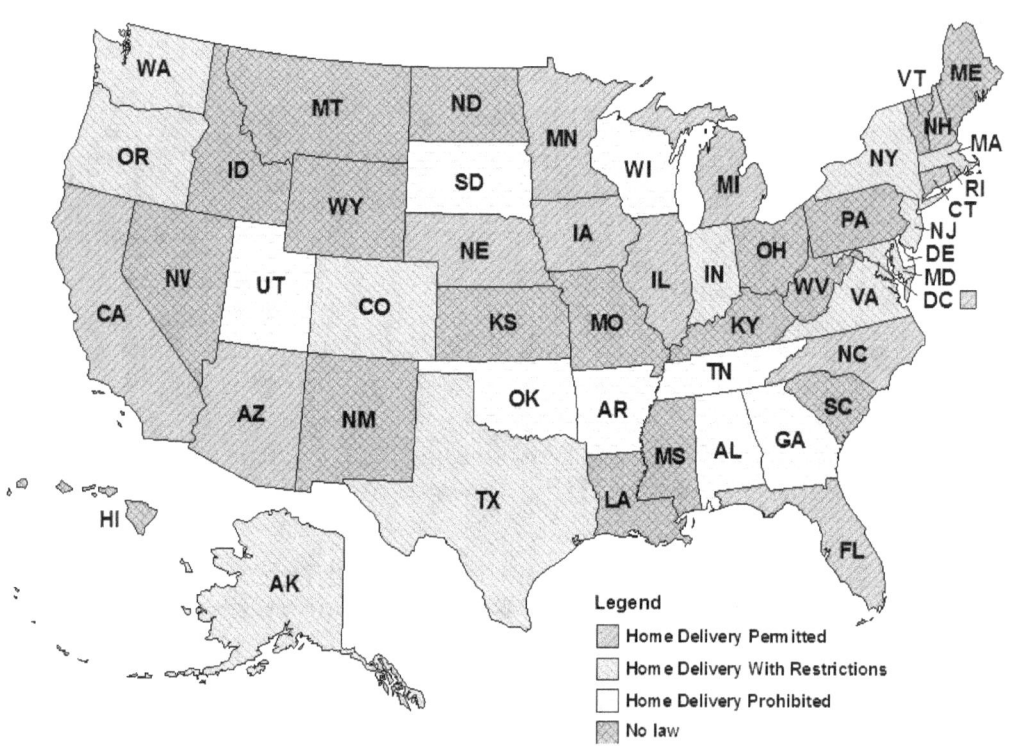

WA
MT
ND
MN
VT
ME
NH
MA
OR
ID
SD
WI
MI
NY
RI
CT
WY
IA
PA
NJ
DE
MD
DC
NE
OH
NV
UT
IL
IN
WV
VA
CA
CO
KS
MO
KY
NC
TN
OK
AR
SC
AZ
NM
MS
AL
GA
TX
LA
HI
FL
AK
Legend
Home Delivery Permitted
Home Delivery With Restrictions
Home Delivery Prohibited
No law

Exhibit 4.3.41: Wine

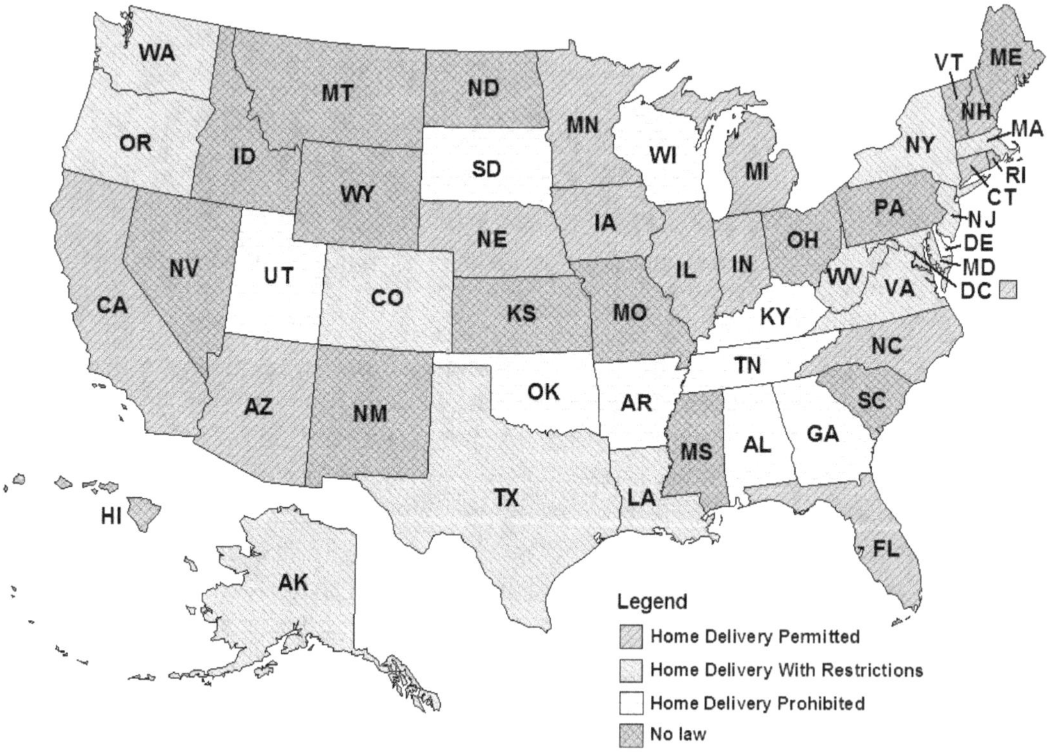

WA
MT
ND
VT
ME
NH
MN
MA
OR
ID
SD
WI
NY
MI
RI
CT
WY
PA
IA
NJ
NE
OH
DE
MD
NV
UT
IL
IN
WV
VA
DC
CA
CO
KS
MO
KY
NC
TN
OK
AR
SC
AZ
NM
MS
AL
GA
TX
LA
HI
FL
AK
Legend
Home Delivery Permitted
Home Delivery With Restrictions
Home Delivery Prohibited
No law

Exhibit 4.3.42: Spirits

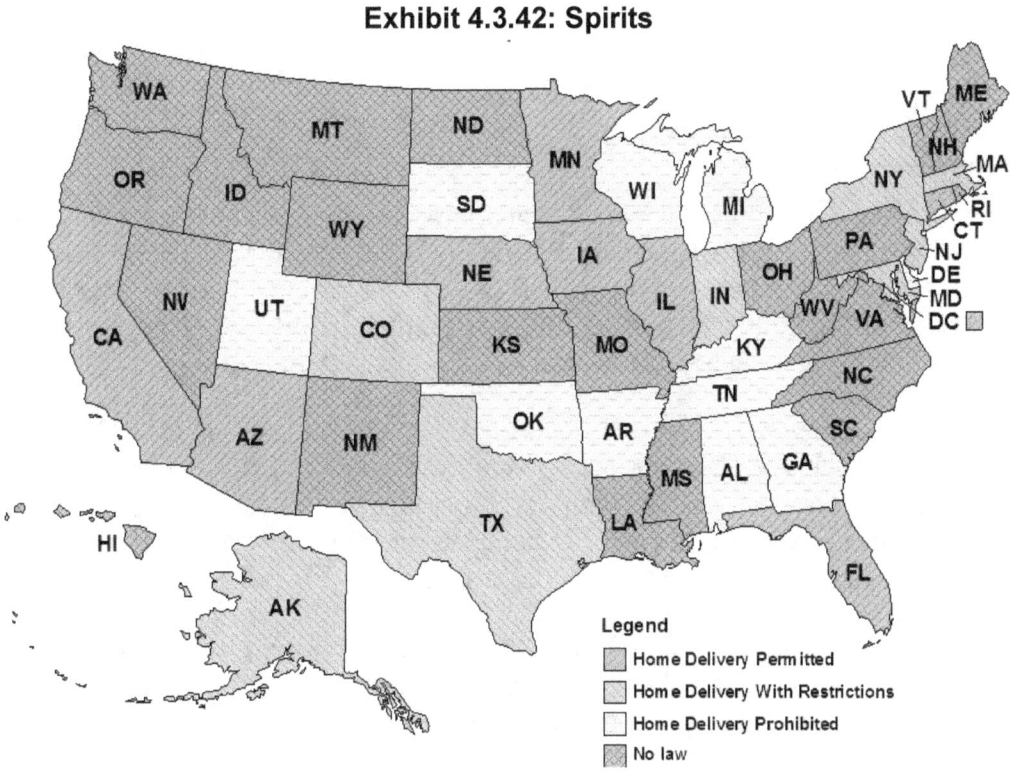

Legend

- Home Delivery Permitted
- Home Delivery With Restrictions
- Home Delivery Prohibited
- No law

Trends in Home Delivery Policies

Between 2010 and 2012, only Louisiana changed its home delivery policies, by permitting wine retailers to deliver to consumers in 2011.

References and Further Information

Legal research and data collection for this topic are planned and managed by SAMHSA and conducted under contract by The CDM Group, Inc. To see definitions of the variables for this policy, go to Appendix B. For further information and background see: http://www.epi.umn.edu/alcohol/policy/homdeliv.shtm.

Fletcher, L.A., Nugent, S.M., Ahern, S.M., & Willenbring, M.L. (1996). Brief report. The use of alcohol home delivery services by male problem drinkers: A preliminary report. *Journal of Substance Abuse, 8(2),* 251–261.

Fletcher, L.A., Toomey, T.L., Wagenaar, A.C., Short, B., & Willenbring, M.L. (2000). Alcohol home delivery services: A source of alcohol for underage drinkers. *Journal of Studies on Alcohol, 61,* 81–84.

Alcohol Pricing Policies

Alcohol Taxes

Policy Description

There is ample evidence that the "economic availability" of alcoholic beverages (i.e., retail price) has an impact on underage drinking and a wide variety of related consequences. The *Surgeon General's Call to Action* includes economic availability as a strategy in the context of increasing the cost of underage drinking, which includes the price, time, effort, and resources required for young people to obtain alcohol as well as penalties associated with its use.

Chaloupka and colleagues (2002) report effects of price on underage drinking, college drinking, and binge drinking (including drinking among youth who show signs of alcohol use disorders). They also report significant effects on youth traffic crashes, violence on college campuses, and crime among people under 21. Although alcohol taxes are an imperfect index of retail prices, tax rates are relatively easy to measure and provide a useful proxy for economic availability.

Based on this and other research, the National Research Council/IOM Report, *Reducing Underage Drinking: A Collective Responsibility*, made the following recommendation: "[S]tate legislatures should raise excise taxes to reduce underage consumption and to raise additional revenues for this purpose."

This policy addresses beer, wine, and distilled spirits taxes. Although some states have separate tax rates for other alcoholic products (e.g., sparkling wine and flavored alcohol beverages), these account for a small market share and are not addressed.

State alcohol taxes fall into four main categories. The names applied to these categories may vary by jurisdiction, but the following terms are commonly used:

- *Specific excise taxes:* Taxes applied per gallon at the wholesale or retail level.
- *Ad valorem excise taxes:* Value-based taxes, usually levied as a percentage of the alcoholic product's retail price (which may also be referred to as gross receipts, gross proceeds, retail receipts, or retail proceeds). Different ad valorem excise tax rates may apply to on- and off-premises sales.
- *Sales tax:* A value-based tax that is not typically specific to alcoholic beverages.
- *Sales tax adjusted retail ad valorem excise tax:* In some states, ad valorem excise taxes are levied in lieu of sales tax (see Exhibit 4.3.43). In these cases, an accurate index of the actual tax reflected in the retail price requires that the retail ad valorem excise tax be adjusted to reflect the fact that sales taxes are not levied. The sales tax adjusted retail ad valorem excise tax = the retail ad valorem excise tax minus the (unlevied) sales tax. As shown in Exhibit 4.3.43, the trade-off between retail ad valorem excise tax and sales tax is not uncommon.

Status of Alcohol Taxation

As of January 1, 2012, all license states have an excise tax for beer, wine, and spirits. The federal government also levies an excise tax of $0.58/gallon for beer, $1.07/gallon for wine, and $13.50/gallon for spirits.

Exhibit 4.3.43: Number and Percentage of States that Levy an Ad Valorem Excise Tax but Do Not Apply General Sales Tax

Beverage type	Type of ad valorem excise tax	Number of states that levy this ad valorem excise tax	Number of states that do not apply general sales tax when the ad valorem excise tax is levied	Percentage of states that do not apply general sales tax when the ad valorem excise tax is levied
Beer	Ad valorem excise tax: onsite	9	6	66
	Ad valorem excise tax: offsite	8	4	50
Wine	Ad valorem excise tax: onsite	9	5	55
	Ad valorem excise tax: offsite	8	4	50
Spirits	Ad valorem excise tax: onsite	12	5	42
	Ad valorem excise tax: offsite	8	4	50

Like the federal excise tax, state excise taxes are generally highest for spirits and lowest for beer, roughly tracking the alcohol content of these beverages. Beer excise taxes range from $0.02 to $1.07/gallon, wine excise taxes range from $0.11 to $2.50/gallon, and spirits excise taxes range from $1.50 to $12.80/gallon. The states with the highest excise tax for one beverage may not be the states with the highest excise taxes for other beverages. States may control for one, two, or three categories (beer, wine, spirits).

Exhibits 4.3.44 through 4.3.46 show the levels of excise taxes for beer, wine, and spirits across the 50 states and the District of Columbia. Exhibit 4.3.47 shows the ad valorem excise tax or sales tax adjusted ad valorem excise tax rates for license states that have ad valorem excise taxes. These may be levied at on- or off-sale outlets and may be for beer, wine, and/or spirits. Beer ad valorem excise tax rates range from 1 to 17 percent for on- and/or off-premises sales. Wine rates range from 1.7 to 15 percent for on- and/or off-premises sales. Distilled spirit rates range from 1.7 to 15 percent for on- and/or off-premises sales.

Trends in Alcohol Taxes

Alcohol taxes have remained relatively constant for several decades. As can been seen in Exhibit 4.3.48, there have been limited tax increases or decreases in beer, wine, or spirits excise taxes since 2003. During this period there have been 28 tax rate increases across all jurisdictions. Eight of these increases occurred from 2011 to 2012, indicating that the rate of increases may be accelerating. Tax rate decreases across all jurisdictions remained stable from 2011 to 2012 (no additional decreases in 2012 were noted).

4.3.44: Beer-Specific Excise Tax

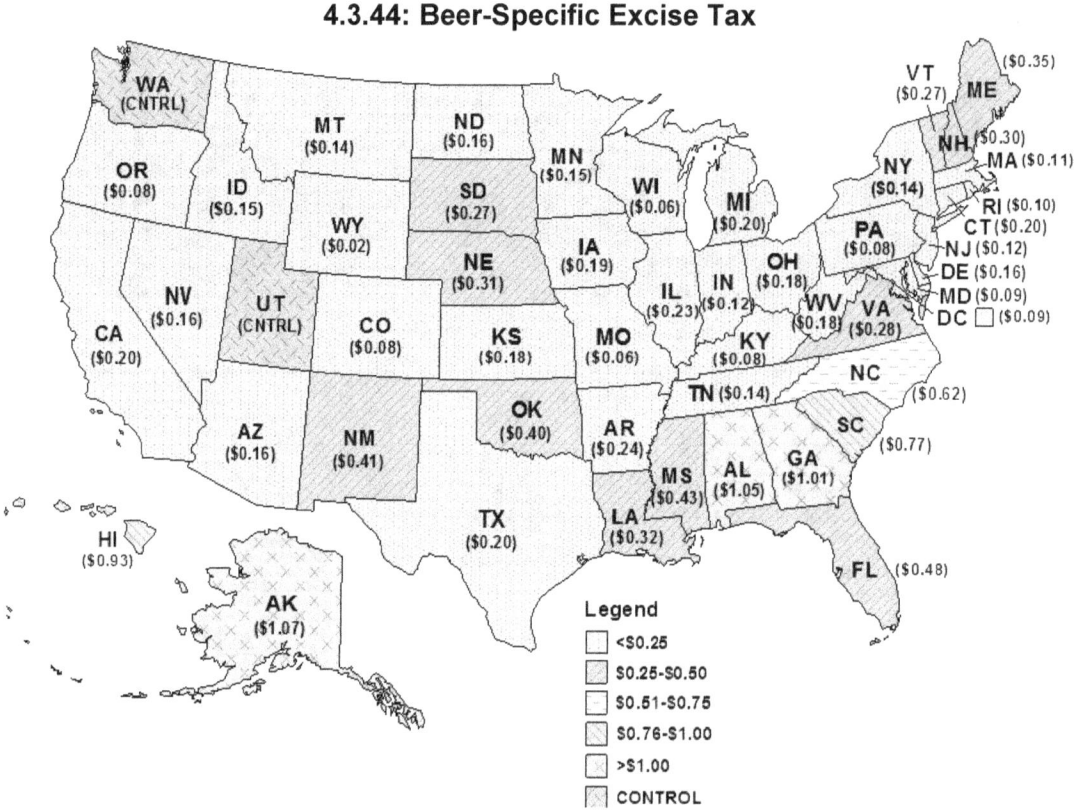

Exhibit 4.3.45: Wine-Specific Excise Tax

Exhibit 4.3.46: Spirits-Specific Excise Tax

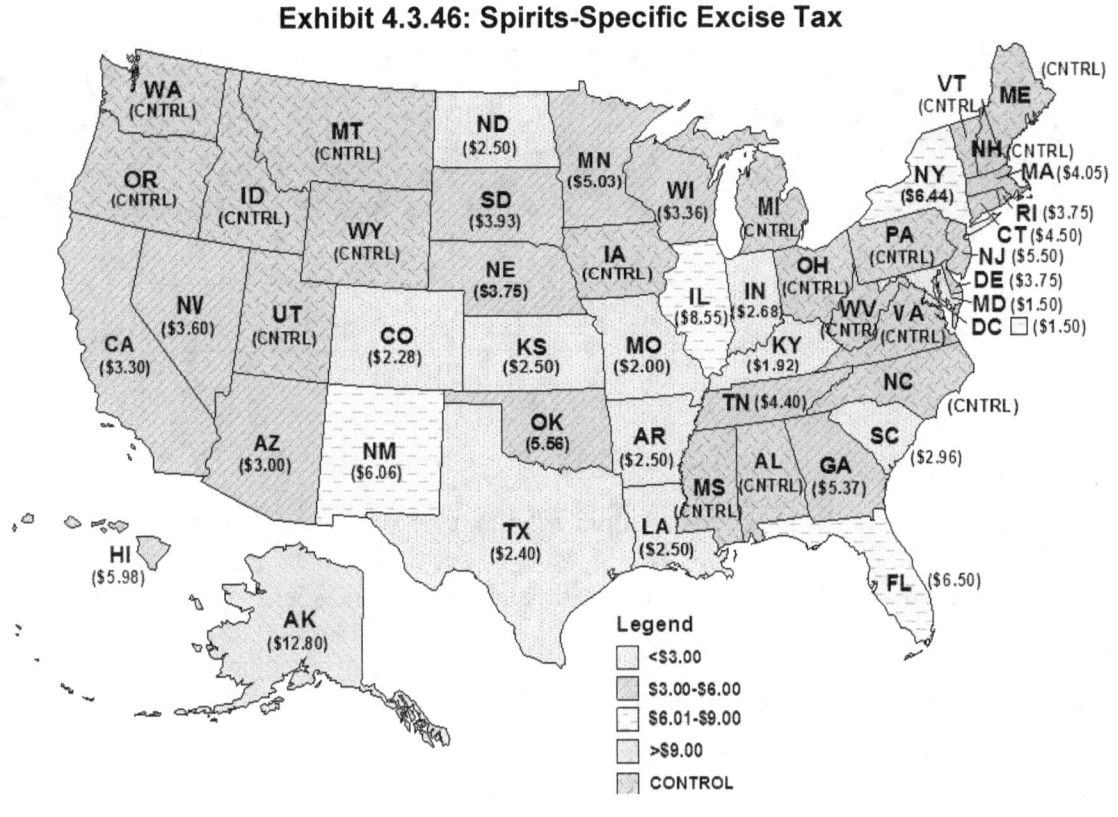

Exhibit 4.3.47: Ad Valorem Excise Tax or Sales Tax Adjusted Ad Valorem Excise Tax Rates as of January 2012

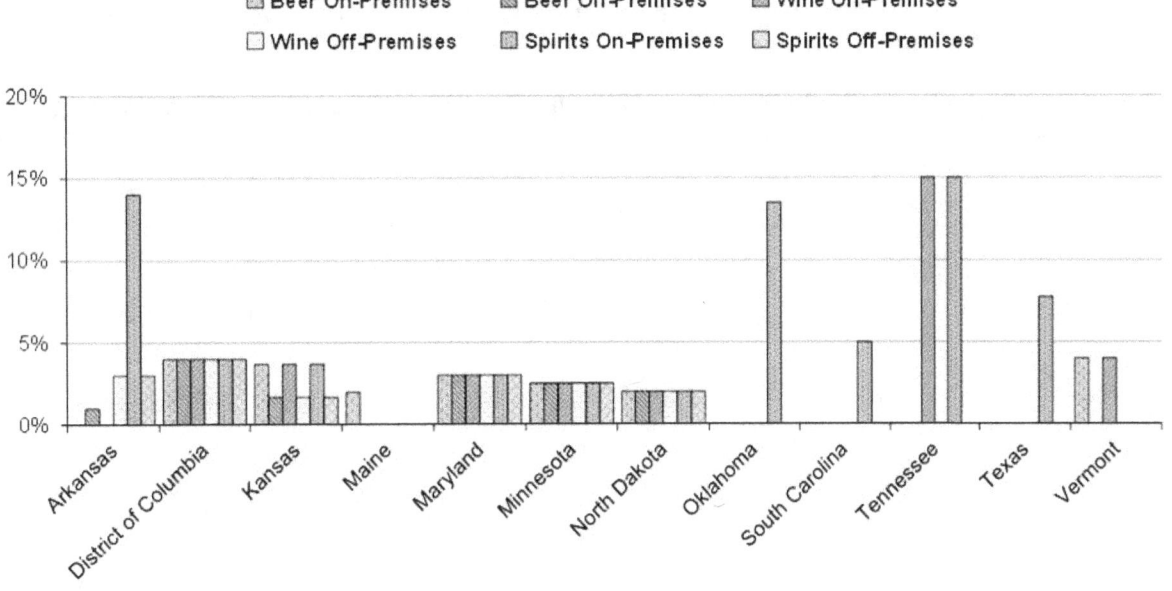

Exhibit 4.3.48: Alcohol Tax Changes 2003–2011

		Beer		Wine		Spirits		
		Specific excise tax	Ad valorem excise tax	Specific excise tax	Ad valorem excise tax	Specific excise tax	Ad valorem excise tax	Total
Number of jurisdictions that:	Increased rates	6	2	7	3	6	4	28
	Decreased rates	1	3	1	3	1	3	13

References and Further Information

Legal research and data collection for this topic are planned and managed by SAMHSA and conducted under contract by The CDM Group, Inc. To see definitions of the variables for this policy, go to Appendix B. For further information and background see:

Chaloupka, F., Grossman, M., & Saffer, H. (2002). The effects of price on alcohol consumption and alcohol-related problems. *Alcohol Research & Health, 26.*

Community Preventive Services Task Force. (2010). Increasing alcohol beverage taxes is recommended to reduce excessive alcohol consumption and related harms. *American Journal of Preventive Medicine, 38,* 230–232.

Department of Health and Human Services. (2007). *The Surgeon General's call to action to prevent and reduce underage drinking.* Rockville, MD: HHS, Office of the Surgeon General. Available at: http://www.surgeongeneral.gov/topics/underagedrinking/calltoaction.pdf

Elder, R.W., Lawrence, B., Ferguson, A., Naimi, T.S., Brewer, R.D., Chattopadhyay, S.K., Toomey, T.L., & Fielding, J.E. (2010). The effectiveness of tax policy interventions for reducing excessive alcohol consumption and related harms. *American Journal of Preventive Medicine, 38,* 217–229.

National Research Council and Institute of Medicine. (2003). *Reducing underage drinking: A collective responsibility.* Washington, DC: National Academies Press.

Low-Price, High-Volume Drink Specials

Policy Description

Low-price, high-volume drink specials restrictions prohibit or limit the ability of on-premises retailers from using various price-related marketing tactics such as happy hours, two-for-one specials, or free drinks that encourage heavier consumption. These promotions are particularly prevalent in college communities, where large numbers of underage students are present.

Research has examined the impact of on-premises retail drink specials on binge drinking among college students. For example, one study measured self-reported binge-drinking rates among college students from 119 colleges, conducted an assessment of marketing practices of on-premises outlets in neighboring communities, and determined whether these communities restricted low-price, high-volume drink specials. The results demonstrated that price-related promotions were significantly correlated with higher binge drinking and self-reported drinking and driving rates among students (Wechsler et al., 2003).

Based on this and other research, the *Surgeon General's Call to Action* concluded that "increasing the cost of drinking can positively affect adolescent decisions about alcohol use," and recommended "[e]limination of low price, high-volume drink specials, especially in proximity to college campuses, military bases, and other locations with a high concentration of youth."

A state low-price, high-volume drink specials law may prohibit or restrict the following practices:

1. Providing customers with free beverages either as a promotion or on a case-by-case basis (e.g., on a birthday or anniversary, as compensation for poor services)
2. Offering additional drinks for the same price as a single drink (e.g., two-for-ones)
3. Offering reduced-price drinks during designated times of day ("happy hours")
4. Instituting a fixed price for an unlimited amount of drinks during a fixed period of time (e.g., "beat the clock" and similar drinking games)
5. Offering drinks with increased amounts of alcohol at the same price as regular-sized drinks (e.g., double shots for the price of single shots)
6. Service of more than one drink to a customer at a time

Status of Low-Price, High-Volume Drink Specials Law

Exhibit 4.3.49 shows the number of states that prohibited the six low-price, high-volume specials listed above.

Seventeen states prohibited *free beverages*. Five additional states (New Jersey, New Mexico, South Carolina, Texas, and Washington) allowed a licensee to offer a free drink on a case-by-case basis only (e.g., on a birthday or anniversary, as compensation for poor services).

Four states prohibited *multiple servings at one time*. In one of these states (Tennessee), this prohibition applied only after 10 p.m. Nineteen states prohibited *multiple servings for single*

Exhibit 4.3.49: Number of States Prohibiting Various Low-Price, High-Volume Drink Specials

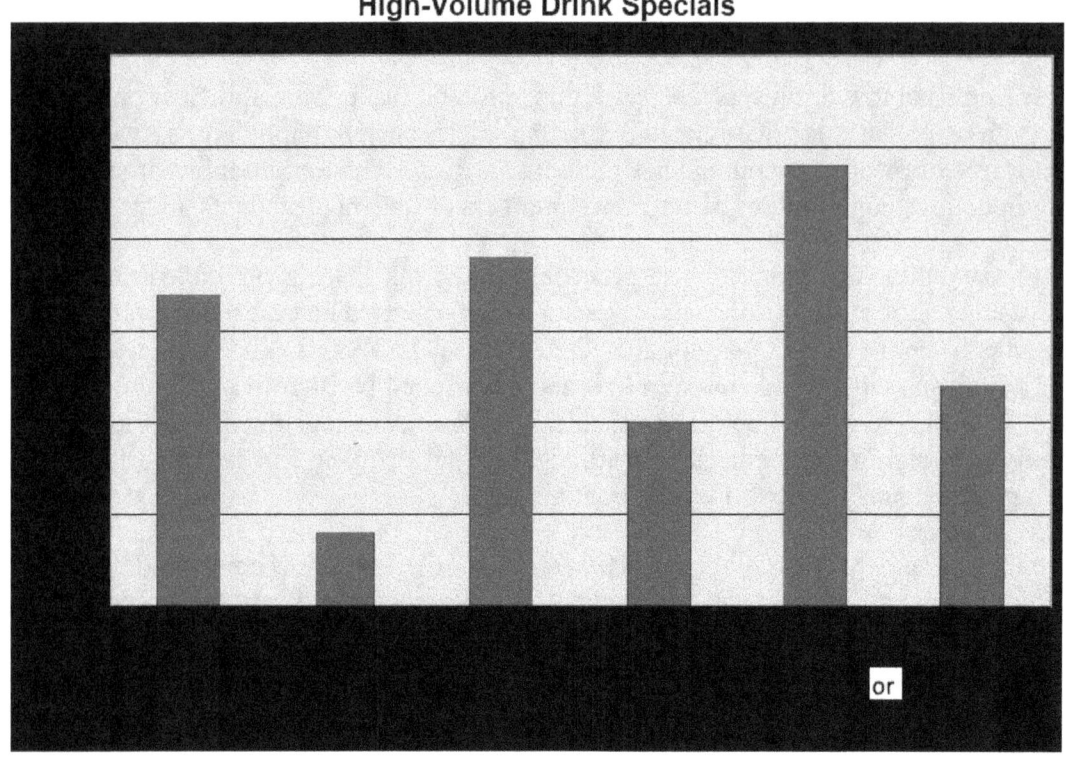

serving price. Twenty-four states prohibited *unlimited beverages for a fixed price or period.* In one of these (Louisiana), this prohibition applied only after 10 p.m. Twelve states prohibited *increased volume without increase in price*, with Tennessee making it unlawful after 10 p.m.

As can be seen in Exhibit 4.3.50, 10 states prohibited *happy hours (reduced prices).* Eight additional states allowed happy hours but restricted the hours in which they may be offered.

Trends in Low-Price, High-Volume Drink Specials Law

Between 2010 and 2011, only one small change occurred in low-price, high-volume drink specials law. One state expanded its definition of "drink" to include two different drinks customarily served at the same time. Such a change created a decrease by one state in "multiple servings at one time." Between 2011 and 2012, one state (Pennsylvania) increased the number of hours during which discounts may be offered. No other changes occurred.

References and Further Information

Legal research for this topic is planned and managed by SAMHSA and conducted under contract by The CDM Group, Inc. To see definitions of the variables for this policy, go to Appendix B. For further information and background, see:

Babor, T., et al. (1978). Experimental analysis of the 'happy hour': Effects of purchase price on alcohol consumption. *Psychopharmacology, 58,* 35–41.

Beverage Information Group, Fact Book. (2010). Norwalk, CT: Beverage Information Group (annual publication).

Exhibit 4.3.50: Happy Hours 2012

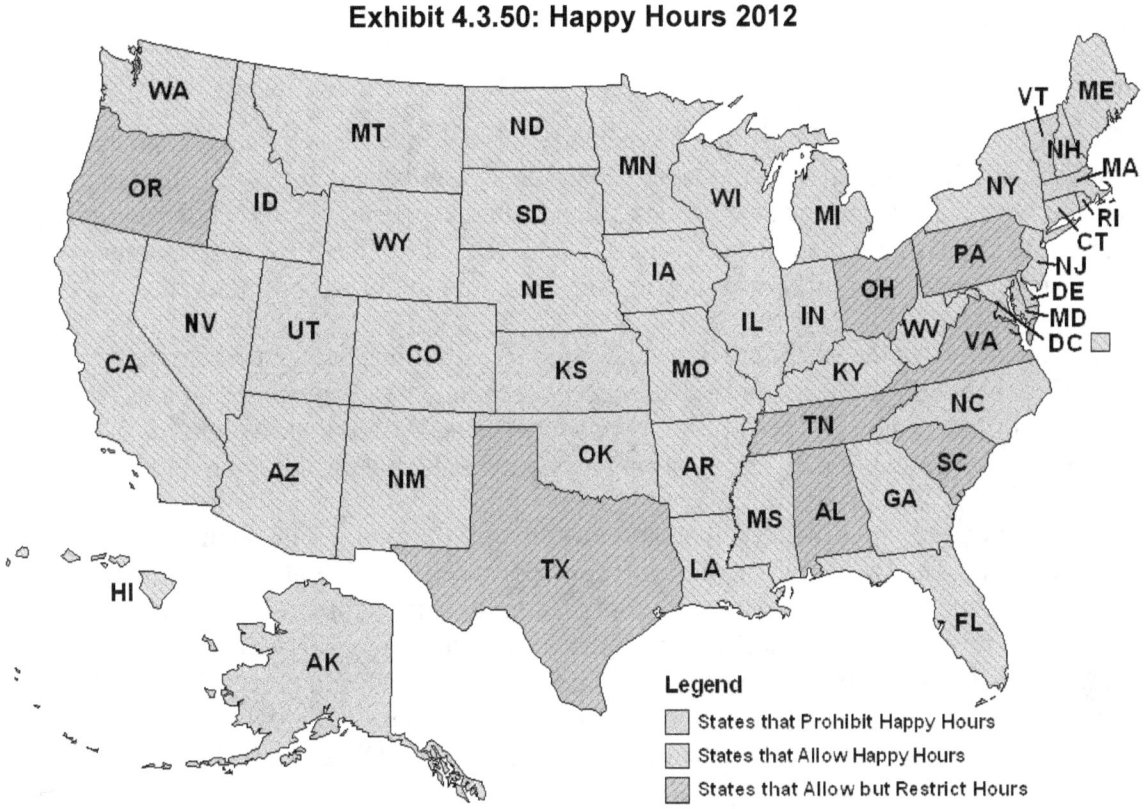

Legend
- States that Prohibit Happy Hours
- States that Allow Happy Hours
- States that Allow but Restrict Hours

Chaloupka, F., et al. (2002). The effects of price on alcohol consumption and alcohol-related problems. *Alcohol Research & Health, 26(1)*, 22–34.

Department of Health and Human Services. (2007). *The Surgeon General's call to action to prevent and reduce underage drinking.* Rockville, MD: HHS, Office of the Surgeon General. Available at: http://www.surgeongeneral.gov and at http://www.hhs.gov/od

Kuo, M., Wechsler, H., Greenberg, P., & Lee, H. (2003). The marketing of alcohol to college students: The role of low prices and special promotions. *American Journal of Preventive Medicine, 25(3)*, 1–8.

National Highway Traffic Safety Administration. (2005). *Research report: Preventing over-consumption of alcohol – sales to the intoxicated and "happy hour" (drink special) laws.* Springfield, VA: National Technical Information Service, DOT HS 809 878, February 2005.

Wechsler, H., Lee, J., Nelson, T., & Lee, H. (2003) Drinking and driving among college students: The influence of alcohol control policies. *American Journal of Preventive Medicine, 25(3)*, 212–218.

Wholesaler Pricing Restrictions

Policy Description

The 21st Amendment to the Constitution repealed Prohibition and gave states broad authority to regulate alcohol sales within their borders. Most states established a three-tier structure: producers, wholesalers, and retailers. Many states included restrictions on wholesaler pricing practices intended to strengthen the three-tier system, reduce price competition among wholesalers and retailers, and combat corruption and crime in the alcohol market.

Research suggests that the specific wholesaler pricing restrictions described below increase the price of alcohol to consumers. Research also shows that underage consumption and problems are strongly influenced by alcohol prices. One study has suggested that restrictions on certain wholesale pricing practices may have a stronger effect on alcohol pricing than do alcohol taxes.

Some states operate alcohol wholesale operations directly through a state agency, usually limited to distilled spirits, beer with high alcohol content, and wine with high alcohol content.[43] In these cases, the state sets wholesaler prices as part of its administrative function, and statutory provisions are relevant only to that portion of the wholesaler market in the control of private entities. For this policy, an index beverage has been selected: beer (5 percent), wine (12 percent), and spirits (40 percent). If the index beverage is controlled, in whole or in part, by the state at the wholesale level, the state is coded as CONTROL and no additional coding is displayed.

Types of Wholesaler Pricing Policies

In general, wholesaler pricing policies fall within four types: (1) restrictions on volume discounts; (2) restrictions on discounting practices; (3) price posting requirements; and (4) restrictions on the ability of wholesalers to provide credit extensions to retailers. These policy categories are closely interrelated but may operate independently of each other. Each is described briefly below.

Volume Discounting Restrictions

Large retailers often have an advantage over smaller retailers due to the large volumes they are able to purchase at once. This purchasing power allows them to negotiate lower prices on most commodities and therefore offer items at lower prices to consumers. Many states have imposed restrictions on the ability of wholesalers to provide volume discounts—the same price must be charged for products regardless of the amount purchased by individual retailers. The primary purpose of these laws is to protect small retailers from predatory marketing practices of large-volume competitors and to prevent corruption. They have a secondary effect of increasing retail prices generally by making retail price discounting more difficult.

Minimum Pricing Requirements

States may require wholesalers to establish a minimum markup or maximum discount for each product sold to retailers based on the producer's price for the product, or states may enact a ban against selling any product below cost. These provisions are designed to maintain stable prices

---

[43] For a state-by-state review of control state wholesaler systems, see http://www.apis.niaaa.nih.gov.

on alcohol products by limiting price competition at both retail and wholesale levels. In most cases, this increases the retail price to consumers, and thus affects public health outcomes.

Post-and-Hold Provisions

This policy requires wholesalers to publicly "post" prices of their alcohol products (i.e., provide a list of prices to a state agency for review by the public, including retailers and competitors) and hold these prices for a set amount of time, allowing all retailers the opportunity to make purchases at the same cost. Post-and-hold requirements are typically tied to minimum pricing and price discounting provisions and enhance the states' ability to enforce those provisions. The wholesalers' submissions can be reviewed easily to determine whether wholesalers are paying the proper taxes on their products and whether they are providing any illegal price inducements to retailers. Post-and-hold provisions reduce price competition among both retailers and wholesalers because the posted prices are locked in for a set amount of time. They also promote effective enforcement of other wholesaler pricing policies. Some states require wholesalers to post prices but have no "hold" requirement—that is, posted prices may be changed at any time. This is a weaker restriction.

Credit Extension Restrictions

Wholesalers often provide retailers with various forms of credit (e.g., direct loans or deferred payment of invoices). Many states restrict alcoholic beverage wholesalers' ability to provide credit to retailers, typically by banning loans and limiting the period of time required for retailers to pay invoices. The primary purpose of the restrictions is to limit the influence of wholesalers on retailer practices. When a retailer is relying on a wholesaler's credit, the retailer is more likely to promote the wholesaler's products and to agree to the wholesaler's demands regarding product placement and pricing. The restrictions have a secondary effect of limiting the retailer's ability to operate on credit, indirectly increasing retail prices.

Federal Court Challenges to State Wholesaler Pricing Restrictions

As noted earlier, in general, states have broad authority under the 21st Amendment to the Constitution to regulate alcohol availability within their boundaries. That authority has been constrained by U.S. Supreme Court and Federal Court of Appeals cases, which have interpreted the Interstate Commerce Clause (ICC) and Sherman Antitrust Act[44] to prohibit certain state restrictions on the alcohol market.[45,46] These cases have led to considerable uncertainty regarding the validity of state restrictions on alcohol wholesaler prices, and additional challenges to those restrictions are anticipated. In the meantime, this uncertainty has prompted states to reexamine their alcohol wholesaler practices provisions.

---

[44] July 2, 1890, ch. 647, 26 Stat. 209, 15 U.S.C. § 1-7.

[45] See, e.g., California Retail Liquor Dealers Ass'n v. Midcal Aluminum, Inc., 445 U.S. 97, 100 S.Ct. 937 (1980).

[46] Several federal and state courts have addressed the constitutionality of selected wholesaler pricing practices, with conflicting results. For example, in *Costco Wholesale Corp. v. Maleng*, 522 F.3d 874 (9th Cir. 2008), the plaintiff challenged nine distinct Washington state restrictions governing wholesaler practices, including policies in all four categories described above. The court upheld the state's volume discount and minimum markup provisions but invalidated the post-and-hold requirements. In *Manuel v. State of Louisiana*, 982 So.2d 316 (3ʳᵈ Cir. 2008), a Louisiana appellate court rejected six separate challenges to the Sherman Act, including the ban on volume discounts. It upheld the state's ability to regulate alcoholic beverages within the state and concluded that the Sherman Act had to yield to the state's authority granted under the 21st Amendment. Maryland's post-and-hold law and volume discount ban were challenged in *TFWS, Inc. v. Franchot*, 572 F.3d 186 (4th Cir. 2009), a complicated case involving multiple appeals and rehearings. On Maryland's fourth appeal, the court upheld its previous decisions to strike down the two policies.

Status of Wholesaler Pricing Restrictions

Federal Law

Federal law addresses restrictions on wholesaler credit practices:

> The Federal Alcohol Administration Act provides for regulation of those engaged in the alcohol beverage industry and for protection of consumers (27 U.S.C. § 201 et seq). Under the Act, wholesalers may not induce retailers to purchase beverage alcohol by extending credit in excess of 30 days from the date of delivery (27 U.S.C. § 205(b)(6), 27 C.F.R. § 6.65).

Some states allow wholesalers to extend credit to retailers for a longer period than is permitted under federal law.

State Law

Exhibits 4.3.51 through 4.3.54 show summary distributions of volume discounts, minimum markup/maximum discount, post and hold, and retailer credit for the license states (beer = 49 license states; wine = 41 license states; spirits = 33 license states).[47] Only two license states (Alaska and Rhode Island) have no wholesaler pricing restrictions. Among the remaining states, bans on extending credit and post and hold (excluding post only) are the most common wholesaler pricing restrictions (ranging from about a fifth to about half the states depending on beverage type). Other restrictions range from under 10 percent of the license states to about a quarter of the states depending on beverage type.

Trends in Wholesaler Pricing Restrictions

Between 2010 and 2011, only one state (South Dakota) changed its wholesaler pricing restriction policies, adopting a price-posting requirement. No additional changes occurred between 2011 and 2012.

Exhibit 4.3.51: Volume Discounts

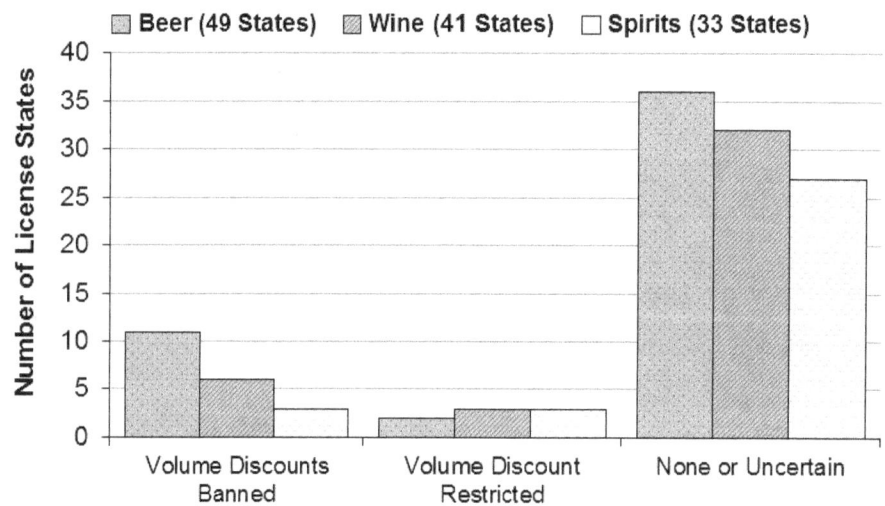

---

[47] Comparisons among beverage types must be made with some caution, because the number of license states differs for each beverage.

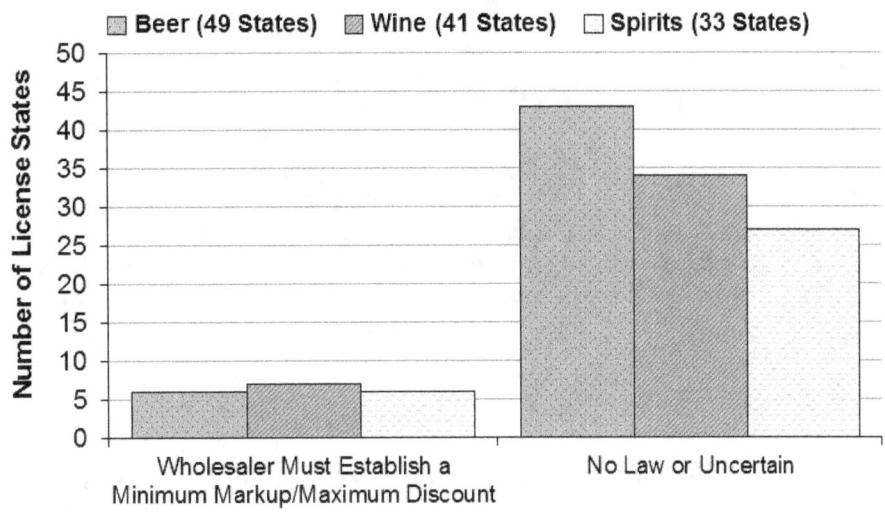

Exhibit 4.3.52: Minimum Markup/Maximum Discount

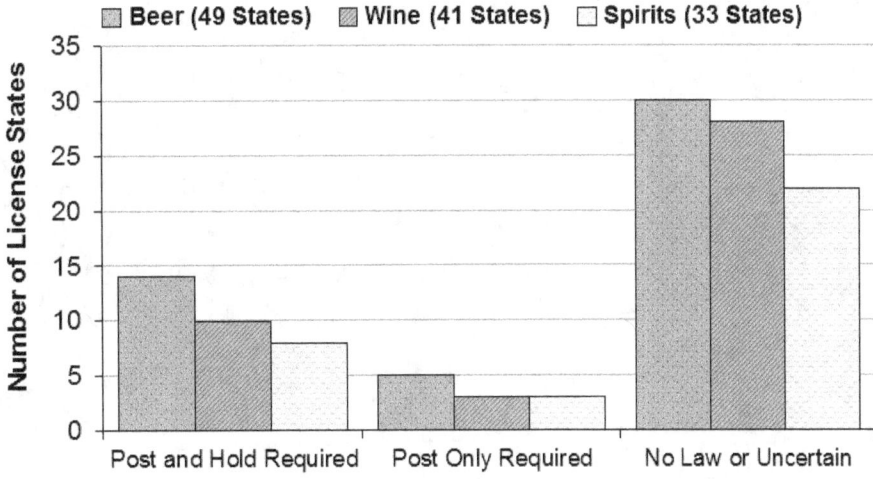

Exhibit 4.3.53: Post and Hold

Exhibit 4.3.54: Retailer Credit

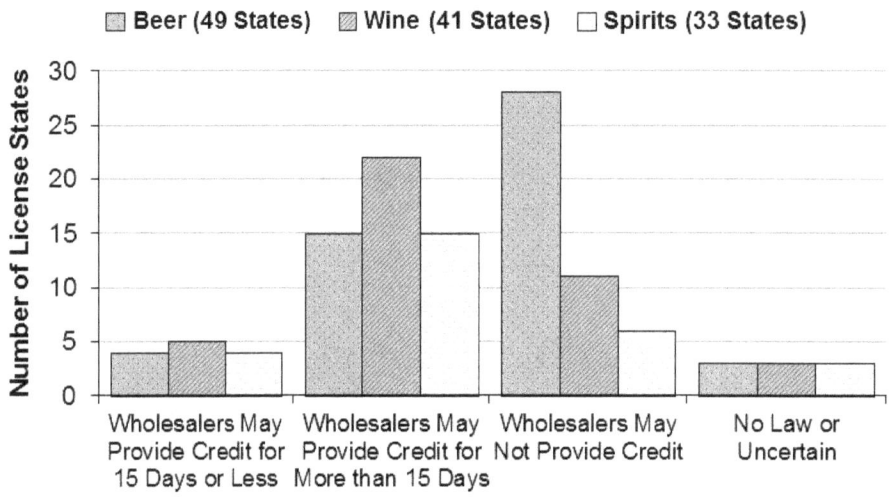

Beer (49 States) Wine (41 States) Spirits (33 States)

Exhibit 4.3.55: Volume Discounts for Beer as of January 1, 2012

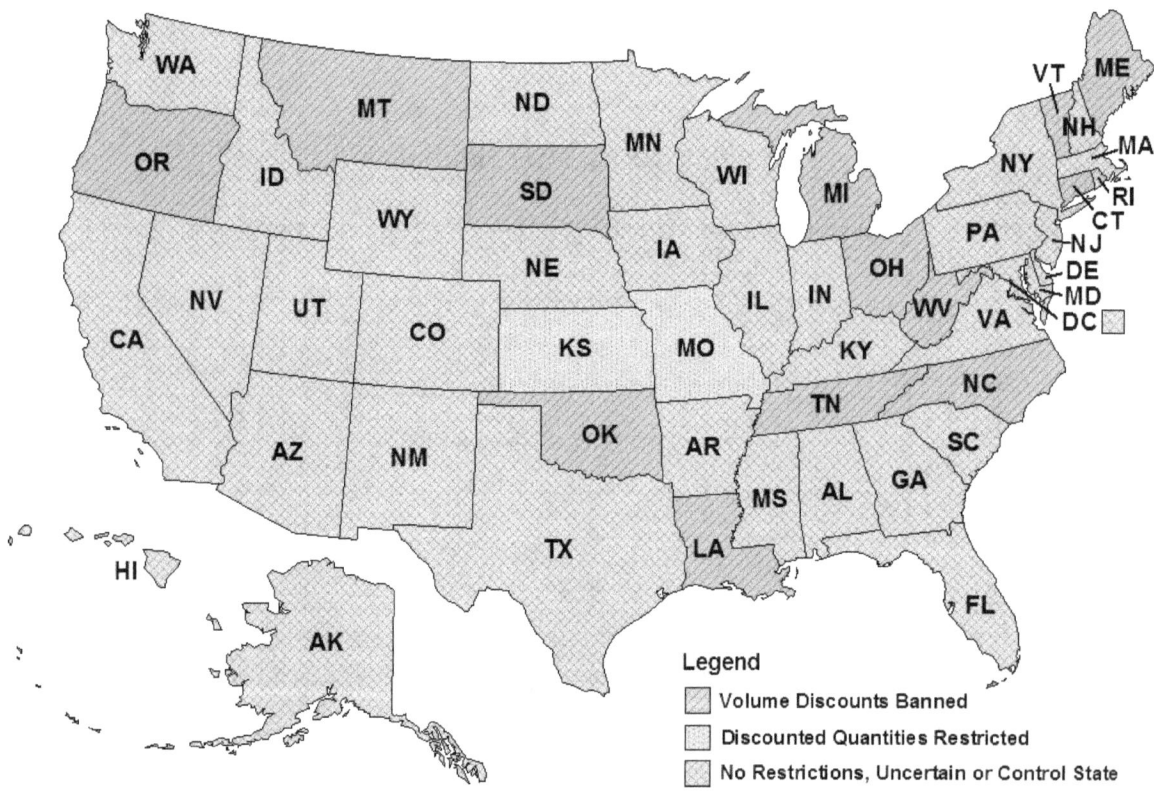

Exhibit 4.3.56: Minimum Markup, Maximum Discount for Beer as of January 1, 2012

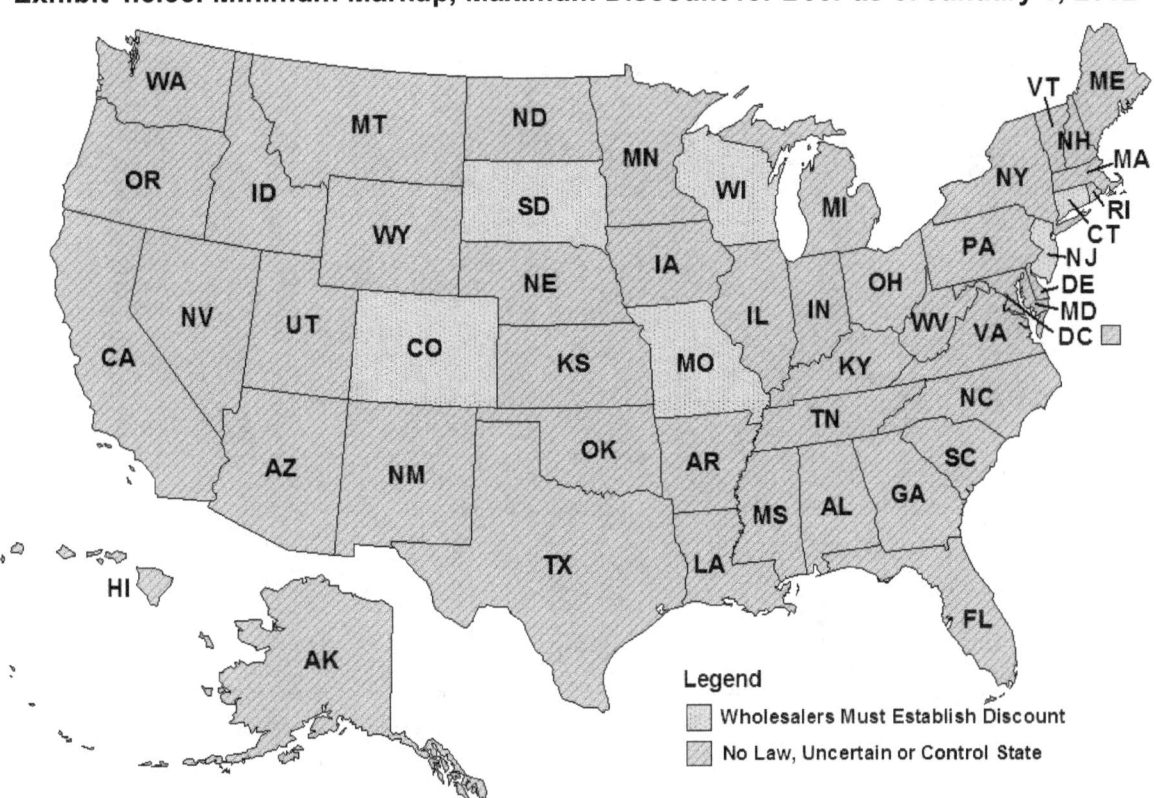

Legend

Wholesalers Must Establish Discount

No Law, Uncertain or Control State

Exhibit 4.3.57: Post-and-Hold Requirements for Beer as of January 1, 2012

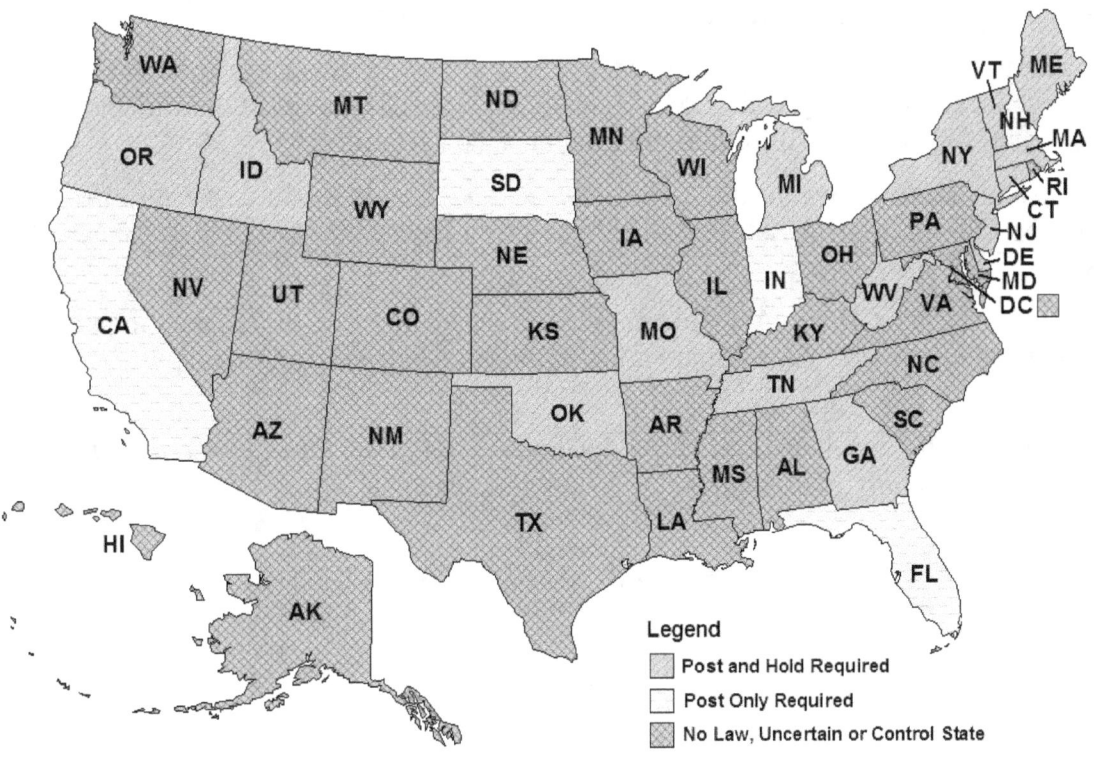

Legend

Post and Hold Required

Post Only Required

No Law, Uncertain or Control State

Exhibit 4.3.58: Retail Credit for Beer as of January 1, 2012

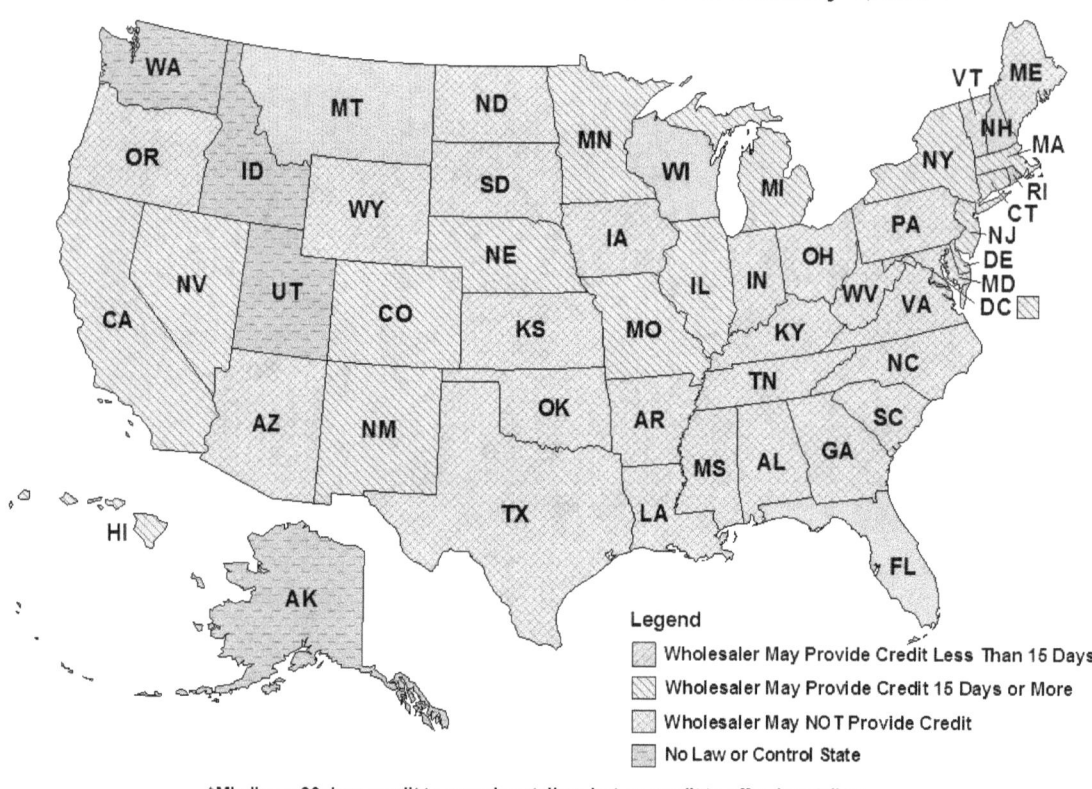

Legend

- Wholesaler May Provide Credit Less Than 15 Days
- Wholesaler May Provide Credit 15 Days or More
- Wholesaler May NOT Provide Credit
- No Law or Control State

*MI allows 30 days credit to on-sale retailers but no credit to off-sale retailers

References and Further Information

Legal research and data collection for this topic are planned and managed by SAMHSA and conducted under contract by The CDM Group, Inc. To see definitions of the variables for this policy, go to Appendix B. For further information and background see:

Chaloupka, F. (2008). *Legal challenges to state alcohol control policy: An economist's perspective.* Presentation at the Alcohol Policy 14 Conference, San Diego, CA, January 28, 2008.

Gruenwald, P., et al. (2006). Alcohol prices, beverage quality, and the demand for alcohol: Quality substitutions and price elasticities. *Alcoholism: Clinical and Experimental Research, 30,* 96–105.

National Research Council and Institute of Medicine. (2003). *Reducing underage drinking: A collective responsibility.* Washington, DC: National Academies Press.

www.ingramcontent.com/pod-product-compliance
Lightning Source LLC
Chambersburg PA
CBHW081346280526
45788CB00009B/2788